Essentials
of Medical
Transcription

A Modular Approach

Essentials of Medical Transcription

A Modular Approach

CINDY DESTAFANO, BSBa, RT(R)
Consolidated School of Business
Lancaster, Pennsylvania

FRAN M. FEDERMAN, MSEd
Central York High School
York, Pennsylvania

Second Edition

SAUNDERS
An Imprint of Elsevier

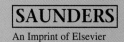

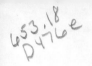
SAUNDERS
An Imprint of Elsevier

11830 Westline Industrial Drive
St. Louis, Missouri 63146

NOTICE

Medical transcription is an ever-changing field. Standard safety precautions must be followed, but as new research and clinical experience broaden our knowledge, changes in treatment and drug therapy may become necessary or appropriate. Readers are advised to check the most current product information provided by the manufacturer of each drug to be administered to verify the recommended dose, the method and duration of administration, and contraindications. It is the responsibility of the licensed prescriber, relying on experience and knowledge of the patient, to determine dosages and the best treatment for each individual patient. Neither the publisher nor the authors assume any liability for any injury and/or damage to persons or property arising from this publication.

Previous edition copyrighted 2001

ISBN-13: 978-0-7216-1015-3
ISBN-10: 0-7216-1015-3

Acquisitions Editor: Susan Cole
Associate Developmental Editor: Lisa M. Neumann
Publishing Services Manager: John Rogers
Project Manager: Doug Turner
Designer: Gail Morey Hudson

Printed in the United States of America

Last digit is the print number: 9   8   7   6   5   4

Reviewers

SHARON B. ALLRED, BRE, CMT
Instructor
Guilford Technical Community College
Jamestown, North Carolina

JANICE LYNN BARKER, MS
Instructor, Information Technology and Office Systems
Lansing Community College
Lansing, Michigan

CHRISTINE A. DUNDAS, RHIT
Assistant Professor
Miami-Dade Community College
Miami, Florida

CAROLYN COLLINS-GATES, MT
Instructor and Program Coordinator
Medical Transcription
Midlands Technical College
Columbia, South Carolina

Medical Transcription Department Manager
Lexington Medical Center
West Columbia, South Carolina

MELISSA LaCOUR, RHIA
Program Director
Health Information Technology
Delgado Community College
New Orleans, Louisiana

PAMELA J. LANDERS-HELMS, BA, CMT
Medical Transcription Quality Assurance Specialist
Lexington Medical Center
West Columbia, South Carolina
Instructor, Midlands Technical College
Columbia, South Carolina

SUSAN D. STEINRIEDE, EdD
Office Information Technology Department Head
Trident Technical College
Charleston, South Carolina

BOBBYE GOODWIN
Medical Transcriptionist
Auburn Memorial Hospital
Auburn, New York

JEANNE GRIFFITH, BS
Director of Training
OIC Training Academy
Fairmont, West Virginia

Dedication

I give special thanks to the most important person in my life—my husband, Izzy; without his unending devotion, support, and encouragement, this textbook would not have been realized. I also want to thank my children, Gwenn, Ben, and Lea, and Allan and Susan, for their encouragement; my mother-in-law, Anna; Central York High School students and staff; and my many friends and family members who have lent their support as well. Of course, one of the most wonderful experiences that resulted from this project is the warm friendship and comradeship that developed between my coauthor, Cindy, and me.

Thank you all.

Finally, this textbook is also dedicated to the memories of special people who had a profound influence on me: my mother and father, Albert and Cynthia Dobbins, and my father-in-law, Morris Federman.

Fran M. Federman

In the ocean of life, we constantly battle the storms and occasionally ride the waves, but mostly we tread water. Deep appreciation and much love go to my family and friends who keep my boat afloat: Dave, my husband, my cocaptain, and my anchor; Matthew and Kate, my children, who always rock the boat but are the wind behind my sails; Jenny, my great stepdaughter, who is about to set sail on her own adventure; my parents, my lighthouse in a storm; my friends, who are the rudders in my life and who help keep my oars in the water (or try at least to); Fran, my friend and shipmate in this uncharted adventure; and you, the student, the reason for the journey.

A medal of valor goes to my good friend, Bunny Best, who withstood my endless torrents of frustration, elation, tedium, and hope.

A very special note of love to my grandmother, Ida M. Davis, for her unfathomable strength, optomism, and love against all odds.

This textbook is dedicated to Richard T. Geiger, my mentor, my guide, my father (December 6, 1928, to July 19, 1999).

Cindy Destafano

Preface

Essentials of Medical Transcription: A Modular Approach, second edition, is a skill development textbook that was conceived as a result of actual classroom experiences with students whose frustrations with other textbooks were evident. Most textbooks provide either a foundational understanding of medical transcription or skill-building exercises, but not both. Therefore, this textbook has been designed as a stand-alone introduction to the beginning competencies of medical transcription. It focuses on the development of transcription skills through a building block format. After providing a foundational understanding of medical documents, proofreading, and transcription necessary for medical transcription practice, later chapters allow students to build their skills in three areas: medical terminology, proofreading, and transcription. This method uses a student-driven approach to learning in which the instructor assumes the role of a coach and facilitates the learning process. Students can evaluate their own progress as they work through the material. This approach creates confidence and competence in preparation for work as entry-level medical transcriptionists through tests, activities, and scenario drills.

PREREQUISITES

Before beginning this course, students should be proficient in keyboarding and have a strong background in medical terminology, basic anatomy and physiology, pharmacology, and laboratory and diagnostic tests and procedures. Students must also understand and be able to use computer word processing software.

OBJECTIVES

Upon successful completion of this course, students should be able to do the following:

1. Understand the content and purpose of chart notes, history and physical examination reports, letters, x-ray reports, and consultations.
2. Use reference resources.
3. Transcribe medical reports using correct capitalization, numbers, punctuation, abbreviations, symbols, and metric measurement rules according to *The AAMT Book of Style for Medical Transcription.**
4. Correctly spell the English and medical terms and abbreviations presented in the dictation tapes and textbook.
5. Produce correct and accurate medical transcription reports within given time constraints.
6. Proofread and edit medical documents.
7. Demonstrate critical thinking and decision-making skills.

---

*Hughes P (editor): *The AAMT book of style for medical transcription,* ed 2, Modesto, CA, 2002, American Association for Medical Transcription.

DISTINCTIVE FEATURES OF OUR APPROACH

This textbook uses a unique interactive approach to build students' skills. Pretests, exercises, and activities are available in the textbook and on the accompanying CD-ROM to reinforce information as it is presented. Progression in competence is easily measured, and further practice is available.

Unit I: Fundamentals of Medical Transcription

Chapters 1 through 4 present the fundamental skills and knowledge necessary for medical transcription practice. They discuss the medical transcription field, medical terminology, keyboarding, proofreading, formatting of different types of reports, and guidelines for transcription. Periodic evaluations and activities reinforce concepts and ensure competency.

Unit II: Skill Building and Simulation in Medical Transcription

Chapters 5 through 11 use an innovative approach by integrating visual and auditory learning to develop transcription skills. These skills are built through keyboarding exercises rather than the traditional approach of simply reading through the chapter. The learning activities move the students from visual keyboarding exercises to auditory transcription exercises. Concepts and skills are presented one at a time, which allows the students to progress sequentially from one skill to the next instead of immediately being thrust into a situation that requires the use of multiple skills and concepts to produce a medical report. The content of Unit II includes the following:

- **Seven Different Specialties.** Each chapter focuses on a specialty students are likely to encounter in the workplace: family practice, orthopedics, urology, pulmonary medicine, gastroenterology, cardiology, and diagnostic imaging. Each chapter gives the students the opportunity to develop the skills presented in the first part of the book. The chapters can be worked through in any order of interest.
- **Medical Terminology Skills.** The students master the fundamentals by keyboarding medical terms and their definitions, spelling medical terms, and transcribing medical sentences.
- **Proofreading Skills.** The students proceed to transcribe reports and develop proofreading skills.
- **Transcription Simulation.** The students take on the role of a medical transcriptionist employed at the fictitious FedDes Wellness Center. The case studies

are developed from actual medical records. After transcribing a report, students will proofread their work and correct any errors. The self-correcting feature of the software will categorize all errors and tabulate the errors on the error analysis chart. The Production for Pay Summary correlates student production to the FedDes Wellness Center pay scale. The scale is also linked to a grading system.

- **Error Analysis Chart.** The error analysis chart was developed to categorize and track undetected errors. A transcription error analysis chart for each document helps each of the students and the instructor prescribe a remedy for every error. Observation of the occurrence of repeated mistakes through charting will improve each student's transcription skills. The chart is divided into two major categories: Medical Language and English Language. Medical language errors are weighted heavier because medication and allergy errors and incorrect patient identification adversely affect patient care.
- **Production for Pay Summary.** The traditional evaluation process is replaced with a motivational Production for Pay Summary sheet linked to a grading grid. Net words of production are calculated to a monetary value. Students experience the real-world accountability of earning a paycheck.

NEW FEATURES IN THE SECOND EDITION

- Narrative and corresponding transcripts comply with *The AAMT Book of Style for Medical Transcription.*
- Illustrations demonstrating the correlation between positioning of the patient for diagnostic examination and the resulting anatomical image have been moved to the related chapter.
- Formatting figures have been moved to the appendix.
- The book's design has been significantly improved in order to make the presentation easier to follow.
- The names of chapter sections have been changed to clarify the organization of the content.
- Dictated transcriptions are now available on the CD-ROM.
- The CD-ROM has been significantly updated in programming, design, and ease of use.
- The CD-ROM allows for use of a foot pedal that is integrated with the computer, which eliminates the need for a transcription machine.
- Additional word processing instructions within Chapter 2 on formatting headers and footers in medical transcription have been included.
- Dictations and supplemental dictations are still available on audiocassette if the instructor wishes to use them instead of the CD-ROM.

SUPPLEMENTAL RESOURCES

A variety of supplemental materials are available to the instructor:

- **Instructor's Manual.** Twenty-five transparency masters, model lesson plans, enrichment activities, and supplemental proofreading and transcribing activities enhance the educational process.
- **Supplemental Transcriptions.** An additional practice transcription not included in the book is offered for each chapter. This supplemental transcription is available on the CD-ROM and the audiocassettes.
- **Audiocassettes.** All of the transcriptions are also available on audiocassette. This is a set of 8 tapes that includes over 300 minutes of transcriptions.
- **Evolve Learning Resource.** For instructors only, this is an on-line course management tool. This resource also lets you link to Web sites carefully chosen to supplement the content of the textbook. These links are regularly updated.

Continuing Education with *Advanced Medical Transcription: A Modular Approach*

Based on the same modular, building block approach, the advanced textbook will guide students through progressively more difficult scenario drills and office simulations. It is an ideal resource to complement the foundational textbook. It uses the same software, error analysis chart, and Production for Pay Summary sheets, with more challenging medical transcriptions in 16 new specialties.

ACKNOWLEDGMENTS

This textbook is a result of the combined talents of many outstanding individuals. We are deeply grateful to Susan Cole, Senior Acquisitions Editor, and Lisa Neumann, Associate Developmental Editor, for their vision, encouragement, and patience in working with us to create this textbook. We also wish to acknowledge the helpful and talented Elsevier production team, including Doug Turner, Project Manager, John Rogers, Publishing Services Manager, Gail Morey Hudson, Designer, and Dave Murphy, Executive Producer. It has been an exciting adventure for us.

We extend tremendous appreciation for the support of Charlotte DiCola, Karen Branner, Sandy Deitz, Dr. Bruce Frantz, and Rachel Damoth.

Contents

Fundamentals of Medical Transcription

Chapter 1

What Is Medical Transcription?

OBJECTIVES

At the completion of Chapter 1, you should be able to do the following:
1. Identify the skills and knowledge necessary to be a successful medical transcriptionist.
2. Identify the personal attributes of a medical transcriptionist.
3. Understand the career outlook and overall job environment for a medical transcriptionist.
4. Understand the job description of the medical transcriptionist.
5. Evaluate your own skills, knowledge, and personal attributes for a career in medical transcription.

What's Ahead

According to *Occupational Outlook Handbook*, the demand for medical transcriptionists is expected to increase with the growth of healthcare services and the industries that provide these services. Growing numbers of medical transcriptionists will be needed to amend patients' records, edit for grammar, and discover discrepancies in medical records.[1]

Transcriptionists work in hospitals, physicians' offices, insurance companies, clinics, government medical facilities, and medical transcription services. An increasing number of medical transcriptionists work from home-based offices as subcontractors for hospitals and transcription services. Many medical transcriptionists work a standard 40-hour week, although one in four transcriptionists works part-time. A substantial number of medical transcriptionists, however, are self-employed, which may result in irregular working hours. Earnings depend on education, experience, and geographic location.[2]

The career outlook for experienced medical transcriptionists includes a wide choice of opportunities, including supervisor or manager, quality assurance expert, instructor, author, editor, consultant, as well as business entrepreneur. You are now ready to step through the door into the exciting world of medical transcription.

■ PROFILE OF THE MEDICAL TRANSCRIPTIONIST

The healthcare team includes many of the obvious professionals—physicians, nurses, technicians, and therapists—as well as the not-so-obvious accountant, social worker, and medical transcriptionist.

Medical transcriptionists transcribe dictated medical information that describes the condition, care, and treatment of a patient. Such documents may include office chart notes, history and physical examinations, consultations, letters, memos, admission notes, operative reports, discharge summaries, and many laboratory and diagnostic tests. All these documents make up the patient's medical record, which becomes the communication medium for patient treatment and care, insurance and reimbursement, legal documentation, and research support. Figure 1-1 shows several model reports typically used in an outpatient facility.

The American Association for Medical Transcription (AAMT) is a membership organization for the medical transcription profession. Although it does not offer program accreditation or evaluation, AAMT does publish

---

CHART NOTE

Patient Name: Felter, Michael
Date of Birth: July 3, 1954
Examination Date: *Current date*

SUBJECTIVE
Patient complains of right elbow pain for past 3 months. He has been playing tennis once a week over the summer with gradually worsening pain.

OBJECTIVE
Tenderness over right medial epicondyle. Pain radiates to the forearm and back of the hand with flexion and supination.

ASSESSMENT
Epicondylitis.

PLAN
Advised patient to stop playing tennis for 3 weeks and rest elbow until inflammation subsides. Prescribed Motrin, 200 mg p.o. q.i.d. Urged the patient to wear an elastic strap for support, when playing tennis in the future.

Harry A. Medulla MD
Harry A. Medulla, MD

ham:cd
D: *current date*
T: *current date*

A

X-RAY REPORT

Patient Name: Farley, Cassandra
File Number: 5690341
Date of Birth: February 1, 19xx
Examination Date: *Current date*
Ordering Physician: Izzy Sertoli, MD

EXAMINATION
PA and Lateral Chest X-Ray.

HISTORY
This is a 57-year-old female with a history of lung cancer and increased shortness of breath for 1 week.

FINDINGS
CHEST: There is mild fibrotic change at both lung bases, over the left lung apex, and along the left chest wall laterally. There is some deformity to the left rib cage, apparently reflecting several old, healed rib fractures. There are some increased markings at the left lung base.

IMPRESSION
Early pneumonia, superimposed upon the underlying fibrotic changes. The heart size is normal.

Adam Valence MD
Adam Valence, MD

av:cd
D: *current date*
T: *current date*

B

Figure 1-1 Medical reports typically used in outpatient facilities. **A,** Sample chart note using SOAP style. **B,** Sample x-ray report.

HISTORY AND PHYSICAL EXAMINATION REPORT

Patient Name: Rouf, Andrea
File Number: 2348901
Date of Birth: April 10, 19xx
Examination Date: *Current date*
Physician: Gwenn Maltase, MD

HISTORY

CHIEF COMPLAINT
Abdominal pain, right lower quadrant for 3 days.

HISTORY OF PRESENT ILLNESS
The patient is a 27-year-old legal secretary, who first noted the onset of colicky lower abdominal pain situated slightly to the right of midline, below the umbilicus and above the pubic bone 3 days ago.

PAST HISTORY
The patient had varicella at age 2 and the mumps at age 4. She had a tonsillectomy and adenoidectomy at age 11. There is no family history of diabetes.

REVIEW OF SYSTEMS
HEENT: Mild upper respiratory infection 2 weeks prior to present illness manifested by rhinitis and sore throat.
GENITOURINARY: Gravida 2, para 2, AB 0. No frequency, hematuria, or nocturia.

PHYSICAL EXAMINATION
GENERAL: The patient is alert, oriented, and in moderate distress. BP 120/80, pulse 106 and regular, temperature 37.2° C, respirations 14/min.
LUNGS: Clear to P&A.
HEART: Normal sinus rhythm, no cardiomegaly, no murmurs, gallops, or thrills.
ABDOMEN: Flat. Tenderness with muscle guarding in right lower quadrant. Rebound tenderness was present. Bowel sounds are normal. No organomegaly.
PELVIC: Bartholin's, urethral, and Skene's glands normal. Adnexa normal. Uterus not enlarged.

EXTREMITIES: Within normal limits. No edema. Good range of motion.
NEUROLOGICAL: Grossly intact.

IMPRESSION
Acute appendicitis.

PLAN
Refer to John Smithson, MD, for surgical consult.

Gwenn Maltase MD
Gwenn Maltase, MD

gm:cd
D: *current date*
T: *current date*

C

CONSULTATION REPORT

Patient Name: McWilliams, Betty
File Number: 5678123
Date of Birth: February 2, 1949
Examination Date: *Current date*
Requesting Physician: Charles P. Davis, MD

HISTORY OF PRESENT ILLNESS
Ms. McWilliams appears to be more stable with the supportive measures already instituted. The respiratory rate is still rapid, but her color is better. There are no signs of congestive heart failure.

IMPRESSION/RECOMMENDATIONS
Review of the clinical picture, chest x-ray, and lung scan point definitely toward a pulmonary embolus. I would recommend checking the blood gases, maintaining the oxygen and supportive measures, and starting her on anticoagulation with heparin. She should be maintained on the ECG monitor.

I feel she also has evidence of thrombophlebitis of the left leg and should be treated with elevation and soaks to this extremity. Thank you. I will follow.

Adam Valence MD
Adam Valence, MD

av:cd
D: *current date*
T: *current date*
c: June Smith, MD

D

DIAGNOSTIC IMAGING LETTER

Current date

Charles P. Davis, MD
FedDes Wellness Center
Family Practice Division, Suite 300
101 Wellness Way Drive
New York, NY 10036

Re: Betty McWilliams
    Date of Birth: February 2, 1949
    Examination: RIGHT BREAST SONOGRAM.

Dear Dr. Davis

Comparison is made to the prior mammogram dated January 25, 20xx. An 18 3 8 3 20 mm well-demarcated simple cyst is demonstrated within the central 12-o'clock position of the right breast corresponding to the well-demarcated density noted on mammography in this region.

IMPRESSION: The two densities noted in the right breast on the recent mammogram correspond to simple cysts as described.

Thank you for this referral.

Sincerely yours

Potter T. Bucky MD
Potter T. Bucky, MD

xx

E

Figure 1-1—cont'd C, Sample history and physical examination report.
D, Sample consultation report (informal style with headings). **E**, Sample diagnostic imaging letter.

Continued

```
Current date


Charles P. Davis, MD
FedDes Wellness Center
Family Practice Division, Suite 300
101 Wellness Way Drive
New York, NY 10036

Re: Betty McWilliams
    Date of Birth: February 2, 1949

Dear Dr. Davis

Ms. McWilliams appears to be more stable with the supportive
measures already instituted. The respiratory rate is still rapid, but
her color is better. There are no signs of congestive heart failure.

Review of the clinical picture, chest x-ray, and lung scan point
definitely toward a pulmonary embolus. I would recommend
checking the blood gases, maintaining the oxygen and supportive
measures, and starting her on anticoagulation with heparin. She
should be maintained on the ECG monitor.

I feel she also has evidence of thrombophlebitis of the left leg and
should be treated with elevation and soaks to this extremity. Thank
you. I will follow.

Sincerely yours


Adam Valence MD
Adam Valence, MD
xx
c: June Smith, MD
```

Figure 1-1—cont'd F, Sample consultation letter (formal style without headings).

recommendations for model curricula and code of ethics, journals, reference materials such as *The AAMT Book of Style for Medical Transcription*, and other items of interest to the medical transcriptionist. A model job description developed by AAMT is shown in Figure 1-2.

AAMT awards the voluntary designation of *certified medical transcriptionist* (CMT) to those who earn passing scores on written and practical examinations. As in many other fields, certification is recognized as a sign of competence in medical transcription. To retain this credential, CMTs must obtain at least 30 continuing education credits every 3 years.[3] Further information about AAMT and its certification process can be obtained by contacting AAMT directly.

American Association for Medical Transcription
PO Box 576187
Modesto, CA 95357-6187
Tel: (209) 551-0883
Fax: (209) 551-9317
E-mail: aamt@sna.com; http://www.aamt.org

Although medical transcriptionists do not have the glamour of emergency room physicians or hold the spotlight in popular TV shows, they provide a vital service to the patient and medical community.

PERSONAL ATTRIBUTES, SKILLS, AND KNOWLEDGE

Successful medical transcriptionists are organized, work independently with little or no supervision, are interested in medical language, are disciplined to work within time constraints, are inquisitive and enjoy learning new concepts, can concentrate for long periods, possess common sense and sound judgment, enjoy detail and precision, and are discreet in handling confidential information.

Medical transcription is both a skill-based and a knowledge-based profession. Skills needed include keyboarding, computer literacy, and English language mastery. Specifically, you need the following:
- Excellent grammar, spelling, and punctuation skills
- Computer and word processing skills
- Fast and accurate keyboarding skills
- Proofreading skills
- Critical thinking skills
- Hearing acuity

The act of listening to an oral dialogue of a person's medical condition and then transcribing it requires the transcriptionist to have an extensive understanding of the following medical subjects:
- Medical terminology
- Anatomy and physiology
- Pharmacology
- Human diseases and conditions
- Surgical procedures
- Diagnostic studies
- Therapeutic treatments
- Laboratory tests

Many of us are visual learners, so the act of listening and then transcribing what we hear is a new and very different course of study. Most students have never encountered a class where they were required to coordinate multiple mental and physical skills to produce a document. It requires the coordination of your eyes, ears, fingers, and foot as you transcribe medical terms that are presented in terse phrases and a seemingly incoherent style of prose. It often frustrates even the most enthusiastic and earnest student. The presentation of this textbook allows you to build your medical transcription skills sequentially. This method still requires your commitment and effort, but it should make learning a positive experience. You have chosen a noble profession that plays a vital role in providing quality patient care.

AMERICAN ASSOCIATION FOR MEDICAL TRANSCRIPTION

> # AAMT Model Job Description: MEDICAL TRANSCRIPTION
> ## PROFESSIONAL LEVELS 1, 2, AND 3

PROFESSIONAL LEVEL 1

Position Summary

Medical language specialist who transcribes dictation by physicians and other healthcare providers in order to document patient care. The incumbent will likely need assistance to interpret dictation that is unclear or inconsistent, or make use of professional reference materials.

Nature of Work

An incumbent in this position is given assignments that are matched to his or her developing skill level, with the intention of increasing the depth and/or breadth of exposure; OR the nature of the work performed (type of report or correspondence, medical specialty, originator) is repetitive or patterned, not requiring extensive depth and/or breadth of experience.

Knowledge, Skills, & Abilities

1. Basic knowledge of medical terminology, anatomy and physiology, disease processes, signs and symptoms, medications, and laboratory values. Knowledge of specialty (or specialties) as appropriate.
2. Knowledge of medical transcription guidelines and practices.
3. Proven skills in English usage, grammar, punctuation, style, and editing.
4. Ability to use designated professional reference materials.
5. Ability to operate word processing equipment, dictation and transcription equipment, and other equipment as specified.
6. Ability to work under pressure with time constraints.
7. Ability to concentrate.
8. Excellent listening skills.
9. Excellent eye, hand, and auditory coordination.
10. Ability to understand and apply relevant legal concepts (e.g., confidentiality).

PROFESSIONAL LEVEL 2

Position Summary

Medical language specialist who transcribes and interprets dictation by physicians and other healthcare providers in order to document patient care. The position is also routinely involved in research of questions and in the education of others involved with patient care documentation.

Nature of Work

An incumbent in this position is given assignments that require a seasoned depth of knowledge in a medical specialty (or specialties); OR the incumbent is regularly given assignments that vary in report or correspondence type, originator, and specialty. Incumbents at this level are able to resolve nonroutine problems independently, or to assist in resolving complex or highly unusual problems.

Figure 1-2 AAMT model job description.

Continued

Knowledge, Skills, & Abilities

1. Seasoned knowledge of medical terminology, anatomy and physiology, disease processes, signs and symptoms, medications, and laboratory values. In-depth or broad knowledge of a specialty (or specialties) as appropriate.

2. Knowledge of medical transcription guidelines and practices.

3. Excellent skills in English usage, grammar, punctuation, and style.

4. Ability to use an extensive array of professional reference materials.

5. Ability to operate word processing equipment, dictation and transcription equipment, and other equipment as specified, and to troubleshoot as necessary.

6. Ability to work independently with minimal or no supervision.

7. Ability to work under pressure with time constraints.

8. Ability to concentrate.

9. Excellent listening skills.

10. Excellent eye, hand, and auditory coordination.

11. Proven business skills (scheduling work, purchasing, client relations, billing).

12. Ability to understand and apply relevant legal concepts (e.g., confidentiality).

13. Certified medical transcriptionist (CMT) status preferred.

PROFESSIONAL LEVEL 3

Position Summary

Medical language specialist whose expert depth and breadth of professional experience enables him or her to serve as a medical language resource to originators, co-workers, other healthcare providers, and/or students on a regular basis.

Nature of Work

An incumbent in this position routinely researches and resolves complex questions related to health information or related documentation; AND/OR is involved in the formal teaching of those entering the profession or continuing their education in the profession; AND/OR regularly uses extensive experience to interpret dictation that others are unable to clarify. Actual transcription of dictation is performed only occasionally, as efforts are usually focused in other categories of work.

Knowledge, Skills, & Abilities

1. Recognized as possessing expert knowledge of medical terminology, anatomy and physiology, disease processes, signs and symptoms, medications, and laboratory values related to a specialty or specialties.

2. In-depth knowledge of medical transcription guidelines and practices.

3. Excellent skills in English usage, grammar, punctuation, and style.

4. Ability to use a vast array of professional reference materials, often in innovative ways.

5. Ability to educate others (one-on-one or group).

6. Excellent written and oral communication skills.

7. Ability to operate word processing equipment, dictation and transcription equipment, and other equipment as specified, and to troubleshoot as necessary.

8. Proven business skills (scheduling work, purchasing, client relations, billing).

9. Ability to understand and apply relevant legal concepts (e.g., confidentiality).

10. Certified medical transcriptionist (CMT) status preferred.

Figure 1-2—cont'd For legend, see previous page.

BECOMING A MEDICAL TRANSCRIPTIONIST USING THE *ESSENTIALS OF MEDICAL TRANSCRIPTION* METHOD

This textbook introduces you to medical transcription skills that are basic to the profession. In Unit I you will become familiar with medical reports fundamental to ambulatory care, related medical terminology, appropriate formatting styles, select specialized rules of grammar and punctuation for dictated medical reports, proofreading techniques, and the transcription process. You will learn how to use a variety of reference materials. All formatting and style are based on the *AAMT Book of Style for Medical Transcription*.

In Unit II, each chapter is presented as an independent module, allowing your instructor to present the material in any order. Therefore, instructions and transcription tips are repeated in each chapter. You will apply principles discussed in Unit I as you transcribe medical reports from seven different specialties relating to a fictitious outpatient healthcare facility, "FedDes Wellness Center." Accompanying audiocassettes and the CD-ROM provide a list of medical terms that are pronounced, spelled, and defined, followed by keyboarding exercises. It is important for you to listen to the pronunciation of the terms before starting to transcribe the report. You also may want to practice spelling the terms as you listen

to each term pronounced. Listening to a medical term and then correctly spelling it are critically necessary skills. A list of the patient's name and the type of report, transcription tips, and error analysis and production pay charting are included for each specialty. You will be able to assess your mastery of transcription skills in a real-world scenario.

Checkpoints are included in each chapter to allow you to assess your mastery of each presented skill. As a programmed learning textbook, answers to all exercises are found on the CD-ROM.

So you are interested in becoming a medical transcriptionist—let's begin our journey using the *Essentials of Medical Transcription* as your guide.

REFERENCES

1. US Department of Labor, Bureau of Labor Statistics: *Occupational outlook handbook, 2003*. Available online at www.bls.gov/oco/ocos271.htm
2. US Department of Labor, Bureau of Labor Statistics: *Occupational outlook handbook, 2003*. Available online at www.bls.gov/oco/ocos271.htm
3. US Department of Labor, Bureau of Labor Statistics: *Occupational outlook handbook, 2003*. Available online at www.bls.gov/oco/ocos271.htm

ACTIVITY 1-1
So You Want to Be a Medical Transcriptionist

Directions: Let's assess your knowledge, aptitude, and ability to become a successful medical transcriptionist. Answer "yes" (Y) or "no" (N) to the following questions. If most of your answers are "yes," you are well on your way to becoming a medical transcriptionist.

1. Y or N   Do you have proficient keyboarding skills? Can you type at least 50 words per minute (wpm)?
2. Y or N   Do you have excellent English usage, punctuation, grammar, and spelling skills?
3. Y or N   Are you able to use dictionaries and reference books? Could you find the correct spelling and classification of a prescription drug?
4. Y or N   Do you have a mastery of anatomy and medical terminology? Do you know that the "prostrate" is not an organ of the male anatomy and that the word *mole* could be a pigmented nevus or a uterine neoplasm?
5. Y or N   Are you competent in word processing software?
6. Y or N   Do you have excellent proofreading skills?
7. Y or N   Can you sit in one place for extended periods of time?
8. Y or N   Do you like medical topics?
9. Y or N   Do you have hearing acuity and medical language discrimination skills? Can you distinguish words that sound alike and then select the one with the correct meaning, or catch and correct inconsistencies within a report?

10. Y or N   Are you detail oriented?
11. Y or N   Are you able to work with little supervision?
12. Y or N   Are you able to work under time constraints and production demands (quantity and quality)?
13. Y or N   Are you logical and organized?
14. Y or N   Do you have critical thinking and decision-making skills?
15. Y or N   Are you able to concentrate for long periods of time?
16. Y or N   Do you have excellent eye, hand, and auditory coordination?
17. Y or N   Do you want to be a member of a professional healthcare team?
18. Y or N   Can you be discreet in handling confidential information?
19. Y or N   Do you perform tasks completely and comprehensively?
20. Y or N   Do you take pride in your work?

Chapter 2
Understanding Medical Documents

OBJECTIVES

At the completion of Chapter 2, you should be able to do the following:
1. List the basic information found in chart notes, history and physical examination reports, diagnostic reports, and procedure reports.
2. Identify the types of information that appear in chart notes, history and physical examination reports, consultation letters, diagnostic reports, and procedure reports.
3. Apply a statement to the correct medical report or portion of a chart note.
4. Make a template for the major medical reports.
5. Format and type model medical chart notes, history and physical examination reports, consultation letters, diagnostic imaging reports, and procedure reports.

What's Ahead

Let's find out if you understand medical documents.

TEXTBOOK USERS

Select the best answer for each question or statement concerning medical reports. Refer to the answer key (Appendix E) for immediate feedback.

SOFTWARE USERS

Click on *Chapter 2, Pretest*, and follow the directions.

PRETEST

Directions: Select true (T) or false (F) and the best multiple-choice answer for each question or statement concerning medical reports.

1. T or F   There are three parts in a SOAP note.

2. T or F   A history and physical examination format may be used in a chart note.

3. T or F   Findings from a consultation can be dictated in letter format.

4. T or F   Allergies in a medical report are formatted in such a way as to draw attention to their importance.

5. T or F   The medical record is a legal record.

6. T or F   Templates are never used in medical transcription.

7. T or F   All medical reports include the patient's name.

8. T or F   Ultrasound uses low-frequency sound waves to image the body.

9. T or F   The average chart note is four pages in length.

10. T or F   Abbreviations and phrases are used often in a chart note to save space.

11. T or F   Many healthcare facilities have their own manual of style.

12. T or F   CAT is also referred to as *computerized axial tomography*.

13. T or F   Chart notes do not include a signature line.

14. T or F   Usually, 1-inch margins are used to format a consultation letter.

15. T or F   Dictation for medical reports usually is cryptic.

16. T or F   Complete sentences are normally found in history and physical examination reports.

17. T or F   History and physical examination reports are divided into three sections.

18. T or F   The abbreviation *HEENT* means *head, ears, eyes, nose, and throat*.

19. T or F   In a history and physical examination report, lifestyle habits would be dictated under the "Family History" section or topic.

20. T or F   *Noncontributory* means nothing significant was discovered when the physician performed a review of systems (ROS).

21. T or F   The abbreviation *HPI* means *health program information*.

22. T or F   The first page of statistical data in a diagnostic imaging report is the same as in other reports.

23. T or F   The military-style dateline is never used in consultation letters.

24. T or F   Minimally, three perpendicular projections are taken during a medical imaging procedure.

25. T or F   Templates are identified with the *.dot* file extension.

26. Medical reports are vital in which of the following?
    (a) Research
    (b) Compiling statistics
    (c) Evaluating the healthcare delivery system
    (d) All the above

27. Which of the following are the basic four medical reports in medical offices?
    (a) Consultation letter, chart note, history and physical, and pathology
    (b) Chart note, history and physical, diagnostic, and consultation
    (c) Chart note, history and physical, SOAP, and consultation
    (d) Consultation letter, SOAP, history and physical, and pathology

28. The acronym *SOAP* includes which four topics?
    (a) Symptom, objective, assessment, progress
    (b) Symptom, objective, assessment, plan
    (c) Subjective, objective, assessment, plan
    (d) Subjective, objective, assessment, progress

PRETEST *(cont'd)*

29. The dictated sentence, "Discontinue use of perfumed body lotion," would be found in a chart note under which topic?
    (a) Subjective
    (b) Chief complaint
    (c) Plan
    (d) Assessment

30. The dictated sentence, "Smooth, erythematous rash over neck extending over trunk and back," would be found in a chart note under which topic?
    (a) Subjective
    (b) Objective
    (c) Assessment
    (d) None of the above

31. The dictated sentence, "My head and throat hurts," would be found in a chart note under which topic?
    (a) Subjective
    (b) Objective
    (c) Assessment
    (d) Symptom

32. The dictated sentence, "BP 120/82," would be found in a chart note under which topic?
    (a) Subjective
    (b) Objective
    (c) Assessment
    (d) Progress

33. The dictated sentence, "Acute otitis," would be found in a chart note under which topic?
    (a) Subjective
    (b) Objective
    (c) Assessment
    (d) Plan

34. The dictated sentence, "Bactrim b.i.d. × 10 days," would be found in a chart note under which topic?
    (a) Subjective
    (b) Objective
    (c) Progress
    (d) Plan

35. Which of the following is the usual spacing between each heading in a history and physical examination report?
    (a) Single spacing
    (b) Double spacing
    (c) Triple spacing
    (d) Quadruple spacing

36. The dictation style of a history and physical examination report includes which of the following?
    (a) Recurrent phrases and terms
    (b) More negative than positive statements
    (c) Clipped sentences
    (d) All the above

37. The history section of a history and physical examination report includes which of the following?
    (a) Chief complaint
    (b) Medications
    (c) Review of systems
    (d) All the above

38. In a history and physical examination report, the physician's comments concerning a guaiac test would be found under which topic?
    (a) Neck
    (b) Heart
    (c) Rectal
    (d) Pelvic

39. Most transcriptionists create a template to include which of the following?
    (a) Margins
    (b) Commonly used topics
    (c) Tab stops
    (d) All the above

40. In a history and physical examination, the dictated sentence, "The patient is a 2-year-old female," would be found under which topic?
    (a) Past history
    (b) Treatment/plan
    (c) History of present illness
    (d) None of the above

PRETEST *(cont'd)*

41. In a history and physical examination, the dictated sentence, "She had lower back/spine surgery in 1979," would be found under which topic?
    (a) Past history
    (b) History of present illness
    (c) Chief complaint
    (d) None of the above

42. In a history and physical examination, the dictated sentence, "Her father died at age 75 of what sounded like a heart aneurysm," would be found under which topic?
    (a) Heart
    (b) Family history
    (c) Social history
    (d) Past history

43. In a history and physical examination, the dictated sentence, "Nasal and oral mucosa was normal with oral mucosa pink and moist," would be found under which topic?
    (a) HEENT
    (b) Abdomen
    (c) Would not be included in this report
    (d) Would be included in an x-ray report

44. In a history and physical examination, the dictated sentence, "Both tympanic membranes are clear," would be found under which topic?
    (a) HEENT
    (b) Heart
    (c) Neck
    (d) None of the above

45. In a history and physical examination, the dictated sentence, "Micronase 2.5 mg b.i.d., Voltaren 75 mg daily, and Lescol 20 mg daily," would be found under which of the following?
    (a) HPI topic
    (b) HEENT topic
    (c) Would not be included in a history and physical examination report
    (d) None of the above

46. In a history and physical examination, the dictated sentence, "DJD of the left hip," would be found under which topic?
    (a) Lab
    (b) HEENT
    (c) Impression
    (d) Plan

47. In a chart note, the dictated sentence, "With his left hand occupied, he slipped and fell backward striking the dorsum of his left hand with the wrist flexed," would be found under which topic?
    (a) Subjective
    (b) Objective
    (c) Assessment
    (d) Plan

48. In a history and physical examination, the dictated sentence, "Early osteoarthritis affecting mainly the right hip but also the left hip and lumbar spine," would be found under which topic?
    (a) Impression
    (b) Plan
    (c) Objective
    (d) Treatment

49. In a chart note, the dictated sentence, "This patient presents with pain, redness, and tenderness in the right great toe," would be found under which topic?
    (a) Chief complaint
    (b) Lab
    (c) Assessment
    (d) Plan

50. In a history and physical examination, the dictated sentence, "There is a slight tenderness to palpation over the left trapezius," would be found under which topic?
    (a) Heart
    (b) Neck
    (c) Lungs
    (d) Extremities

To become proficient in transcribing medical reports, it is important that you understand the format of the transcribed reports. You also should be able to identify the various sections of a report and understand the link between the sections or topic headings and their contents. Some physicians do not dictate a report into its correct sections, or they fail to identify the headings. As you read through this chapter, take particular note to the design, headings, and formats of the different medical documents.

Although various institutional formats are acceptable, standardized formats for many report types have been developed by the Healthcare Informatics Committee of the American Society for Testing and Materials (ASTM). A standard called E2184, *Standard Specification for Healthcare Document Formats*, specifies the requirements for the sections and subsections and their arrangement in an individual's healthcare documents.

The transcribed medical report is a legal medical document that communicates the patient's health status to others. It must be transcribed accurately and completely. Any error, no matter how small, may jeopardize the patient's health. The attending physician and any involved specialist, therapist, or technician will base their assessment and recommendations for care and treatment of the patient on the medical transcripts they receive and review.

Medical records also provide documented evidence of a patient's medical treatment to insurance companies, along with information necessary for federal and state regulatory requirements. Records play a vital role in research, compiling statistics, and evaluating the healthcare delivery system. Quality assurance issues and consumer concerns about access to care rely heavily on statistics and data acquired from medical records to address these problems.

Medical records are vital records for your employer's accounting department. Procedure codes (CPT) and diagnostic codes (ICD-9-CM) reported on the patient's health insurance claim form are based on the documentation in the medical record and are used in billing.

Medical reports are dictated by physicians in all medical specialties, including ophthalmology, dentistry, chiropractic, pathology, psychiatry, and veterinary medicine.

Medical reports dictated in office practice, hospital, and inpatient facilities have similarities and differences. The four reports that form the basis of a patient's medical record in the inpatient setting, such as a hospital or rehabilitation center, are the (1) history and physical examination, (2) operative report, (3) consultation, and (4) discharge summary. These records are frequently referred to as the "big four."

Consultation, letters, chart notes, history and physical examination reports, diagnostic imaging reports, and procedure reports form the fundamental group that make up a patient's medical record in the outpatient setting, such as a private or group practice.

Each report always must include patient identifying information, such as the patient's legal name, date of birth (DOB), and a file number. Healthcare facilities that adhere to standards of the Joint Commission on Accreditation of Healthcare Organizations (JCAHO) must include the patient's name and identification number on all medical reports. It is critical to spell the patient's name correctly and document the patient's birth date accurately. Many facilities assign a unique identification number to each patient that is used each time that patient seeks care at the facility.

Typical Formatting of Medical Reports

All medical reports include the title of the report (chart note, history and physical, x-ray, etc.), statistical data (patient's name, identification number, DOB, date of examination, physician's name, etc.), and signature line. In addition, chart notes, procedure reports, and diagnostic imaging reports contain sections or headings. History and physical examination reports contain section headings and subsection headings. In clinical practice, however, you may see a variety of formatting styles. Therefore you always should refer to your employer's own manual of style before transcribing medical reports.

For the purpose of this textbook, you will be asked to format all medical reports in block style using 1-inch margins, single spacing, and blank lines separating the sections/headings, which are capitalized. You will be asked to format consultation letters with a 2-inch top margin to accommodate a letterhead. Using a standard format for medical documents will allow you to concentrate on developing your transcription skills. Refer to the model medical documents based on *The AAMT Book of Style for Medical Transcription* included in Appendix C.

- Block format is preferred; all lines flush left.
- Use 1-inch margins, top and bottom, left and right, for reports. Use 2-inch top margins for letters.
- Ragged right margins are preferred.
- Avoid end-of-line hyphenation.
- Double-space between major sections of reports.
- Single-space between subheadings contained in the physical examination section.
- Use all capital letters for major section headings.
- Use initial capital letters for subsection headings.
- In medical reports, key the content on the next line following the section or subsection heading, if possible.
- When headings are included in letters, key the content on the same line following the headings. Use all capital letters for headings and a colon after each heading.
- Content included in the physical examination section of a medical report is keyed on the same line following the subheading. Use a colon after each subheading.

- Capitalize the word following the heading.
- Paragraphs are used to separate narrative blocks within sections.
- End each entry with a period unless it is a date or the name of a person.
- When a medical report is longer than one page, the word *continued* is keyed in the footer pane on each printed page before the last page.
- When a medical report is longer than one page, the name of the report, patient's name, file number, and page number are keyed in the header pane on each printed page.
- When a letter is longer than one page, the name of the patient, date, and page number are keyed in the header pane on each printer page.
- Do not carry a single line of a report onto a continuation page.
- Do not allow a continuation page to include only the signature block and the data following it.

Formatting Signature Lines (Medical Reports)

The physician's or dictator's name and title is entered four lines below the final line of text, flush left. Common practice often includes the dictator's and transcriptionist's initials placed at the end of each report. Enter the initials, flush left and two lines below the physician's name. Use either all capitals or all lowercase letters for both sets of initials with a colon or diagonal between them, without the use of periods. The date of the dictation, indicated by the letter D, and date the document was transcribed, indicated by the letter T, are entered flush left below the initials of the dictator and transcriptionist (Figure 2-1).

Physicians should not use rubber stamps or initials to sign dictation because it is difficult to prove legal authenticity without a complete signature. Rubber stamps can be stolen, and initials can be forged.

Outpatient Medical Documents

As a novice medical transcriptionist, you will probably begin your career in a private or group physician practice. For this reason, this textbook devotes its content to

developing your transcription skills by familiarizing you with the medical documents commonly found in the private or group physician practice. Each component of the transcription process will be explained step by step. An emphasis on developing fundamental transcription skills, and not requiring you to discern between multiple formatting and guideline rules that exist in current practice, should simplify the learning process for a beginning medical transcriptionist. To assist you in this learning process, you will be asked to follow a specific format for each report based on *The AAMT Book of Style* as presented in this chapter and Appendix C.

CHART NOTES

The physician dictates the chart note after talking, examining, or meeting with the patient. Remember that speaking with a physician over the phone still involves the patient's healthcare, and as such, this information needs to be documented in the medical record. The physician also must sign the report.

The chart note contains a precise description of the patient's major presenting problem (chief complaint), physical findings, and the physician's plan of treatment. It also may include the results of laboratory and x-ray tests. Chart notes can vary in length from a mere sentence or two to several pages, with the average length being two to four paragraphs. The items dictated into a chart note will vary depending on the severity of the patient's problem and brevity of the dictator.

Abbreviations and phrases are used often in a chart note to save space. It is imperative that all abbreviations are correctly transcribed and that no ambiguity exists as to their exact meaning. An example would be *Ca*, which could be interpreted as *calcium* or *cancer*. When in doubt, spell out the word and verify its meaning with the dictator. Many healthcare facilities have an approved list of abbreviations with clearly defined definitions that are acceptable to all practitioners of the organization, whereas other facilities may not allow the use of abbreviations. Healthcare facilities owned by hospital organizations are required to follow JCAHO rules and regulations, including having an approved abbreviation list on site.

Formatting Statistical Data

As with other medical reports, chart notes require the patient's statistical data on the first and succeeding pages. The patient's statistical data on the first page include the patient's full name, date of birth, and examination visit. The same information is included on the document if it extends beyond one page. The patient's full name, date of birth, and page number appear on continuation sheets.

```
_____

Potter T. Bucky, MD


ptb:cd
D: 11/20/xx (date the report was dictated)
T: 11/21/xx (date the report was transcribed)
```

Figure 2-1 Example of a signature block.

Statistical data for the first page:
   Patient Name: Doe, Jane
   Date of Birth: December 21, 1952
   Examination Date: April 1, 20xx
Statistical data for continuation pages:
   Patient Name: Doe, Jane
   Date of Birth: December 21, 1952
   Page 2

Formatting Chart Notes

A common chart note format is the *SOAP* method, which is an acronym for *subjective, objective, assessment,* and *plan.* The SOAP format is illustrated in Appendix C, Figure C-1. Each heading has a distinctive meaning, as follows:

S: Subjective findings are typically associated with what prompted the patient to seek medical care. A patient will describe feelings and symptoms to the physician.

   Example: My head and throat hurt, and I have been throwing up all day.

O: Objective findings are measurable findings discovered by the physician or by the results of diagnostic studies or laboratory tests.

   Example: Temperature is 103.2°F, and throat culture is positive.

A: Assessment is the physician's diagnosis or diagnoses of the patient's disease or condition, based on subjective and objective findings.

   Example: Strep throat.

P: Plan is the treatment plan developed by the physician relative to the findings of the subjective and objective assessment of the patient.

   Example: Amoxicillin 250 mg t.i.d. × 10 days.

When physicians are dictating chart notes using the SOAP format, they may say the headings or just give the first letter. Whether the heading is spelled out or only the first letter is typed depends on your employer's formatting guidelines. In such cases, a physician may dictate one of the following:

"Subjective: Patient complains of shortness of breath on exertion, with occasional pain radiating down left arm."

"S: Patient complains of shortness of breath on exertion, with occasional pain radiating down left arm."

Another format for chart notes uses the history and physical style and may include sections found in a history and physical examination report (see Appendix C, Figure C-2). Exercises provided later will help you identify dictated sentences and their headings.

HISTORY AND PHYSICAL EXAMINATION REPORTS

The dictation style of history and physical examination (H&P) reports contains recurrent phrases and terms.

It also contains more negative than positive statements. The major headings do not vary much and are used repeatedly in almost every report, as illustrated in Box 2-1. However, sometimes not all headings are needed, and the standard format is modified according to the dictator's needs.

A characteristic of both the H&P report and the chart note is the tendency to condense and abbreviate whenever possible. Students who first encounter chart notes or H&P reports often become frustrated because of the short, cryptic style of dictation. Clipped sentences, which often lack a subject or verb, are a common and acceptable dictating style. When you are listening to such dictation, you will find that words may be omitted or a subject or verb may not be included, yet the meaning of the sentence will be clear to you even though some words are unspoken. The following are some

---

BOX 2-1 History and Physical Examination Report Headings

History
Chief complaint
History of present illness (or present illness)
Past medical history
Allergies
Medications
Family history
Social history
Habits
Review of systems

Physical Examination
General (this includes vital signs)
HEENT (head, eyes, ears, nose, throat)
Neck
Chest (includes thorax, breasts, and axillae)
Heart
Lungs
Abdomen
Pelvic (sometimes listed as *genitalia*)
Rectal
Extremities
Neurological (includes mental status)

Laboratory Tests
(When available)

Diagnostic Tests
(When available)

Impression

Plan
(Or recommendation)

---

examples of clipped sentence structure:

CHEST: Clear to percussion and auscultation. Heart regular rate and rhythm.

ABDOMEN: Flat, soft, nontender, nondistended, normoactive bowel sounds.

RECTAL: No masses. Guaiac negative.

This means: The chest was clear to percussion and auscultation. The heart rate and rhythm were regular. The abdomen was soft and nontender, was not distended, and had normal bowel sounds. The rectal exam was negative in that no masses were found, and the guaiac test found no occult blood in the feces.

Formatting Statistical Data on the H&P Report

In this textbook, H&P reports, like chart notes, are formatted in block style using 1-inch margins, single spacing, and blank lines separating the headings, which are capitalized as illustrated in Appendix C, Figure C-3. The patient's statistical data are required on the first and continuation pages and include the patient's full name, identification number, date of birth, examination date, and physician's name. An employer's transcription guidelines may expand the requirements to suit the needs of the individual facility and its staff members.

History and Physical Examination Report

Statistical data for the first page:

    Patient Name: Doe, Jane

    File Number: 00912

    Date of Birth: December 21, 1952

    Examination Date: April 1, 20xx

    Physician: Potter T. Bucky, MD

History and Physical Examination Report

Statistical data for continuation pages:

    Patient Name: Doe, Jane

    File Number: 00912

    Page 2

The physical examination of a patient is an exact and involved process, and the headings in an H&P report are more numerous than on chart notes. The H&P report is divided into two major headings, "History" and "Physical Examination."

Headings in the "History" Section of the H&P Report

Headings within the "history" section of the history and physical examination report follow a specific format. In this textbook, topic headings are formatted in all capital letters. These major headings are as follows:

- *Chief complaint* (CC) is the specific reason for which the patient sought medical care, stated in the most concise terms or sometimes quoted in the patient's own words.
- *History of present illness* (HPI) contains all historical information that was given by the patient concerning the illness. This information includes all relevant symptoms and their duration and any remedies that have been attempted. Depending on the illness, this information may be stated in a concise sentence, or it may occupy a page or more of information if the problem is the culmination of weeks or even months of a chronic evolving illness.
- *Past medical history* (PMH) includes information about previous illnesses, injuries, surgeries, and chronic conditions that a patient may have had, along with any allergies to medications. This topic also may include immunizations.
- *Allergies* are a list of the patient's allergies. Allergies are keyed in all capitals, boldfaced, or underlined to call attention to their importance. The format varies by facility. Medications may be included in this section or under a separate heading.
- *Medications* are a list of medications that the patient is currently taking. Sometimes this information is not listed as a separate topic but included under "Past Medical History" or "Allergies."
- *Family history* consists of information about any hereditary or familial diseases.
- *Social history* is included if the physician believes this information is pertinent to the patient's treatment plan. This topic may include lifestyle habits such as smoking and drinking, as well as the patient's occupation, hobbies, family structure, and living arrangements.
- *Review of systems* (ROS) includes a brief review of any relevant information about each major body system. Depending on the patient's problem, this topic may be very comprehensive and divided into subheadings (e.g., HEENT, cardiovascular, respiratory, gastrointestinal, genitourinary, gynecologic, neuropsychiatric, musculoskeletal), or it may be combined into one paragraph or may simply be a brief statement such as "noncontributory" when all systems are negative.

Headings in the "Physical Examination" Section of the H&P Report

The "Physical Examination" heading of the report is exactly what its name implies. The physician completes a physical examination of the patient, and the findings are transcribed under the pertinent topic. In this textbook, subheadings are formatted in all capital letters. Information following the subsection heading continues on the same line. A colon is used after each subheading. The major subheadings for the physical examination of the report include the following:

- The *general* section discusses the appearance of the patient, such as pallor, gait, mood, and personal hygiene. It also includes a statement of the patient's vital signs (blood pressure, temperature, pulse, and respiration).
- *HEENT* is an abbreviation for the *head*, *eyes*, *ears*, *nose*, and *throat*.
- The *neck* is palpated for enlargement of the lymph nodes or thyroid gland, assessment of the carotid pulses, and distention of the jugular veins.

- The *chest* also includes the thorax, breasts, and axillary areas.
- The *lungs* are evaluated by auscultation, during which the physician listens with a stethoscope to air moving in and out of the lungs. Diseases or injury can produce abnormal changes in the quality and volume or loudness in breath sounds. The physician also may perform the percussion (tapping) maneuver.
- The *heart* is evaluated with a stethoscope for any abnormal sounds, such as murmurs or bruits (sound or murmur heard in auscultation), clicks (brief, sharp sounds, especially any of the short, dry clicking heart sounds during systole), rubs (sounds caused by rubbing together of two serous surfaces), thrills (vibrations), and gallops (disordered heart rhythms).
- The *abdomen* is assessed by auscultation, in which the physician listens for any abnormal bowel sounds, and percussion, in which the physician palpates the abdomen for tenderness, guarding, and masses.
- The *pelvic* region or genitalia are examined. Women may undergo a bimanual pelvic exam and Papanicolaou (Pap) smear.
- The *rectal* exam involves a digital evaluation of the rectum for deformity or masses. The physician also may comment on the results of a guaiac test (for occult blood) or colonoscopy (fiberoptic instrument) in this topic of the report. Men may undergo a digital rectal examination of the prostate. Digital palpation is a useful method for detection of early prostatic carcinoma.
- The *extremities* are examined for developmental or traumatic deformities, muscle wasting, and stiffness. The bones, joints, and muscles of all extremities are evaluated.
- The *neurological* examination is a systematic evaluation of the nervous system, including mental status, functioning of the cranial nerves and reflexes, and sensory and neuromuscular function. The Babinski reflex and deep tendon reflexes (DTRs) are usually checked.
- *Laboratory data* include laboratory test results, such as complete blood count (CBC), white blood cell count (WBC), and urinalysis (UA).

The H&P report concludes with the *impression* and *plan* headings. These two headings are formatted in all capital letters with the content information keyed on the following line.

- The *impression* is the physician's diagnosis or diagnoses of the patient's clinical condition or disease based on the findings of the physical examination and diagnostic tests.
- The *plan of treatment* is developed by the physician based on the findings of the physical examination and diagnostic tests.

DIAGNOSTIC IMAGING REPORTS AND LETTERS

Diagnostic imaging reports typically include clinical radiology (x-ray), ultrasonography (US) or sonography, computed tomography (CT), nuclear medicine (NM), and magnetic resonance imaging (MRI). Each area is classified as a separate imaging modality because each uses a different type of energy and recording device to image the body.

A computer is involved in the imaging process of almost all these different modalities. The image can be displayed on a video monitor and then digitally stored or printed on traditional x-ray film. All modalities except diagnostic x-ray have cross-sectional image recording capabilities. Each modality has its own unique features and capabilities for anatomic imaging. A certain body structure is imaged better with one modality than with another. The physician chooses the best, most effective imaging modality to evaluate the anatomy of interest.

Diagnostic x-rays use low levels of radiation to record images of the body on x-ray film. Newer methods sometimes allow the image to be digitized and stored in a computer.

Ultrasound or sonography uses high-frequency sound waves to image the body. It is unique in that it does not expose patients to ionizing radiation and therefore is the modality of choice to evaluate maternal or fetal anatomy in pregnant women.

In nuclear medicine the energy source is a radioactive isotope that is injected into the patient's body. Specialized computers and cameras then record and store the image.

Computed tomography uses a combination of radiation and computerized imaging techniques to record and display an individual's anatomy. It is sometimes referred to as a *CAT scan* (computerized axial tomography). This term is technically incorrect because current CT scanners can image the body in more than the axial plane.

In magnetic resonance imaging a sophisticated machine uses a magnetic field and radio frequency waves to generate an image. MRI does not use ionizing radiation and often produces sharper soft tissue images than other modalities.

Typical Formatting of Diagnostic Imaging Reports and Letters

Medical imaging reports look very different from SOAP notes, consultation letters, or H&P reports. The title of the report reflects the imaging modality chosen and the anatomy of interest. The report often includes a statement about various anatomic projections. To best visualize an anatomic part, the patient is imaged in many different positions, called *projections*.

At least two perpendicular projections are taken during a medical imaging procedure. Because the human body is three-dimensional and most imaging techniques are one-dimensional, multiple projections are required to evaluate the anatomy of interest thoroughly. For example, multiple views of the lumbar spine are routinely taken in diagnostic x-ray. If the patient is supine, the resulting projection is termed an *anteroposterior* or *AP projection*. If the patient is imaged when lying on the left side, the projections are termed a *left lateral projection*. If the patient is rotated 45 degrees toward the left when in the supine position, this is termed a *left posterior oblique projection* or *LPO*.

The body of the medical imaging report uses this positioning terminology because the physician, typically a radiologist, interprets the film. Your success in this area depends on a firm grasp of medical terminology and a solid understanding of positional terms, body planes, and basic radiological science terminology.

Physicians in the community typically refer patients to imaging centers. The transcribed report is sent back to the referring physician in a letter format. Hospital reports usually are not converted to letter format.

Formatting Statistical Data on the Diagnostic Imaging Report

In this textbook, diagnostic imaging reports are formatted in block style using 1-inch margins, single spacing, and blank lines separating the headings, which are capitalized (see Appendix C, Figure C-4). The statistical data on the first page should include the patient's full name, identification or file number, date of birth, examination date and ordering physician. The employer's transcription guidelines may expand the requirements to suit the needs of the facility and staff members.

X-ray Report
Statistical data for the first page:
    Patient Name: Doe, Jane
    File Number: 45231
    Date of Birth: December 21, 1952
    Examination Date: April 1, 20xx
    Ordering Physician: Izzy Sertoli, MD
X-ray Report
Statistical data for continuation pages:
    Patient Name: Doe, Jane
    File Number: 45321
    Page 2

The diagnostic imaging letter is formatted as illustrated in Appendix C, Figure C-5. The patient's name and date of birth are included in the reference line of the diagnostic imaging letter.

Headings Included on the Diagnostic Imaging Report

History comprises the technologist's observations and remarks concerning the chief complaint. These findings provide clinical information helpful to the radiologist in interpreting the films. This is a relatively new topic of the report and may not be included. Use of computerized medical records necessitates that the radiologist dictate this information into the report.

The *findings* are the physician's interpretation in regard to the disorder and disease processes shown on the hard-copy film or monitor.

The *impression* is the physician's assessment of the patient's health status as determined by the diagnostic images. This is usually a brief summary of the findings.

PROCEDURE REPORTS

With current sophisticated computerized medical technology, many procedures once performed exclusively in the hospital setting are now routinely performed in the medical office environment. Compact, low-cost, and technologically sophisticated medical machines are common diagnostic tools in ambulatory medical practices. Transcriptionists employed in medical offices often find procedure reports such as electrocardiograms (ECGs), sigmoidoscopy, and colposcopy as standard components of a dictation.

The format and headings used for these reports are similar to those used in diagnostic imaging reports, as illustrated in Appendix C, Figure C-6. Identification of headings such as the patient name and identification data (usually date of birth and file number), date of procedure, ordering physician, and name of procedure will accurately associate the physician's findings with the correct patient.

Formatting Statistical Data on the Procedure Report

In this textbook, procedure reports are formatted in block style using 1-inch margins, single spacing, and blank lines separating the headings, which are capitalized. Statistical data on the first page should include the patient's full name, date of birth, practice-specific file number, examination visit, and ordering physician. The employer's transcription guidelines may expand the requirements to suit the needs of the facility and staff members.

Procedure Report
Statistical data for the first page:
    Patient Name: Kleine, Ann
    File Number: 186-00-6810
    Date of Birth: March 7, 19xx
    Examination Date: January 1, 20xx
    Ordering Physician: Izzy Sertoli, MD
Procedure Report
Statistical data for continuation pages:
    Patient Name: Kleine, Ann
    File Number: 186-00-6810
    Page 2

OPERATIVE REPORTS

Operative reports are detailed and descriptive and allow the reader to visualize the operation. The operative reports here are of relatively simple operations. The preoperative and postoperative diagnoses are dictated in the report and may be the same, but it is not acceptable to type *same* under the postoperative topic. The transcriptionist must key the diagnostic statement. Abbreviations should be avoided.

Formatting Statistical Data on the Operative Report

The format of this report is similar to procedure and diagnostic imaging reports. The differences are two additional headings in the statistical section (see Appendix C, Figure C-7).

Operative Report
Statistical data for the first page:
 Patient Name: Mason, Charles
 File Number: 00123
 Date of Birth: March 27, 19xx
 Operation Date: February 1, 20xx
Operative Report
Statistical data for continuation pages:
 Patient Name: Mason, Charles
 File Number: 00123
 Page 2

CONSULTATION REPORTS

The consultation report advises the referring physician of the status of a patient who has been referred to a specialist. Because the patient usually returns to the primary care physician, documentation of the patient's assessment, care, and progress must be sent within a short time. The consultation report format uses headings associated with the history and physical examination (see Appendix C, Figure C-8).

Formatting Statistical Data on the Consultation Report

In this textbook, consultation reports are formatted in the same manner as other medical reports, in block style using 1-inch margins, single spacing, and blank lines separating the headings, which are capitalized. Statistical data on the first page should include the patient's full name and date of birth, along with practice-specific file number, examination visit, and requesting physician. The employer's transcription guidelines may expand the requirements to suit the needs of the facility and staff members.

Statistical data for the first page:

Patient Name: Kleine, Ann
File Number: 186-00-6810
Date of Birth: March 7, 19xx
Examination Date: May 1, 20xx
Requesting Physician: Izzy Sertoli, MD
Statistical data for continuation pages:
 Patient Name: Kleine, Ann
 File Number: 186-00-6810
 Page 2

BUSINESS AND CONSULTATION LETTERS

Both business letters and consultation letters are written in formal style. The consultation report can be presented in a letter format (see Appendix C, Figure C-9). The business letter is usually used for nonpatient correspondence such as supply orders, collection reminders, requests for information, and making travel arrangements.

The two common formats for letters are the block format and modified block format. In the block format with open punctuation, all information begins at the left margin. This textbook will present and provide exercises using the block format.

All letters are printed on 8.5 × 11–inch paper and contain most, if not all, of the following components:

- *Dateline*: The dateline is positioned 2 inches from the top of the page to allow for a printed letterhead. The dateline includes the month (no abbreviations), date, and year.
   Example: December 21, 20xx.
- *Inside address*: The inside address is comprised of the addressee's name, title, street address, city, state (two-letter state abbreviation), and zip code.
   Example
   Adam Valence, MD
   FedDes Wellness Center
   Cardiology Division, Suite 413
   101 Wellness Way Drive
   New York, NY 10036
- *Reference line*: The reference line is commonly used in medical correspondence. It saves time by giving the addressee a specific named reference. It also is very helpful when filing the document. The reference line is introduced by the abbreviation *Re* and followed by a colon. The reference line is double spaced and placed above the salutation line in a letter.
   Example
   Re: Betty McWilliams
    Date of Birth: February 2, 1949
    Examinations:
    Video Esophagram and GI Series.
    Flat Plate of the Abdomen.
- *Salutation*: The salutation line is the greeting line for all correspondence and begins with the word *Dear*.

The recipient's last name only is used in the salutation. A colon (mixed punctuation) or no punctuation mark (open punctuation) follows the name. In some geographic locations, the title *Dr.* is spelled out.

Example of mixed punctuation: Dear Dr. Valence:
Example of open punctuation: Dear Dr. Valence

- *Body*: Business and consultation may be one or more pages. Paragraphs are single-spaced. Double spacing is used to separate paragraphs.
- *Closing line*: The complimentary close is the closing line for all correspondence and begins with words such as "Sincerely, "Sincerely yours," or "Very truly yours." Only the first word of the closing line begins with a capital letter. A comma (mixed punctuation) or no punctuation (open punctuation) follows the last word of the closing.

Example of mixed punctuation: Sincerely yours,
Example of open punctuation: Sincerely yours

- *Signature line*: The signature line is composed of the writer's full name and title (if applicable). A handwritten signature would appear above the typed signature line. Physicians should not use rubber stamp signature pads.
- *Reference initials*: The reference initials identify the typist or transcriptionist.
- *Enclosure line*: This line alerts the addressee that items are enclosed with the letter.
- *Copy line*: This line informs the addressee that a copy of the correspondence will be sent to someone else. Use the abbreviation *c*, followed by a colon, and the complete name of the recipient. The abbreviation *cc* (carbon copy) is no longer used.

Example: c: John Smith

- *Continuation sheet*: If the letter is longer than one page, a heading must appear on the succeeding pages. The heading is placed 1 inch from the top of the page. The heading includes the patient's name, date, and page number.

Example
Betty McWilliams
December 21, 20xx
Page 2

The placement of the letter parts in a business letter is illustrated in Appendix C, Figure C-10.

USING TEMPLATES IN MEDICAL TRANSCRIPTION

To increase production speed, some transcriptionists will make a template or macro of a standard chart note, H&P report, and diagnostic imaging report and then add or delete the headings as needed. Another advantage to using a template is that along with the presented outline, the page margins and tab stops are established.

Because transcriptionists' pay may be based on word count or line count, it becomes even more important to use templates. Selected activities in this textbook require the creation and use of templates.

There are a variety of standard headings, headings, and subheadings found on the different medical documents. You may find certain headings are more applicable to one specialty than another and that these headings can be easily added or modified to the template.

A template is a document file that allows customized formats, content, and features. Templates can contain a host of customized features, such as text, graphics, styles, macros, abbreviations, toolbars, and menu bars. Templates are usually identified with the *.dot* file extension.

Directions for Creating a Document Template

1. Click *File, New, Blank Document*.
2. Click *Template* under *Create New*, then click *OK*.
3. Create the template as you would any other medical document, formatting the desired page margins, tab stops, headings, and subheadings. For example, when creating a template for an H&P report, type the headings and subheadings.
4. To save the template, click *File* and *Save As*.
5. In the *Save as type* box, click *Document Template*. This file type will already be selected if you are saving a file that you created as a template.
6. In the *File name* box, type a name for the new template, then click *Save*.
7. Open the template file when needed.
8. After you finish keying in the document, save the file under a new name.

NOTE: If you save a template in the Templates folder, the template appears on the General tab when you click *New* on the File menu. If you want to create custom tabs for your templates in the New dialog box, create a new folder in the Templates folder and save your templates in that folder. The name you give that folder will appear on the new tab.

An example of a template for an H&P report is shown in Figure 2-2.

USING HEADERS AND FOOTERS IN MEDICAL TRANSCRIPTION

Headers and footers are useful additions to multiple-page medical reports. The text in the top margin of a page is a *header*; the text in the bottom margin of a page is a *footer*. Headers can also contain descriptive information about a document, such as the date, title of the report, the physician's and the patient's name, and page number. For example, the statistical data for

```
HISTORY AND PHYSICAL EXAMINATION REPORT

Patient Name:
File Number:
Date of Birth:
Examination Date:
Physician:

HISTORY

CHIEF COMPLAINT

HISTORY OF PRESENT ILLNESS

PAST HISTORY

REVIEW OF SYSTEMS

GENITOURINARY:

PHYSICAL EXAMINATION
GENERAL:
HEENT:
LUNGS:
HEART:
ABDOMEN:
PELVIC:
EXTREMITIES:
NEUROLOGICAL:

IMPRESSION

PLAN



Gwenn Maltase, MD

gm:xx
D:
T:
```

Figure 2-2 Template for a history and physical examination report.

continuation pages of procedure reports include the patient name, file number, and page number. This tool adds to the document a header, which prints the same information at the top of each page. Footers can be used to add the word "continued" at the end of the page in a multiple-page medical report.

Directions for Using Headers and Footers

1. First, insert a Next Page Section break to begin page 2 of your document. To do this, choose *Insert*, *Break*, *Section Break Types*, *Next Page*. Click *OK*.
2. Choose *View, Header/Footer* (Word), which displays the Header/Footer toolbar. The toolbar selections include Insert Auto Text, Insert Page Number, Insert Number of Pages, Format Page Number, Insert Date, Insert Time, Page Setup, Show/Hide Document Text, Same as Previous, Switch Between Header and Footer, Show Previous, Show Next, and Close buttons.
3. Click *Same as Previous* button on the Header and Footer toolbar so that the Header does not appear on the first page of your document.
4. Key in the statistical information in the Header pane.
5. Click the *Switch Between Header and Footer* button to display the footer pane.
6. Click *Same as Previous* button on the Header and Footer toolbar so that the Footer does not appear on the first page of your document.
7. Key the word *continued* in the Footer pane.
8. Click *Close*.

REMEMBER: The default page setup for headers and footers is 0.5 inch. The default setting is used for headers and footers in all medical documents, except letters. Letters do not contain a footer. The header in a letter is formatted at 1 inch, and the top margin for the second page of a letter is also formatted at 1 inch.

Understanding the contents of medical documents is the first step to becoming an accomplished transcriptionist. Assess your knowledge of medical document content by completing these two activities.

TEXTBOOK USERS

Select the best answer for each question or statement concerning medical reports. Refer to the answer key (Appendix E) for immediate feedback.

SOFTWARE USERS

Click on *Chapter 2, Activity 2-1,* and follow the directions.
Follow the same process for *Chapter 2, Activity 2-2.*

ACTIVITY 2-1
Understanding Medical Documents

Directions: Select true (T) or false (F) and the best multiple-choice answer for each question or statement concerning medical reports.

1. T or F   Medical reports dictated in office practices differ from those dictated in hospital settings.

2. T or F   The most common medical reports found in outpatient facilities are chart notes, consultation letters, history and physical examination reports, diagnostic imaging reports, and procedure reports.

3. T or F   The medical report must include patient identification information.

4. T or F   The assessment of the Babinski reflex is found under the "HEENT" topic.

5. T or F   Most beginning medical transcriptionists obtain their first job at hospitals.

6. T or F   A chart note can also be referred to as a *follow-up note*.

7. T or F   CC is the abbreviation for *chief complaint*.

8. T or F   Abbreviations and phrases are not used in chart notes.

9. T or F   Medical reports require that the patient's statistical data appear on the first page but not on succeeding pages.

10. T or F   The assessment of the thorax is found under the "Chest" topic.

11. T or F   The letter *O* in the acronym *SOAP* stands for *objective*.

12. T or F   HPI is the abbreviation for *history of present illness*.

13. T or F   The history and physical format of a chart note contains no variations in headings.

14. T or F   UA is the abbreviation for *urinalysis*.

15. T or F   The dictation style of a history and physical examination report contains more negative than positive statements.

16. T or F   PMH is the abbreviation for *premenstrual history*.

17. T or F   Headings found on the H&P are more numerous than on chart notes.

18. T or F   All the patient's relevant symptoms and their duration are found under the "Past Medical History" topic.

19. T or F   The patient's information about previous illness, injuries, and surgeries is found under the "Past Medical History" topic.

20. T or F   The patient's medication history can be found under the "Past Medical History" topic.

21. T or F   The assessment of the carotid pulses is found under the "Neck" topic.

22. T or F   The assessment of the deep tendon reflexes is found under the "Neurological" topic.

23. T or F   Consultation findings can be dictated in letter and report style.

24. T or F   Abbreviations are acceptable in the dateline of a letter.

25. T or F   The salutation line is the greeting line for all correspondence.

26. In a chart note, the dictated word *epicondylitis* would be found under which topic?
    (a) Subjective
    (b) Objective
    (c) Assessment
    (d) Plan

27. In a chart note, the dictated sentence, "Prescribe Motrin 200 mg q.i.d.," would be found under which topic?
    (a) Subjective
    (b) Objective
    (c) Assessment
    (d) Plan

ACTIVITY 2-1 *(cont'd)*

28. The dictated sentence, "Severe pain in the second and third fingers on the right hand," would be found under which topic?
    (a) Review of systems
    (b) Chief complaint
    (c) General
    (d) Extremities

29. The dictated sentence, "BP 120/80, pulse 106 and regular, temperature 37.2°C, respirations 14/min," would be found under which topic?
    (a) General
    (b) Genitourinary
    (c) Lungs
    (d) Heart

30. The dictated sentence, "Gravida 2, para 2," would be found under which topic?
    (a) HEENT
    (b) Genitourinary
    (c) Lungs
    (d) Heart

31. The dictated sentence, "Clear to P&A," would be found under which topic?
    (a) HEENT
    (b) Genitourinary
    (c) Lungs
    (d) Heart

32. The dictated sentence, "No frequency, hematuria, or nocturia," would be found under which topic?
    (a) HEENT
    (b) Genitourinary
    (c) Lungs
    (d) Heart

33. The dictated sentence, "Uterus not enlarged," would be found under which topic?
    (a) HEENT
    (b) Genitourinary
    (c) Pelvic
    (d) Heart

34. The dictated sentence, "She is currently under therapy for hyperthyroidism," would be found under which topic?
    (a) HEENT
    (b) Genitourinary
    (c) Pelvic
    (d) History of present illness

35. The dictated sentence, "She has multiple filled caries," would be found under which topic?
    (a) HEENT
    (b) Genitourinary
    (c) Pelvic
    (d) History of present illness

ACTIVITY 2-2
Understanding Medical Documents

Directions: Select true (T) or false (F) and the best multiple-choice answer for each question or statement concerning medical reports.

1. T or F   The letter *S* in the acronym *SOAP* stands for *symptoms*.

2. T or F   The number of headings found on the H&P is less than found on chart notes.

3. T or F   The patient is imaged in numerous different positions called *projections*.

4. T or F   Headings in medical documents are typically keyed in all capital letters.

5. T or F   Double spacing is used to separate headings.

6. T or F   To increase production speed, transcriptionists rely on templates.

7. T or F   All imaging modalities have cross-sectional image recording capabilities.

8. T or F   Diagnostic x-rays use low levels of radiation to record images of the body on x-ray film.

9. T or F   Ultrasound uses low-frequency sound waves to image the body.

10. T or F   Computed tomography uses a combination of radiation and computerized imaging techniques to record and display anatomy.

11. T or F   The physician always dictates the letters of the acronym *SOAP*.

12. T or F   Magnetic resonance imaging uses radio frequency waves to generate an image.

13. T or F   Left lateral projection describes the patient with the left side closest to the film.

14. T or F   The physician specialist who typically interprets films is the radiologist.

15. T or F   The "History" topic is a relatively new topic found in diagnostic imaging reports.

16. T or F   Ultrasound uses high-frequency sound waves to image the body.

17. T or F   The H&P report is used in both outpatient and inpatient facilities.

18. T or F   Magnetic resonance imaging produces sharper soft tissue images than other modalities.

19. T or F   Medical imaging reports are formatted similar to H&P reports.

20. T or F   In this textbook all medical reports are formatted in block style using 1 inch margins.

21. T or F   The complimentary closing is the closing line for all correspondence.

22. T or F   The letter *A* in the acronym *SOAP* stands for *allergies*.

23. T or F   A template is a document file with customized format, content, and features.

24. T or F   *AP projection* is the abbreviation for *anteroposterior projection*.

25. T or F   The assessment of the thorax is found under the "Neck" topic.

26. In a chart note, the dictated sentence, "BP 120/70, weight 150 lb, height 5 ft 7 in," would be found under which topic?
    (a) Subjective
    (b) Objective
    (c) Assessment
    (d) Plan

27. In a chart note, the dictated sentence, "Patient complains of left elbow pain for the past 2 weeks," would be found under which topic?
    (a) Subjective
    (b) Objective
    (c) Assessment
    (d) Plan

ACTIVITY 2-2 *(cont'd)*

28. In a chart note, the dictated sentence, "Tenderness over right medial epicondyle," would be found under which topic?
    (a) Subjective
    (b) Objective
    (c) Assessment
    (d) Plan

29. The dictated sentence, "Supple without thyromegaly or lymphadenopathy," would be found under which topic?
    (a) HEENT
    (b) Genitourinary
    (c) Pelvic
    (d) Neck

30. The dictated sentence, "Clear to auscultation anteriorly and posteriorly," would be found under which topic?
    (a) Chest
    (b) Genitourinary
    (c) Pelvic
    (d) Neck

31. The dictated sentence, "Nontender, no hepatomegaly," would be found under which topic?
    (a) Chest
    (b) Neurological
    (c) Pelvic
    (d) None of the above

32. The dictated sentence, "She denies fever, chills, hematemesis, or change in bowel habits," would be found under which topic?
    (a) Lungs
    (b) Genitourinary
    (c) History of present illness
    (d) None of the above

33. Diagnostic imaging reports include which of the following?
    (a) Ultrasonography
    (b) Nuclear medicine
    (c) Magnetic resonance
    (d) All the above

34. In a chart note, the dictated sentence, "She has vomited five times during the last 24 hours," would be found under which topic?
    (a) Subjective
    (b) Objective
    (c) Assessment
    (d) Plan

35. In a history and physical examination, the dictated sentence, "Gravida 1, para 1," would be found under which topic?
    (a) Physical examination
    (b) HEENT
    (c) Genitourinary
    (d) None of the above

The ability to format medical documents is the second step to becoming an accomplished transcriptionist. You are to create a template for Figures C-1, C-3, and C-5 in Appendix C, then type the documents.

TEXTBOOK USERS

Open your word processing package.
Create a template for Figure C-1.
Save the template on your student disk for further use throughout the text.
Follow the same process to create templates for Figures C-3 and C-5.
Using your created templates, type the model medical documents shown in
   Figures C-1, C-3, and C-5.
Identify and correct all errors.
Save each typed model document under a new file name on your student disk.

SOFTWARE USERS

Click on *Chapter 2, Activity 2-3*, and follow the directions.
Follow the same process for *Activity 2-4* and *Activity 2-5*.

Let's pause and see how well you have mastered the information in this chapter. This section allows you to evaluate your understanding of medical documents and their contents.

TEXTBOOK USERS

Select the best answer for each question or statement concerning medical reports. Refer to the answer key (Appendix E) for immediate feedback.

SOFTWARE USERS

Click on *Chapter 2, Check Your Progress*, and follow the directions.

CHECK YOUR PROGRESS

1. T or F   The left posterior oblique projection describes the patient in the supine position who is rotated 45 degrees toward the left.

2. T or F   The medical reports found in the office practice are chart notes, history and physical examination reports, consultation letters, diagnostic imaging reports, and procedure reports.

3. T or F   Continuation sheets for letters and reports require a page number.

4. T or F   The assessment of the deep tendon reflexes can be found under the "Extremities" topic.

5. T or F   Creating templates is a difficult process.

6. T or F   The assessment of the Babinski reflex is found under the "Neurological" topic.

7. T or F   A computer is involved in the imaging process of most medical imaging modalities.

8. T or F   ROS is the abbreviation for *review of systems*.

9. T or F   In this textbook all medical reports are formatted in block style using 1 inch margins.

10. T or F   Medical imaging reports are formatted similar to chart notes.

11. T or F   AP projection describes a patient who is imaged in the supine position.

12. T or F   To conserve space, chart notes are formatted with wide margins.

13. T or F   Medical reports should end with a signature line.

14. T or F   The letter *P* in the acronym *SOAP* stands for *procedure*.

15. T or F   *CBC* is the abbreviation for *complete blood count*.

16. T or F   The dictation style of a history and physical examination report contains more positive than negative statements.

17. T or F   The dictation style of chart notes contains cryptic sentences.

18. T or F   The assessment of the carotid pulses is found under the "Chest" topic.

19. T or F   The reference line in a business letter appears after the salutation line.

20. T or F   The copy line appears above the enclosure line.

21. T or F   Reference initials in a medical transcription document identify the typist or transcriptionist.

22. T or F   The abbreviation *Ca* means either calcium or cancer.

23. T or F   Headings are keyed in such a way as to indicate their importance.

24. T or F   Diagnostic x-rays use high levels of radiation to record images of the body on x-ray film.

25. T or F   The abbreviation *CC* means *chief complaint*.

26. T or F   Ultrasound is the modality of choice to evaluate maternal anatomy.

27. T or F   In nuclear medicine the energy source is a radioactive isotope that is injected into the patient's body.

28. T or F   Consultation letters are written in a formal style.

29. T or F   Pathology reports are one of the basic four medical reports.

30. T or F   Chart notes are also referred to as *progress notes*.

31. T or F   There is more than one format style for a chart note.

CHECK YOUR PROGRESS *(cont'd)*

32. T or F   The reference line is commonly used in consultation letters.

33. T or F   A chart note using the history and physical examination format may include diagnosis, laboratory, and treatment headings.

34. In a chart note, the dictated sentence, "Bobby vomited five times during the last 24 hours," would be found under which topic?
    (a) Subjective
    (b) Objective
    (c) Assessment
    (d) Plan

35. In a history and physical examination report, the dictated sentence, "gravida 2, para 2" would be found under which topic?
    (a) Physical examination
    (b) HEENT
    (c) Genitourinary
    (d) None of the above

36. In an H&P report, the dictated sentence, "BP 120/72, pulse 105 and regular, temperature 37.2°C," would be found under which topic?
    (a) Physical examination
    (b) HEENT
    (c) General or Vitals
    (d) Heart

37. In an H&P report, the dictated sentence, "Acute appendicitis," would be found under which topic?
    (a) Physical examination
    (b) General
    (c) Impression
    (d) Plan

38. What are the basic four medical reports in medical offices?
    (a) Consultation letter, chart note, history and physical, and pathology
    (b) Chart note, history and physical, diagnostic, and consultation
    (c) Chart note, history and physical, SOAP, and consultation
    (d) Consultation letter, SOAP, history and physical, and pathology

39. What four headings are in the acronym *SOAP*?
    (a) Symptom, objective, assessment, progress
    (b) Symptom, objective, assessment, plan
    (c) Subjective, objective, assessment, plan
    (d) Subjective, objective, assessment, progress

40. In a history and physical examination report, the dictated sentence, "Clear to P&A," would be found under which topic?
    (a) HEENT
    (b) General
    (c) Lungs
    (d) Heart

41. In an H&P report, the dictated sentence, "No murmurs, gallop, or thrills," would be found under which topic?
    (a) Impression
    (b) Neurological
    (c) Pelvis
    (d) Heart

42. In an H&P report, the dictated sentences, "Bowel sounds are normal. No organomegaly," would be found under which topic?
    (a) Impression
    (b) Abdomen
    (c) Rectal
    (d) None of the above

43. Medical reports are vital in which of the following?
    (a) Research
    (b) Compiling statistics
    (c) Evaluating healthcare delivery system
    (d) All the above

44. Reference initials must be included on which of the following?
    (a) Chart notes
    (b) History and physical examination reports
    (c) Consultation letters
    (d) All the above

45. The findings of an ECG would be included in which of the following?
    (a) Diagnostic imaging report
    (b) Procedure report
    (c) Business letter
    (d) None of the above

CHECK YOUR PROGRESS *(cont'd)*

46. The dictated sentence, "Discontinue use of perfumed body lotion," would be found in a chart note under which topic?
    (a) Subjective
    (b) Chief complaint
    (c) Plan
    (d) Assessment

47. The dictated sentence, "Smooth, erythematous rash over neck extending over trunk and back," would be found in a chart note under which topic?
    (a) Subjective
    (b) Objective
    (c) Assessment
    (d) None of the above

48. The dictated sentence, "My head and throat hurt," would be found in a chart note under which topic?
    (a) Subjective
    (b) Objective
    (c) Assessment
    (d) Symptom

49. The dictated sentence, "BP 120/82," would be found in a chart note under which topic?
    (a) Subjective
    (b) Objective
    (c) Assessment
    (d) Progress

50. The dictated sentence, "Acute otitis," would be found in a chart note under which topic?
    (a) Subjective
    (b) Objective
    (c) Assessment
    (d) Plan

Chapter 3

Proofreading

OBJECTIVES

At the completion of Chapter 3, you should be able to do the following:
1. Explain the importance of accurate proofreading in medical transcription.
2. Identify common errors found in medical documents.
3. Proofread from a computer screen.
4. Improve proficiency at creating and using templates in medical documents.
5. Reinforce spelling and keyboarding skills.

Pretests 3-1 through 3-3
The Proofreading Process
Guidelines to Proofreading Success
Error Analysis Chart
Basic English Usage Review
Activities
  3-1 through 3-3: Proofreading Worksheet Exercises
  3-4 through 3-6: Keyboarding and Proofreading Exercises
Check Your Progress 3-1 through 3-3

What's Ahead

Let's find out if you are able to type and proofread three medical documents that contain various errors.

TEXTBOOK USERS

Open your word processing package.
Type and proofread the medical documents shown in *Chapter 3, Pretest 3-1*, using the formatting guidelines established in Chapter 2.
Identify and correct all errors.
Save your work on your student disk.
After completing the Pretest, refer to the answer key (Appendix E).
Manually complete the error analysis chart.
Follow the same process for *Chapter 3, Pretests 3-2 and 3-3*.

SOFTWARE USERS

Click on *Chapter 3, Pretest 3-1*, and follow the directions.
Follow the same process for *Chapter 3, Pretests 3-2 and 3-3*.

PRETEST 3-1

Directions: Type and proofread this medical document, which contains multiple errors. Use open punctuation and all other formatting guidelines established in this textbook.

current date

Arthur Guttenberg, MD
5723 North Front Street
New York, New York 10010
RE: Martha Ultress
    Date of birth: 6/19/59

Dear Dr. Cuttenberg

Thank you for seeing Mary for her right rotator cuff tendinitis. She has has intermittent pain of the right shoulder during the past two months. Over the passed few days the pain has gotten very severe. On examination she could barely abduct past thirty degrees. Thee x ray was notable for some calcific tendinitis. I injected the subacromial bursa with Steroids and obtained a rather dramatic improvement in her bursitis only to have it return again; one wk later. I started her on a physical-therapy program and would appreciate you evaluation concerning the continuing care and treatment of this patient.

Very Truly Yours,

Harry A. Medulla, MD/xx

PRETEST 3-2

Directions: Type and proofread this medical document, which contains multiple errors. Use open punctuation and all other formatting guidelines established in this textbook.

CHART NOTE
Patient Name: Jose Ramirez
DOB: 5/23/xx
Examination Date: *current date*

History of present illness
This fifteen year old male is seen for a follow-up on his acne He has been using clearasil medicated astringent and oxy wash for about two months with no improvement He is on no orale medications denies any alergies and is in good health.

Physical esamination
Todays exam reveal inflammatory systic lesions along the jaw line and upper back. Some deep systs are palpable on the chin and over the right shoulder area.

Plan
She is to start E-Mycin two hundred fifty milligrams bid and ten percent Benzac topically hs after washing. He is to contine washing with oxy wash up to 3x a day as tolerated. He has been cautioned not to pick-at the lessions. We discussed the need to keep her hands away from his face as much as possible and to stop leaning on his elbow with his chin in his hand. It is a bad habit that only promotes the spread of bacteria and should be continued. He will be seen again in four to six weeks.

Allan Pore, MD

ap: xx
D: *current date*
T: *current date*

PRETEST 3-3

Directions: Type and proofread this medical document, which contains multiple errors. Use open punctuation and all other formatting guidelines established in this textbook.

CHART NOTE

Linda Smithers

DOB: August 13, XX

Examiantion Date: *current date*

CHEIF COMPLANT
Itching and a rash.

SUBJECTION
The patient is a pleasant, 26 year old female who is quiet cooperative and in no a cute distress. She complains a rash that began about 2 week's ago. She's taken benadryl at bedtime with no relief. Upon questioning he admits to using a new perfumed body lotion after her shower.

OBJECTION
Vital Signs: Temperature 98.6 blood pressure 136/72 weight 165 lbs height 5 3 pulse 74 respirations 22. Smooth erythematous rash over neck extending over trunk and back. On the upper extremities she has a erythematous rash extending to her wrists.

ASESMENT
Contact dermatits, secondary to allergy to perfume

PLAN
1. Discontine use of perfumed body lotion.
2. Wash all clothing and bed linen that were exposed to the perfumed lotion.
3. Take benadryl twenty five milligrams q6hx3 days

Allan Pore, MD

xx
D: *current date*
T: *current date*

To become an accomplished medical transcriptionist, proofreading is an essential skill. Too often, this skill is neglected in the learning process. As computer technology rapidly advances, the potential role of the medical transcriptionist may change to that of a document manager and editor. The shift to this role is foreseeable as voice technology takes a foothold in document preparation. However, according to the American Association for Medical Transcription (AAMT), "In spite of the advances in this technology, there will continue to be a need for skilled medical language specialists."

THE PROOFREADING PROCESS

The process of proofreading involves multiple steps that include reading, correcting, and revising a document to produce a final copy. Each document must be proofread word for word, figure for figure, and thought for thought.

Medical dictation can be highly technical and complex, and the potential for transcribing errors is high. The skills essential to good proofreading are spelling, knowledge of punctuation rules, and knowledge of grammar. You should proofread a document three times. The first step is reading for spelling, typographic errors, and repeated words. To obtain the fundamental skills in medical transcription, it is advisable to find the errors yourself and not rely on spell-check software. Professional medical transcriptionists use electronic medical dictionaries and spellers from numerous publishing companies, such as *Dorland's* and *Stedman's* electronic dictionaries, to increase their production speed and accuracy.

The second step in proofreading is looking for punctuation and grammar errors. Use your word processing software features to check your grammar.

The third step is reading the document for meaning. Does the sentence make sense within the content of the report? You need to learn the meaning of words, not just their spellings. In addition, you should be familiar with common English and medical sound-alike words. Play back the dictation at normal speed. Listen and follow along with the dictator as you check for errors. You should never change the meaning or intent of the dictation. As a novice transcriptionist, proofreading accuracy may require you to listen to the dictation more than once.

Proofreading requires excellent critical thinking skills. Paramount among these skills is the ability to know and use reference books. The transcription process is discussed in Chapter 4.

GUIDELINES TO PROOFREADING SUCCESS

Do not proofread too quickly. Proofreading is not a haphazard event but a sequential, detailed process.

Proofread on the screen as you type. This is a good habit to develop now, because professional medical transcriptionists are under production deadlines. Check for typographic, spelling, grammar errors, and incongruities in meaning or style. After correcting these errors, print a copy. It is easier to correct a document on paper than on a computer screen.

When in doubt, "look it up." Use every available reference material to clarify the meaning or spelling or grammar rule in question. If your investigation is futile, leave a blank space that approximates the length of the misunderstood word. Then attach a flag (usually an adhesive note) that indicates where the problem is found within the transcription and includes its phonetic spelling. You should be able to defend grammatically every comma, period, and hyphen that you have placed in your document.

Let time elapse between when you complete the document and when you proofread it for the final time. Errors seem to stand out after a waiting period has elapsed. Another trick is to read the document backward, which forces you to slow down and focus on each word. Also, look for any illogical words and phrases, such as, "The right hand was draped and prepped," when later in the report is the statement, "Sutures in left hand."

ERROR ANALYSIS CHART

The error analysis chart was developed as a tool to categorize and track undetected errors. A transcription error analysis chart for each document will help you and your instructor prescribe a remedy for each error. Observing the occurrence of repeated mistakes through charting will improve your transcription skills.

The chart is divided into two major categories, Medical Language and English Language, as shown in Figures 3-1 and 3-2. The medical language errors have a higher "error value" than the English errors. Because medication and allergy errors and incorrect patient identification adversely affect patient care, medical transcriptionists are heavily penalized if such errors are found during quality assurance audits. Some institutions strip incentive pay regardless of when the error is discovered, even if it is weeks later. An error follows you!

Analyzing Errors
Wrong Words
Failure to catch wrong words indicates the transcriptionist lacks knowledge of the medical terminology. It is important that the sentence makes sense. Sound-alike words cause many of these errors. An unfamiliar word should never be transcribed before it is referenced. Physicians may also dictate *nonwords*, especially by

NAME _____		DOCUMENT NO. _____	
TYPE OF ERROR	**ERROR VALUE**	**NUMBER OF ERRORS**	**TOTAL ERROR VALUE***
Medical Language			
Add/omit word(s)			
Misspelled word(s)			
Incorrect date(s) or number(s)			
Total Medical Language Errors	3 ×	=	
English Language			
Add/omit word(s)			
Misspelled word(s)			
Grammatical error(s)			
Punctuation error(s)			
Total English Language Errors	1 ×	=	
Total Language Errors			

*To compute total error value, multiply the number of errors by the error value (number of errors × error value = total error value).

Figure 3-1 Error analysis chart.

using an incorrect prefix or suffix, such as "nonavoidable" instead of "unavoidable."

Added or Omitted Letters and Words

Errors in which letters are added or omitted at the end of a word are overlooked if the addition or omission does not make the typed word meaningless. Failure to catch this type of error indicates the copy is being read word by word rather than for meaning.

Misspelled Words

Failure to catch misspelled words indicates the transcriptionist did not use the word processing software and reference materials effectively.

NAME Mary Jones		DOCUMENT NO. 1	
TYPE OF ERROR	**ERROR VALUE**	**NUMBER OF ERRORS**	**TOTAL ERROR VALUE***
Medical Language			
Add/omit word(s)			
Misspelled word(s)		3	
Incorrect date(s) or number(s)			
Total Medical Language Errors	3 ×	3 =	9
English Language			
Add/omit word(s)			
Misspelled word(s)		2	
Grammatical error(s)			
Punctuation error(s)			
Total English Language Errors	1 ×	2 =	2
Total Language Errors			11

*To compute total error value, multiply the number of errors by the error value (number of errors × error value = total error value).

Figure 3-2 Completed error analysis chart.

Grammatical Errors

Failure to catch grammatical errors indicates the transcriptionist did not use the word processing software effectively or missed common sentence errors, such as subject-verb agreement, pronoun-antecedent agreement, number usage, word division, and capitalization.

Punctuation Errors

Failure to catch punctuation errors indicates the transcriptionist did not use the word processing software effectively or failed to recognize the essential uses of the marks of punctuation. However, do not spend too much time pondering the proper placement of commas, semicolons, and other marks.

Let's look at the completed error analysis chart in Figure 3-2. Student Mary Jones has completed her transcript and proofread the document. On checking her work against the answer key, she finds three medical language errors and two English language errors. Because the errors are weighted differently, the total error value for her document is 11.

MARK	EXPLANATION	EXAMPLE	RESULT
?	is this correct?	I saw your patient Janée Brun.	I saw your patient Jean Brun.
℀ or —	delete	Jean Brun, your patient, came in.	Jean Brun came in.
\	delete or change	Jean Brue, your patient, came in.	Jean Brun, your patient, came in.
#	space	JeanBrun, your patient, came in.	Jean Brun, your patient, came in.
tr ∽	transpose	Jean Brun, your patient, came in.	Your patient, Jean Brun, came in.
◡	close up space	Jean Brun, your patient, came in.	Jean Brun, your patient, came in.
stet	let it alone	Jean Brun, your patient, came in.	Jean Brun, your patient, came in.
⌐	move left	Jean Brun, your patient, came in.	Jean Brun, your patient, came in.
⌐	move right	Jean Brun, your patient, came in.	Jean Brun, your patient, came in.
⌐⌐	move up	Jean Brun, your patient, came in.	Jean Brun, your patient, came in.
⌴	move down	Jean Brun, your patient, came in.	Jean Brun, your patient, came in.
lc or /	use lower case	Jean Brun, your Patient, came in.	Jean Brun, your patient, came in.
℀	delete and close up	I can see it's surface now.	I can see its surface now.
sp	spell out	There were 2 patients to be...	There were two patients to be...
¶	paragraph	...high fever. On physical exam...	...high fever.
no ¶	no paragraph	On physical exam I found...	On physical exam I found a ...
⊙	change to period	...high fever On physical exam...	...high fever. On physical exam...
∧	insert	Your patient came in to see me	Your patient came in to see me.
⋮	insert semcolon	blood pressure: 130/90 temperature	blood pressure: 130/90; temperature
⌄	insert apostrophe	She doesnt remember asking for...	She doesn't remember asking for...
( )	insert parentheses	(1 Sterile field. 2 Suture materials.	(1) Sterile field. (2) Suture materials.
=	insert hyphen	She was seen in follow up exam on...	She was seen in the follow-up exam on...
∧	insert comma	Jean Brun your patient, came in.	Jean Brun, your patient, came in.
⊙	insert colon	Diagnosis Appendicitis	Diagnosis: Appendicitis
⌄	insert quotation marks	There has been some hurting in my...	There has been some "hurting" in my...
][	center	]Physical Examination[	Physical Examination
cap ≡	use capital letters	Physical Examination	PHYSICAL EXAMINATION
	don't spell out	There was fifty-seven cents.	There was 57 cents.

Figure 3-3 Proofreader marks. (*From Fordney MT, Diehl MO: Medical transcription do's and dont's, ed 2, Philadelphia, 1999, Saunders.*)

Reviewing Proofreading Marks

The standard proofreading marks used by copywriters to make corrections to various types of both medical and general documents are shown in Figure 3-3.

BASIC ENGLISH USAGE REVIEW

Because the medical language is a scientific language, you will encounter discrepancies in usage and punctuation between rules found in an English grammar textbook and the rules found in a medical transcription manual of style. Discrepancies in usage and punctuation rules are also found in the various medical transcription manuals.

To avoid questions when medical transcription manuals of style contradict one another, as well as discrepancies found in your English grammar, word processing, or keyboarding textbooks, use *The AAMT Book of Style for Medical Transcription*, a medical dictionary, and the following guidelines for the activities presented in this textbook.

The Joint Commission on Accreditation of Healthcare Organizations (JCAHO) is an accrediting agency that strives to improve the safety and quality of health care

provided to the public. It has developed standards for quality and safety in the delivery of health care and evaluates health care organizations of all sizes and types based on these standards.

In July of 2002, JCAHO initiated National Patient Safety Goals, which focus on priority safety goals for the health care industry. In 2003, compliance with these goals was assessed at health care facilities undergoing accreditation. The second goal of the six goals established in the National Patient Safety Goals was to "improve the effectiveness of communication among caregivers." Within this goal was a directive to "standardize the abbreviations, acronyms, and symbols used throughout the organization, including a list of abbreviations, acronyms, and symbols not to be used." JCAHO required that each organization develop a list of prohibited or dangerous abbreviations, acronyms, and symbols. In November of 2003, this recommendation was amended, with JCAHO establishing a minimum list of abbreviations, acronyms, and symbols that were not to be used. Starting in January 1, 2004, the following items must be included on each accredited organization's "do not use" list (Table 3-1).

JCAHO has also established an additional list of dangerous abbreviations. Starting April 1, 2004, organizations

TABLE 3.1

SET	ITEM	ABBREVIATION	POTENTIAL PROBLEM	PREFERRED TERM
1.	1.	U (for unit)	Mistaken as zero, four or cc.	Write "unit"
2.	2.	IU (for international unit)	Mistaken as IV (intravenous) or 10 (ten).	Write "international unit"
3.	3. 4.	Q.D., Q.O.D. (Latin abbreviation for once daily and every other day)	Mistaken for each other. The period after the Q can be mistaken for an "I" and the "O" can be mistaken for "I".	Write "daily" and "every other day"
4.	5. 6.	Trailing zero (X.O mg), Lack of leading zero (.X mg)	Decimal point is missed.	Never write a zero by itself after a decimal point (X mg), and always use a zero before a decimal point (0.X mg)
5.	7. 8. 9.	MS MSO_4 $MgSO_4$	Confused for one another. Can mean morphine sulfate or magnesium sulfate.	Write "morphine sulfate" or "magnesium sulfate"

From Joint Commission on Accreditation of Healthcare Organizations: *Setting the standard*, 2002. Available on-line at www.jcaho.org/general + public/patient + safety/settingthestandard_brochure.pdf.

TABLE 3.2

μg (for microgram)	Mistaken for mg (milligrams) resulting in one thousand-fold dosing overdose.	Write "mcg"
H.S.(for half-strength or Latin abbreviation for bedtime)	Mistaken for either half-strength or hour of sleep (at bedtime). q.H.S. mistaken every hour. All can result in dosing error.	Write out "half-strength" or "at bedtime"
T.I.W. (for three time a week)	Mistaken for three times a day or twice weekly resulting in an overdose.	Write "3 times weekly" or "three times weekly"
S.C. or S.Q. (for subcutaneous)	Mistaken as SL for sublingual, or "5 every."	Write "Sub-Q", "subQ", or "subcutaneously"
D/C (for discharge)	Interpreted as discontinue or whatever medications follow (typically discharge meds).	Write "discharge"
c.c. (for cubic centimeter)	Mistaken for U (units) when poorly written.	Write "mL" for milliliters
A.S., A.D., A.U. (Latin abbreviation for left, right, or both ears)	Mistaken for OS, OD, OU, OU, etc.	Write: "left ear", "right ear", or "both ears"

From Joint Commission on Accreditation of Healthcare Organizations: *Setting the standard*, 2002. Available on-line at www.jcaho.org/general + public/patient + safety/settingthestandard_brochure.pdf.

must identify and replace a minimum of three of the abbreviations on that list. In keeping with *The AAMT Book of Style*, the following have been identified for replacement (Table 3-2).

Also, the Institute for Safe Medication Practices (ISMP) has a list of dangerous abbreviations relating to medication use that it recommends should be explicitly prohibited. This list is available on the ISMP Web site, www.ismp.org. Appendix B, "Dangerous Abbreviations and Dose Designations," in *The AAMT Book of Style* provides a more extensive list. This textbook complies with the recommendations found in *The AAMT Book of Style*, Appendix B.

Abbreviations Guidelines

To avoid confusion and improve clarity of communication, avoid the use of abbreviations, acronyms, and brief forms unless they are internationally recognized terms and symbols.

1. Abbreviations are used for all metric measurements with numbers.
   Example: Each kidney weighs 80 gm.
2. Abbreviations are used for chemical and mathematical compounds.
   Examples: Na (sodium), NaCl (sodium chloride), T4 (thyroxine)

3. Abbreviations are used for units of measurement. Units of measurements are typed in lowercase letters without periods and kept on the same line.
   Example: A CBC showed 12,000 WBCs per cu mm.
4. Latin abbreviations are typed in lowercase letters with periods.
   Example: The medication was ordered b.i.d.
5. Abbreviations are used with laboratory test results that use metric measurements.
   Example: The hemoglobin was 13.6 gm% and the hematocrit 42 vol%.
6. Abbreviations are used for many tests, such as CBC (complete blood count), RBC (red blood cell), and SGPT (serum glutamic-pyruvic transaminase). The plural of capitalized abbreviations is formed by adding the letter *s* only (no added apostrophe).
   Example: A CBC showed 12,000 WBCs per cu mm. His WBCs were borderline high.
7. Abbreviations are used in vital signs.
   Example: BP 136/86, pulse 76, and respirations 20/min.
8. Plural abbreviations are formed by adding the letter *s*.
   Example: TMs are within normal limits, with no erythema noted.

9. The letter *x* is used to abbreviate *by* or *times* when it precedes a number or another abbreviation.
   Examples
   The lesion is 1.5 × 1 cm on her leg.
   The patient was prescribed Augmentin 500 mg p.o. t.i.d. × 2 weeks.
10. Abbreviate units of measure, even if dictated in full, if they are accompanied by a numeral.
    Examples
    Dictated as: A 2.5 centimeter laceration was noted on her left anterior forearm.
    Transcribe: A 2.5 cm laceration was noted on her left anterior forearm.
11. Do not use an abbreviation or acronym in the admission, discharge, preoperative or postoperative diagnosis, consultative conclusion, or operative title.
    Examples
    Dictated as: IMPRESSION: HTVD
    Transcribe: IMPRESSION: Hypertensive vascular disease.
12. Do not use an abbreviation, acronym, or brief form when a term is dictated in full, except for *units of measure.*
    Examples
    The lesion is 1.5 × 1 cm on her leg.
    The patient reported a history of transurethral resection of the prostate (not TURP, unless dictated TURP).
13. Do not use an abbreviation for common nonmetric units of measure to express weight, depth, distance, height, length, or width, except in tables.
    Example: The patient was 5 feet 3 inches and weighed 105 pounds.

Capitalization Guidelines
1. Capitalization usually indicates importance.
2. Capitalize the first word of every sentence, the first-person pronoun *I*, the first word of a salutation in a letter, any noun or title in the salutation, and the first word of a complimentary closing.
   Examples
   He responded to treatment.
   Dear Dr. Smith
   Sincerely yours
3. Capitalize the days of the week and months of the year, but not the seasons.
   Examples
   The tests were ordered for Monday, May 8.
   The doctor will attend the convention in the spring.
4. Capitalize personal and business titles when they precede a name.
   Examples
   Dr. Smith will do the consultation.
   The orthopedic physician will do the consultation.

5. Capitalize eponyms, which are surnames teamed with a disease, instrument, or surgical procedure.
   Examples
   The patient presents with symptoms of Dreuw syndrome.
   The patient presents symptoms of alopecia parvimaculata syndrome.
6. Capitalize trade names, brand names of drugs, and trademarked suture materials. Generic drugs and suture materials are not capitalized.
   Examples
   The patient was given Tylenol.
   The patient was given acetaminophen.
7. Capitalize the names of the genus but not the names of the species that may follow it. The genus also may be referred to by its first initial only.
   Example: The patient suffered with *E coli.*
8. Capitalize acronyms.
   Example: The patient was scheduled for MRI (magnetic resonance imaging).
9. Capitalize allergy information to call attention to its importance.
   Example: ALLERGIES: CODEINE.
10. Capital letters are used for electrocardiographic (ECG) leads, waves, and segments. Chest leads are indicated with a *V* for the central terminal, an Arabic number for the chest electrode, and a letter for right or left arm or foot. The leads are *V1* through *V6* and *aVL, aVR,* and *aVF.* Waves include *P, Q, R, S, T,* and *U* and their combinations.
    Example: There is 1 mm of ST-segment depression in leads II, III, and aVF and approximately 1 mm of ST elevation in leads I, aVL.

Number Expression Guidelines
Different disciplines have different rules for spelling out numbers instead of using figures (Arabic numbers). Figures are usually used in medical documents because they are easy to read and stand out in the sentence. Figures are used to express quantities accompanied by a unit of measure, patient age and other vital statistics, and laboratory values, as well as in any other instance when it is important to communicate the information quickly and easily.
1. Numbers are spelled out at the beginning of a sentence.
   Example: Three tests were conducted on the woman.
2. Figures are used almost exclusively as opposed to spelled-out numbers to improve clarity and avoid potential mistakes. There are always exceptions, and

judgment and discretion are needed when deciding whether to use numerals or spell out numbers.

Examples

Mrs. Jones is widowed, but she resides with one of her three children.

Patient complains of right elbow pain for the past 3 weeks.

She had an appendectomy done approximately 4 years ago and had her spleen removed when she was 24 years old.

3. Figures are used to express the day of the month and the year.

Example: The patient underwent prostatic resection in 1998.

4. Figures are used in ranges and ratios.

Examples

The last time he vomited was 4-5 hours ago.
The solution was diluted 1:1000.

5. Figures are used for numbers over ten (unless mixing large numbers).

Example: The new clinic will cost $4.5 million.

6. Figures are used in lists.

Example

IMPRESSION

1. Resolving cellulitis of the right side of abdomen and chest.
2. Right hip pain.
3. Questionable alcohol abuse vs. dementia.

7. Figures are used to indicate the patient's weight, height, blood pressure (BP), pulse, and respiration. Figures are used to indicate the patient's age, except at the beginning of a sentence.

Examples

This is the second admission for this 2-year-old.

Two-year-old patient was admitted for the second time.

Her physical findings are: Weight 25 pounds, height 21 inches, BP 142/72, pulse 117, respirations 20/min.

8. Figures are used for temperature. If the temperature scale name (Farenheit or Celcius) or its abbreviation (F or C) is not dictated, it is not necessary to insert it. The word *degree* or its symbol (if available) is included only if dictated.

Examples

Her temperature was 98.6°F (or 98.6 F).
Her temperature was 98.6 degrees.

9. Figures are used to indicate the dosage and the number of times that the medicine needs to be taken.

Example: His medications include Naprosyn 30 mg t.i.d. × 2 weeks, Dyazide 40 mg daily, and Synthroid 40 mcg p.c.

10. Figures are used for suture materials. Suture materials range in size. The sizes can be transcribed as follows:

• Using the number symbol, figure, and zeros: #1-0, #2-0, #3-0, #4-0.
• Using figure and zeros: 1-0, 2-0, 3-0, 4-0.

Examples

The subcutaneous tissues were closed with interrupted #3-0 plain catgut.

The subcutaneous tissues were closed with interrupted 3-0 plain catgut.

11. Figures with capital letters are used to refer to the vertebral column.

Example: The disk was herniated at L4-5.

12. Figures are used with electrocardiographic leads.

Examples

The intrinsicoid deflection was 0.08 sec in V6.
Use chest leads V1 and V2.

13. Figures and capital letters are used to refer to the vertebral column and spinal nerves.

Examples

There is left-sided point tenderness over the C5-C6 paraspinal areas.

There is evidence of degenerative arthritis involving the L3-4 and L5-S1 facet joints bilaterally.

14. Figures are used to refer to grade, phase, and pregnancy and delivery.

Examples

She was diagnosed with grade 3/6 holosystolic murmur.

The patient is gravida 1, para 1.

15. Figures are used with the + or − symbols.

Example: Rigor mortis is 2+.

16. Figures are used with circular position.

Example: The incision was made at the 2 o'clock position.

17. Figures are used with drug names.

Examples

The patient is taking Humulin 70/30.
The patient received Obetrol 20.

18. Figures are used when keying numbers containing decimal fractions. Place a zero before a decimal that lacks a whole number.

Examples

The physician injected 0.75% of medication in the arm.

Some common decimal equivalents are:
$1/8 = 0.125; 1/4 = 0.25; 1/2 = 0.5; 3/4 = 0.75$

19. Figures are used for measurements and Latin terms. No period follows metric abbreviations unless the abbreviation ends a sentence.

Example: The physician prescribed 80 mEq of potassium.

Common metric abbreviations:

kg	kilogram
g or gm	gram
mg	milligram
mm	millimeter
mcg	microgram
mL or ml	milliliter
mEq	milliequivalent
cm	centimeter
dL	deciliter

Common Latin abbreviations:

a.c.	before meals
ad lib.	as needed
b.i.d.	twice a day
n.p.o.	nothing by mouth
p.c.	after meals
p.o.	by mouth
p.r.n.	as needed
q.	every
q.h.	every hour
q.i.d.	four times a day
q.2h.	every two hours
q.3h.	every three hours
q.4h.	every four hours
t.i.d.	three times a day

20. Figures are used with symbols and abbreviations.
    Example: The patient may take 1 q. 4-6 hours as needed for nausea.
21. Roman numerals are generally used to express stages and clotting factors.
    Examples
    She was diagnosed with stage IV decubitus ulcer.
    Prothrombin time is a test to measure the activity of factors I, II, V, VII, and X, which participate in the extrinsic pathway of coagulation.
22. Roman numerals are used for standard leads and intercostal space positions.
    Example: There is reciprocal depression in leads I and II.
23. Ordinal numbers are used to indicate order or position in a series rather than quantity. As with all numbers in medical reports, AAMT recommends using numerals (figures): 1st, 2nd, 3rd, etc.
    Example: On the 3rd day, the baby's temperature was normal.
24. The use of subscripts and superscripts is often avoided because of the time involved in formatting them, the difficulty in reading them on single-spaced documents, and electronic transmission of documents.
25. The plurals of single-digit numbers, letters, and symbols are formed by adding *s*.

26. The plurals of double-digit numbers and all-capital abbreviations are formed by adding the letter *s*.
    Example: The patient's blood pressure has been relatively well controlled, with systolic pressures running 140-150s.

Punctuation Guidelines
Punctuation marks such as periods, hyphens, commas, and colons signal the reader to stop, pause, hesitate, or anticipate what is to come.

Period
1. A period is used to end a sentence.
    Example: The thyroid and adrenals are normal.
2. A period is used to separate a decimal fraction from the whole number.
    Example: Her white blood count is 6.8.
3. A period is used to take the place of the word *point*.
    Example: Her temperature was 98.6°F.

Hyphen
4. A hyphen is used when joining numbers or letters to form a word, phrase, or abbreviation.
    Examples
    The woman is scheduled for a C-section.
    The x-ray will be scheduled next week.
    She attributes her improvement to B-12 injections.
5. A hyphen is used to join two or more words when used as an adjective before a noun.
    Examples
    On follow-up examination, a lump was felt.
    The patient will follow up with serology.
6. A hyphen is used when two or more words are viewed as a single word.
    Example: The well-behaved child was waiting patiently for his appointment.
7. A hyphen is used between numbers and *year old*.
    Examples
    The patient was a 26-year-old female.
    The patient is a 5-year-old female with an ear infection.
8. A hyphen is used between two "like" vowels.
    Example: We will see him again in three weeks for a re-evaluation.
9. A hyphen is used to take the place of the word *to* or *through* to identify ranges.
    Example: The last time he vomited was 4-5 hours ago.
10. A hyphen is used with words beginning with *ex* and *self*. Words beginning with *pre*, *re*, *post*, and *non* are generally not hyphenated. Words beginning with *co* and *vice* may or may not be hyphenated and should be researched in a dictionary.

Examples

The patient's ex-husband was in the hospital.

Susan conducted a self-examination of her breasts.

His abdomen is soft and nontender.

The patient has postinfarct dementia that requires persistent feeding through the PEG tube.

Patient returns today for a recheck of his left ankle pain.

No pretibial edema was noticed.

11. Hyphens are used to form compound adjectives.

Example: Although the stated age of this patient is 45, his speech is child-like.

Comma

12. A comma is used to join independent clauses separated by *and, but, or, for, nor, yet,* or *so.* Independent clauses can be written as individual sentences.

Example: The ducts appear to be somewhat congested, and there is marked fibrosis of the membranes of the glomeruli.

13. A comma is used after opening clauses that begin with the following words: after, although, as, as if, because, before, for, how, if, once, since, so, so that, than, that, though, unless, when, whenever, where, whereas, whether, *and* while.

Example: As noted above, she has had some nausea and vomiting.

14. A comma is used after an introductory element if it improves the clarity of the sentence.

Example: In cases involving diabetes, an endocrinologist may be consulted.

15. A comma is used to separate items in a series.

Example: The patient denies any hematuria, fever, chills, or dysuria.

16. A comma is used to set off nonessential or extraneous words, phrases, and clauses within a sentence.

Example: A diagnosis of a blood clot in the lung, pulmonary embolism, was made.

17. A comma is used to set off an appositive.

Example: The physician, Dr. Davis, recommended a follow-up visit.

18. A comma is used to set off words in a direct (spoken or written) address.

Example: Dr. Adams, I have your chart notes.

19. A comma is used to separate the parts of the date when the month, day, and year are given.

Example: She was admitted on Monday, May 1, 20xx, and discharged on June 2, 20xx.

20. A comma is used to separate vital signs.

Example: BP 130/80, pulse 112 and regular, and respirations 16/min.

21. A comma is used to separate city and state names used in the address of a letter.

Example
FedDes Wellness Center
101 Wellness Way Drive
New York, NY 10036

22. A comma is used to punctuate large numbers with five or more digits in units of three.

Examples

One hundred boxes of latex gloves cost $1250.50.

The x-ray machine cost $25,000.

City Hospital services more than 1,250,000 patients a year.

Semicolon

23. A semicolon is used to join two sentences together that do not have a joining conjunction.

Example: The heart sounds were normal; there was no gallop.

24. A semicolon is used to separate items in a series when any of the items already contain commas.

Example: The college invited Potter T. Bucky, MD, radiologist; Benjamin Keytone, MD, urologist; Adam Valence, MD, cardiologist; and Allan Pore, MD, dermatologist, to the dedication of the new science lab.

Colon

25. A colon is used to set off headings, topics, and sub-topics in medical documents.

Example: CHIEF COMPLAINT: Persistent right knee pain.

26. A colon may be used in the salutation of a business letter.

Example: Dear Sir:

27. A colon is used in expressions of time.

Example: Her next scheduled appointment is at 2:30 p.m.

28. A colon is used to separate figures in ratios.

Example: The solution was diluted 1:1000.

Apostrophe

29. An apostrophe is used to form the possessive of singular and plural nouns.

Examples

The patient's father is diabetic.

She experienced severe pain in the right side that radiated into the groin for approximately 8 hours' duration.

30. An apostrophe is used to form a contraction of words. However, contractions should be avoided in medical reports.

Examples

It's the physician's recommendation to include regular exercise in her weight control program.

It is the physician's recommendation to include regular exercise in her weight control program.

Quotation Marks

31. Quotation marks are used to indicate a direct quote.

    Example: The patient complained of food "getting caught in her throat" when she eats.

Symbols

32. The diagonal or virgule (/) is used to indicate the words *per, to,* and *over*.

    Examples

    BP 120/80, respirations 20/min.

    His fasting blood sugar was 129 mg/dL.

33. The diagonal or virgule (/) is used to separate the indicators of visual acuity.

    Example: Visual acuity is 20/30 both in the left and right eye but corrected 20/25.

34. The percent sign (%) is used with words and figures.

    Examples

    The patient was injected with 2% Xylocaine.

    Serum electrolytes were as follows: sodium 140 mg%, chloride 101 mg%, potassium 4.6 mg%, carbon dioxide 26 vol%.

35. The number or pound sign (#) is used to abbreviate the word *number* followed by a medical instrument or apparatus.

    Example: The small piece of metal was removed with a #25-gauge needle.

Spacing Guidelines

1. One space following end of sentence punctuation.

    Example: The patient is a 45-year-old computer programmer. He presents with a sinus headache.

2. One space following commas, semicolons, and colons.

    Examples

    She denies associated fever, chills, or hematemesis.

    Pupils are constricted and midline; they react to light.

3. Space once after a period that ends an abbreviation.

    Example: Dr. Smith was called for the consultation.

4. No spaces are used after a period within abbreviation.

    Example: Her medication was ordered t.i.d. by her doctor.

5. No spaces are used before or after a hyphen, apostrophe, or diagonal.

    Example: The patient was a well-developed, well-nourished 29-year-old in mild distress.

6. No spaces are used between symbol and referent.

    Example: Her temperature was 98.6°.

7. Keep the numeral and unit of measure together at line breaks. This is important when transcribing a drug and its corresponding dosage.

    Example: The specimen measured 3 cm in diameter. Erythromycin 250 mg t.i.d. was prescribed.

Activities 3-1 through 3-3

Proofreading Worksheet Exercises

Being able to identify and correct errors in medical documents is a skill that qualifies one as an accomplished transcriptionist. Assess your proofreading skill by completing three worksheets.

TEXTBOOK USERS

Proofread and correct errors in the medical documents shown in *Chapter 3, Activities 3-1 through 3-3*.
After completing the activities, refer to the answer key (Appendix E).
Manually complete the error analysis chart for each document.

SOFTWARE USERS

Click on *Chapter 3, Activity 3-1*, and follow the directions.
Follow the same process for *Chapter 3, Activities 3-2 and 3-3*.

ACTIVITY 3-1
Proofreading Worksheet

Directions: Proofread this medical document, which contains multiple errors. Use open punctuation and all other formatting guidelines established in this textbook.

CHART NOTE
Sue Bernshaw

Date of birth: 9/12/65

Examination Date:

SUBJECTION
Removal of sutures placed 10 days ago.

OBJECTION
The wound on the lateral expect of the left knee look well healed.
The 00000 nylon sutures were removed without difficulty.

ASSESMENT
Laceration of right knee, well healed.

PLAN
Advised applying vitamin e to the area.

Harry A. Medulla, MD

ham:xx
D: *current date*
T: *current date*

ACTIVITY 3-2
Proofreading Worksheet

Directions: Proofread this medical document, which contains multiple errors. Use open punctuation and all other formatting guidelines established in this textbook.

CHART NOTE
Gapolli, Rachi

Date of birth: 2/3/69

Examination Date: *current date*

SUBJECTIVE
Patient complains of sensitive pimplelike bump on right posterior shounder area.

OBJECTIVE
A mole, approximately one centimeter in diameter is visible. It is uniformly brown in color with know iregular borders. Patient denies pain or discharge all though she does amit that the area is quite sensitive for the passed 3 days.

TREATMENT
Nevus.

PLAN
I am referring the patient to a dermatologist for it's removal and biopsy.

Charles Davis, MD

cd:x
D: *current date*
T: *current date*

ACTIVITY 3-3
Proofreading Worksheet

Directions: Proofread this medical document, which contains multiple errors. Use open punctuation and all other formatting guidelines established in this textbook.

CHART NOTE
Heather Brodrick,

DOB: 4/19/89

Charles Davis M.D

OBJECTIVE
Patient complains of warks on palm of right-hand that is becoming bother some.

SUBJECTIVE
Examination of the of both hands reveals a three millimeter growth over the dorsum of the distal 4th and 5th matacarpal of the left hand.

PLAN
Verruca.

ASSESSEMNT
The warks were frosen with liquid Nitrogen without incident. Recheck in two three weeks if problem not resolved.

Charles Davvis, MD

Cd:x
D: *current date*
T: *current date*

Activities 3-4 through 3-6

Keyboarding and Proofreading Exercises

Being able to type and proofread medical documents is a distinguishing character-istic of an accomplished transcriptionist. You are to create a template for a chart note using SOAP format, a history and physical examination report, and a consul-tation letter. Print a copy of the transcribed document after you have proofread and corrected any errors you have found on the computer screen. Once again, proofread the printed copy. It is not sufficient merely to identify any errors; you also must cor-rect the errors you find. This systematic approach will reinforce your understanding of grammar, spelling, and punctuation rules.

TEXTBOOK USERS

Open your word processing package.

Type and proofread the medical document shown in *Chapter 3, Activity 3-4*, using the formatting guidelines established in Chapter 2.

Identify and correct all errors.

Save your work on your student disk.

After completing the activity, refer to the answer key (Appendix E).

Manually complete the error analysis chart.

Follow the same process for *Chapter 3, Activities 3-5 and 3-6*.

SOFTWARE USERS

Click on *Chapter 3, Activity 3-4*, and follow the directions.

Follow the same process for *Chapter 3, Activities 3-5 and 3-6*.

ACTIVITY 3-4
Keyboarding and Proofreading Exercise

Directions: Type and proofread this medical document, which contains multiple errors. Use full block, open punctuation, and all other formatting guidelines established in this textbook.

CHART NOTE
Patient Name: Nathan Wright,
Date of Birth: 11/30/83
Examination Date: *current date*

SUBJECTIVE
Patient presents with typical flu like symptoms of fever, muscular aches and pains, shaking chills, headache, and weakness.

OBJECTIVE
Bi lateral tympanic membranes are clear. Orofarynx is not ejected. Know neck nodes detected. Chest is clear to percusion and auscultation. Temperature 102.3F.

ASSESMENT
Influencza.

PLAN
Symptomatic therapy. Acetaminofen prn. for fever and pain. Re-check in five to twelve days if not improving.

Charles Davis, MD

cd:xx
D: *current date*
T: *current date*

PROOFREADING

ACTIVITY 3-5
Keyboarding and Proofreading Exercise

Directions: Type and proofread this medical document, which contains multiple errors. Use full block, open punctuation, and all other formatting guidelines established in this textbook.

HISTORY AND PHYSICAL EXAMINATION REPORT

Patient Name: Esther Monahan
File Number: 2348901
Date of Birth: September 10, 19xx
Examination Date: *current date*
Physician: Harry A. Medulla, MD

HISTORY

HISTORY OF PRESENT ILLNESS
This 88 –year old lady was admitted to a nursing home with an intensive cellulites involving the right side of the adbomen and the chest. She had been living at home with her daughter, but had become increasingly unable to eat. She developed hypronatremia and dehydration along with the cellulitis. The cause of the cellulitis was never clearly determined. It was felt ultimately to be dew to cracks in the skin from her poor condition and then and infection starting. She received six days of ancef, was put on keflex for follow up. There is some suggestion of possible alcohol use involved, and she did receive some thiamine.

PAST MEDICAL HISTORY
Otherwise fairly benign. Dr. Peebody had provided most of her care.

SOCIAL HISTORY
As above.

FAMILY HISTORY
No pertinent data.

REVIEW OF SYSTEMS
Left hip has bothered her from a hip fracture twelve years ago with pining. Other medical problems include GI bleed, which occurred back in February. Decision was made by the daughter and the patient not to investigate further. She had been on Aspirin at the time, and it was stopped. It sounds like it was a lower GI bleed rather than an upper at that time.

PHYSICAL EXAMINATION

GENERAL: Elderly woman who is a little hard-of-hearing. Her vision is poor. Vital signs are good.
HEENT: No jaundice. Mouth and pharyxn are unremarkable.
NECK: Supple. Carotids are equal. No jvd.
LUNGS: Clear to percusion and auscultation.
HEART: Regular rhythm. No murmurs, no gallops.
BREASTS: Atrophic.
ABDOMEN: Soft with out organomegaly. The right side of the abdomen and chest, particularly underneath the breast, is still a bit irritated and red, but clearly much better than had been previously described.
EXTREMITIES: Ankles show three plus edema up to the knee.

Continued

ACTIVITY 3-5 *(cont'd)*

HISTORY AND PHYSICAL EXAMINATION REPORT
Patient Name: Monahan, Esther
File Number: 2348901
Page 2

IMPRESSION
1. Resolving cellulitis of the right side of abdomen and chest. Continue antibiotics.
2. Ankle edema attributed to congestive heart failure. Prescribed lotensin, 5 milligrams daily along with brief regimen of diuretics. Will monitor progress.
3. Right hip pain.
4. Questionable alcohol abuse versus dementia.

Harry A. Medulla, MD

ham:xx
D: *current date*
T: *current date*

PROOFREADING

ACTIVITY 3-6
Keyboarding and Proofreading Exercise

Directions: Type and proofread this medical document, which contains multiple errors. Use full block, open punctuation, and all other formatting guidelines established in this textbook.

current date

Dr. Katherine Davis
Medical Practice Ltd.
312 Main Street
New York, New York 10010

Re: Kevin Schlitz
    Date of Birth: October 29, 1936

Dear Dr. Davis

I had the opportunity to examine Mr. Schlitz in my office on *current date* in regards too his slow-healing ulceration of his right foot. The wound definitely looks improved from the last time I saw it. She has been doing a good job at not bearing weight upon his right foot.

At this point, I think it would be appropriate to place him in some extra-depth shoes or boots with accomodative insoles to help reduce pressure in the fore foot area. I am concerned that he has a very high potential for ulceration beneath the third metatarsal due to increased loading in this area.

I wrote a prescription and sent him to an orthotic specialist for new shoes and to have accommodative insoles constructed. I think the patient has an unrealistic outlook in regards to what type of insoles will be in her shoes. He is currently wearing a very rigid functional device. This is not the appropriate device to reduce pressure in the fore foot area. The prosthesis I am reccommending should help cushion and distribute his weight evenly in the forefoot area as well as help maintain the rear foot in a better functioning position. Please feel free to contact me if you have any questions in regard to this matter.

Sincerely

Harry A. Medulla M.D

xx

Let's pause a minute and see how well you have mastered typing and proofreading medical documents. This section allows you to evaluate your skills.

TEXTBOOK USERS

Open your word processing package.

Type and proofread the medical document shown in *Chapter 3, Check Your Progress 3-1*, using the formatting guidelines established in Chapter 2.

Identify and correct all errors.

Save your work on your student disk.

After completion, refer to the answer key (Appendix E).

Manually complete the error analysis chart for each document.

Follow the same process for *Chapter 3, Check Your Progress 3-2 and 3-3*.

SOFTWARE USERS

Click on *Chapter 3, Check Your Progress 3-1*, and follow the directions.

Follow the same process for *Chapter 3, Check Your Progress 3-2 and 3-3*.

TERMINOLOGY

CHECK YOUR PROGRESS 3-1

Directions: Type and proofread this medical document, which contains multiple errors. Use full block, open punctuation, and all other formatting guidelines established in this textbook.

current date

Arthur Guttenberg, MD
5723 North Front Street
New York, New York 10010

RE: Martha Ultress
    Date of birth: 6/19/59
Dear Dr. Cuttenberg

Thank you for seeing Mary for her right rotator cuff tendinitis. She has has intermittent pain of the right shoulder during the past two months. Over the passed few days the pain has gotten very severe. On examination she could barely abduct past thirty degrees. Thee x ray was notable for some calcific tendinitis. I injected the subacromial bursa with Steroids and obtained a rather dramatic improvement in her bursitis only to have it return again; one wk later. I started her on a physical-therapy program and would appreciate you evaluation concerning the continuing care and treatment of this patient.

Very Truly Yours,

Harry A. Medulla, MD/xx

CHECK YOUR PROGRESS 3-2

Directions: Type and proofread this medical document, which contains multiple errors. Use full block, open punctuation, and all other formatting guidelines established in this textbook.

CHART NOTE

Patient Name: Jose Ramirez
DOB: 5/23/xx
Examination Date: *current date*

History of Present Illness
This fifteen year old male is seen for a follow-up on his acne He has been using clearasil medicated astringent and oxy wash for about two months with no improvement He is on no orale medications denies any alergies and is in good health.

Physical Esamination
Todays exam reveal inflammatory systic lesions along the jaw line and upper back. Some deep systs are palpable on the chin and over the right shoulder area.

Plan
She is to start E-Mycin two hundred fifty milligrams bid and ten percent Benzac topically nightly after washing. He is to contine washing with oxy wash up to 3x a day as tolerated. He has been cautioned not to pick-at the lessions. We discussed the need to keep her hands away from his face as much as possible and to stop leaning on his elbow with his chin in his hand. It is a bad habit that only promotes the spread of bacteria and should be continued. He will be seen again in four to six weeks.

Allan Pore, MD

ap:xx
D: *current date*
T: *current date*

TERMINOLOGY

CHECK YOUR PROGRESS 3-3

Directions: Type and proofread this medical document, which contains multiple errors. Use full block, open punctuation, and all other formatting guidelines established in this textbook.

CHART NOTE

Linda Smithers
DOB: August 13, XX

Examiantion Date: *current date*

CHEIF COMPLANT: Itching and a rash.

SUBJECTION
The patient is a pleasant, 26 year old female who is quiet cooperative and in no a cute distress. She complains a rash that began about 2 week's ago. She's taken benadryl at bedtime with no relief. Upon questioning he admits to using a new perfumed body lotion after her shower.

OBJECTION
Vital Signs: Temperature 98.6 blood pressure 136/72 weight 165 lbs height 5 3 pulse 74 respirations 22. Smooth erythematous rash over neck extending over trunk and back. On the upper extremities she has a erythematous rash extending to her wrists.

ASSESSMENT
Contact dermatits, secondary to allergy to perfume

PLAN
1. Discontine use of perfumed body lotion.
2. Wash all clothing and bed linen that were exposed to the perfumed lotion.
3. Take benadryl twenty five milligrams q6hx3 days

Allan Pore, MD

xx
D: *current date*
T: *current date*

Chapter 4

Transcription Process

OBJECTIVES

At the completion of Chapter 4, you should be able to do the following:
1. Understand the transcription process.
2. Operate a transcriber.
3. Use reference materials proficiently.
4. Select the appropriate reference material for a medical term.

What's Ahead

Let's find out if you can select the appropriate or best reference material to locate a particular medical term.

TEXTBOOK USERS

Select the best answer for each question or statement concerning reference materials.
Refer to the answer key for immediate feedback (Appendix E).

SOFTWARE USERS

Click on *Chapter 4, Pretest,* and follow the directions.

PRETEST

Directions: Select true (T) or false (F) for each statement concerning reference materials and the transcription process.

1. T or F   The character is the preferred method of measuring productivity.

2. T or F   Document formats often vary from office to office.

3. T or F   Electronic medical dictionaries contain all information found in printed versions.

4. T or F   Electronic spellers can recognize homonyms.

5. T or F   Sources found on the Internet are rarely useful.

6. T or F   The telephone book can be a helpful resource material.

7. T or F   The letter *s* in the word *prednisone* has the sound of *z*.

8. T or F   *A&P* is an abbreviation for *auscultation and percussion*.

9. T or F   It is not necessary to clean the earphones every day.

10. T or F   The center of the foot pedal is the position to press for *play* on a three-position foot pedal.

11. T or F   A transcriber operates similar to a musical cassette player.

12. T or F   The handheld transcriber uses the $3^{15}/_{16} \times 2^{1}/_{2}$–inch standard cassette.

13. T or F   Medical dictation seems to have an incoherent style of dictation.

14. T or F   It is important to study and know the introductory pages in a medical dictionary.

15. T or F   Pronunciation guides are included in medical dictionaries.

16. T or F   Drug books are updated every 2 years.

17. T or F   Eponym word books often include definitions.

18. T or F   There is only one correct way to transcribe a sentence.

19. T or F   A transcriptionist does not need an English dictionary.

20. T or F   Medical words are listed in the same manner as in an English dictionary.

21. T or F   Word books include homonyms.

22. T or F   Anatomy and physiology textbooks are usually not helpful to a medical transcriptionist.

23. T or F   To a beginning transcription student, listening to medical dictation may sound like a foreign language.

24. T or F   Increasing the speed control on the transcriber will help the transcriptionist transcribe the material faster.

25. T or F   Word expanders are an example of a productivity tool.

PRETEST *(cont'd)*

Directions: Which reference book would you select to find the word or phrase to verify spelling, capitalization, punctuation, or definition?

26. Foley catheter
    (a) eponym word book
    (b) English dictionary
    (c) manual of style
    (d) all the above

27. *Discrete* or *discreet*
    (a) standard English dictionary
    (b) eponym word book
    (c) manual of style
    (d) a and c

28. Keflex
    (a) medical dictionary
    (b) anatomy and physiology textbook
    (c) drug book
    (d) none of the above

29. K wire
    (a) English dictionary
    (b) orthopedic word book
    (c) abbreviation book
    (d) b and c

30. Transurethral resection
    (a) surgery word book
    (b) orthopedic word book
    (c) cardiology word book
    (d) none of the above

31. I&D
    (a) cardiology word book
    (b) urology word book
    (c) abbreviation word book
    (d) radiology word book

32. Endoscopic retrograde cholangiopancreatography
    (a) drug book
    (b) radiology word book
    (c) eponym book
    (d) all the above

33. *Follow up* or *follow-up*
    (a) manual of style
    (b) eponym book
    (c) neither a nor b
    (d) a and b

34. *Xanax* or *Zantac*
    (a) eponym book
    (b) surgical book
    (c) drug book
    (d) cardiology book

35. *Parental* or *parenteral*
    (a) homonym book
    (b) PDR
    (c) eponym book
    (d) all the above

36. Tetracycline
    (a) PDR
    (b) drug word book
    (c) neither a nor b
    (d) a and b

37. The plural form of *bronchus*
    (a) medical dictionary
    (b) surgical word book
    (c) eponym book
    (d) none of the above

38. Achilles heel
    (a) abbreviation book
    (b) manual of style
    (c) eponym book
    (d) none of the above

39. *Fogarty catheter* or *Fogarty's catheter*
    (a) eponym book
    (b) manual of style
    (c) medical dictionary
    (d) all the above

40. *e coli* or *E coli*
    (a) manual of style
    (b) eponym book
    (c) surgical book
    (d) cardiology book

PRETEST (cont'd)

Directions: Select the best word that completes the meaning of the sentence.

41. The patient who had _____ went to the dermatologist.
    (a) psoriasis
    (b) cirrhosis
    (c) anuresis
    (d) enuresis

42. The man was experiencing itching of the foreskin and _____.
    (a) ileum
    (b) glands
    (c) glans
    (d) ilium

43. Physical examination revealed erythematous _____ on the chin, just right of midline.
    (a) faucis
    (b) fauces
    (c) macula
    (d) macule

44. Examination of the skin revealed several _____ nodes.
    (a) shoddy
    (b) radical
    (c) shotty
    (d) radicle

45. The physician thought the patient's _____ may be associated with his otosclerosis.
    (a) tinnitus
    (b) neither a nor c
    (c) tendinitis
    (d) all the above

46. After the 10th day, the child finished his complete _____ of antibiotics.
    (a) coarse
    (b) course
    (c) dilation
    (d) dilution

47. The knife wound resulted in _____ bleeding.
    (a) serrious
    (b) perfuse
    (c) cerious
    (d) serous

48. The young man was complaining of _____ after running 6 miles.
    (a) palpitation
    (b) profusion
    (c) perfusion
    (d) palpation

49. There was a green _____ discharge from the child's nose.
    (a) mucas
    (b) malleus
    (c) mucous
    (d) malleolus

50. The physician _____ many good reasons to quit smoking.
    (a) sighted
    (b) sited
    (c) cited
    (d) cighted

The transcription process is the integration of listening, keyboarding, and understanding the dictation. With practice, this skill can be mastered. Your goal is to synchronize your fingers, foot, and brain into one fluid motion. This chapter discusses various transcription tools and their use.

SOUND OF MEDICAL TRANSCRIPTION

Like hearing French or German spoken, listening to medical dictation for the first time may sound like a foreign language. Hearing all those newly learned medical terms dictated at a fast pace, with liberal doses of clinical slang, abbreviations, and assorted acronyms, can intimidate even the most dedicated student. Fear not; we will test the waters one toe at a time. An awareness of the style and phrasing of medical dictation will make it easier to understand and therefore transcribe.

To the inexperienced ear, medical dictation seems to have an incoherent style of prose. The dictation has a terse, staccato sound, and the dictator has a tendency to abbreviate words and condense sentences wherever possible. Because of these challenges, transcriptionists must be familiar with and be able to use the resources and standard reference materials of the industry. Knowledge of how to effectively use reference materials can increase productivity and perhaps your income. If your paycheck is tied to your productivity, knowing what reference materials to choose in a word search should increase your speed, which should boost your income.

Medical transcriptionists are expected to have the ability to correct errors they hear in dictation. For example, the physician may dictate, "The patient's current medications include Evista 60 milligrams po qd." It is the job of the transcriptionist to accurately transcribe the sentence complying with current rules regarding abbreviations, symbols, and acronyms. As you recall from Chapter 3, the abbreviation *qd* was one of several abbreviations listed as dangerous and not to be used. Hence, the sentence should be transcribed as, "The patient's current medications include Evista 60 mg po daily." This textbook will challenge your listening acuity and critical thinking skills.

USING REFERENCE MATERIALS

Reference materials are essential tools that increase productivity, save time, and ultimately increase production pay for the medical transcriptionist. A medical transcriptionist must have immediate access to a medical reference library that consists of a comprehensive medical dictionary, word books or spellers covering a variety of medical specialties, drug books, abbreviation and acronym word books, style guides, textbooks in anatomy and physiology, and an English dictionary.

Medical Dictionary
The medical dictionary holds a wealth of information to the knowledgeable transcriptionist who is familiar with its layout and understands its design. You should study the preface, front matter or introductory pages, color plates, and tables, as well as the appendices. Unlike an English dictionary, medical words are listed under the governing noun in a medical dictionary, with multiple word terms listed as subentries. Each entry includes the word origin, plural form, preferred spellings, cross-reference, and pronunciation guides, as well as definitions of the main entry and subentries. Two popular medical dictionaries are *Dorland's Illustrated Medical Dictionary* and *Stedman's Medical Dictionary*.

Word Books
Word books (or wordbooks) have become very popular in the last 15 years and are available in each major branch of medicine. Surgery, radiology, cardiology, laboratory, and similar word books are designed as alphabetic lists of medical words without definitions to make it easier and quicker to find the terms. These reference books often include the word division and pronunciation aids. However, because the book contains no definitions, a medical dictionary is still needed in conjunction with the word book to check the correct meaning of the term. The use of word books is invaluable, but you should be aware there is usually no indication that a word may have a sound-alike word or homophone, and word books do not differentiate between preferred and alternative acceptable spellings. This is where critical thinking and word discrimination skills come into practice. The "correct" medical term must make sense in the context of the report.

Pharmaceutical References
Drug books are specialized textbooks that contain an alphabetical indexing, a description of the drug, method of administration and dosage, classification, indications for use and contraindications, and differentiation between generic and brand names. Leading drug books are updated monthly, quarterly, or annually. Several popular drug books are *Drake and Drake Pharmaceutical Word Book*, *Quick-Look Drug Book*, *The American Drug Book*, *Physicians' Desk Reference* (PDR), and *Dorland's Illustrated Medical Dictionary*. Various publishing companies offer drug handbooks whose compact size facilitates ease of handling and use, such as *Mosby's Medical Drug Reference* and the *Merck Manual*.

Abbreviation Books
Abbreviations and acronyms are commonly used and are found in their own word books. *Eponyms* are adjectives

taken from a surname used to describe diseases, instruments, procedures, and other terms. In the eponym word book, the entries are listed alphabetically by the adjective, not the noun. For example, you would find *Valsalva maneuver* under *Valsalva* (adjective) rather than *maneuver* (noun). Eponym word books often include brief definitions of the terms. *The AAMT Book of Style for Medical Transcription* includes an excellent appendix on "dangerous" abbreviations and dose designations.

Style Guides

The need for consistency, accuracy, and clarity in preparing medical documents has resulted in the development of many different and acceptable manuals of style that determine proper editing, punctuation, and grammar guidelines. Often there is no one correct way of transcribing a sentence. *The AAMT Book of Style*, Fordney and Diehl's *Medical Transcription Guide: Do's and Don'ts*, and the *American Medical Association Manual of Style* are all respected manuals of style in medical transcription. Even these references differ, however, and may offer varying guidelines. Every good transcriptionist should be familiar with these reference materials and should use them for guidance when technical questions arise. If the sentence is grammatically correct and the meaning of the sentence is not distorted, a variety of different formats are acceptable.

Anatomy and Physiology Textbooks

Anatomy and physiology textbooks are useful reference materials that can help clarify your understanding of the content of the dictation. These textbooks discuss body structure and function in detail and may include disease processes and disorders.

English Dictionary

Medical transcriptionists must possess a good command of the English language and know how to use an English dictionary. An English dictionary is helpful in finding synonyms, antonyms, grammar, spellings, pronunciations, hyphenations, and definitions.

Electronic Reference Materials

Two distinct electronic reference materials, medical dictionaries and medical spellers, are available for purchase. Both are compatible with popular word processing software packages.

Electronic medical dictionaries contain all the information found in the printed version but also can search the entire database of words in seconds. Many electronic dictionaries also contain a thesaurus, which displays a list of words similar to the selected term.

Electronic medical spellcheckers have the capability of working with the existing spell checker and also can be customized to include troublesome medical terms.

You should always use your speller and dictionary features of the word processing package when you proofread your transcription, but be aware of their limitations. Simply running the spell check will not determine if you have selected the correct word, only that all the words in the document are spelled correctly. Homonyms or sound-alike words (soundalikes) are prime examples where the computer will not recognize the word as misspelled or suggest a substitute word. *The AAMT Book of Style* includes an excellent appendix on soundalikes.

Other available electronic reference software use *macros*, which are word processing files containing recorded commands for a series of tasks that will increase speed and accuracy by saving keystrokes and time. These packages incorporate productivity tools such as word expanders, abbreviation exploders, and other customized features. Once you become an experienced medical transcriptionist, you should investigate the benefits of such specialized software packages.

Online Resources

You can find a wealth of information through the Internet. By accessing online resources, you can obtain information on new medical techniques, procedures, drugs, and transcription products. You also can enter a chat room with a medical transcriptionist. This enables you to obtain advice about word usage and spelling questions, which can be particularly helpful if you work out of your home. Using a web browser, you can key in the string, *medical transcription*, to obtain numerous entries. Box 4-1 lists online resources to help you start your exploration of the Internet.

Other Reference Sources

Other reference materials that may be helpful to you include telephone books, current magazines, *Current Medical Terminology*, *American Hospital Association Guide to the Health Care Field*, and *American Medical Association Membership Directory*. Telephone books can be used to verify spelling of names, companies, schools, healthcare facilities, and so on. Keeping abreast of new developments in medicine and products can be achieved through periodical reading of current professional magazines, such as the *Journal of the American Association for Medical Transcription* (JAAMT) and *Perspectives on the Medical Transcription Profession*.

WORD SEARCH

A common frustration of both inexperienced and experienced medical transcriptionists is the difficulty in finding a word in available reference materials. If earnest effort to decipher a word proves futile, you may be *hearing* the wrong word. Many letters sound alike or even share the

BOX 4-1 Online Resources for Medical Transcriptionists

www.aamt.org/aamt: AAMT Web page

www2.ncbi.nlm.nih.gov/medline/query_form.html:
Medline website

www.wwma.com/kamt: Keeping Abreast of Medical
Transcription

www.advanceforhim.com

www.alphabest.com

www.grammarbook.com

www.careerstep.com

www.cvtinc.com

www.dailygrammar.com

www.delmarhealthcare.com/health/products/
medtran.asp

www.us.elsevierhealth.com

www.fadavis.com

www.fortherecordmag.com

www.glencoe.com

www.glossarist.com

www.google.com

www.chompchomp.com/rules

www.ccc.commnet.edu/grammar

www.encarta.msn.com/column/grammarmain.asp

www.horusdevelopment.com

www.hpisum.com: Perspectives on the Medical
Transcription Profession

www.lm-bookstore.com

www.lairdsschool.com

www.thelittlebluebook.com

www.mtecinc.com

www.peacehealth.org/kbase/list/tests

www.medword.com

www.mtdaily.com: MT Daily

www.mtdesk.com

www.mtgab.com

www.mtgiftgallery.bizhosting.com

www.mtjobs.com

www.mtmonthly.com

www.mtwerks.com

www.mt-advisor.com

www.mt-work.com

www.neilmdavis.com

www.owl.english.purdue.edu/handouts/grammar/
index.html

www.prenhall.com

www.rayveproductions.com

www.stedmans.com

www.textware.com

www.transcriptiongear.com

www.whonamedit.com

same sound. For example, the letter *m* may sound like an *n*. The *z* sound you hear in the prescription drug *prednisone* is actually an *s*. You may even miss the first letter of a word if you do not understand its meaning. The word *anomaly* (meaning a marked deviation from normal) may sound like *nomaly* but begins with the letter *a*. *Apposed* (being placed or fitted together) may be incorrectly transcribed as *opposed*. Be alert for medical terms that contain silent letters, such as *exogenous* or *psoas muscle*. Common sound-alike terms are defined in Box 4-2.

You should try to find a medical word under its main entry. Be aware that not all first words in a medical term are the main entry. Medical terms also may be searched under an alternative entry. Diseases may be searched under the category of "syndromes." Procedures may be searched under the category of "operations." Occasionally, medical terms are formed by "back formation," such as a noun used as a verb. Medical terms composed of a noun and adjective, such as eponyms (Valsalva maneuver, Foley catheter), are found under the noun.

In the work environment, if your own word search proves futile, you should ask a co-worker or supervisor for assistance, review the pertinent medical chart, or flag the word and ask the dictator for clarification. It is not acceptable to simply guess at a word.

TRANSCRIPTION PROCESS

As a novice, it is unrealistic to try to keep up with the dictating voice. This is not the time to be worried about speed. This is the time to concentrate on building your medical vocabulary. It is of no value if you have an excellent keyboarding speed but habitually omit some of the dictated words or consistently misspell medical terms. As a beginning transcription student, now is the time to invest in learning the proper transcription techniques and procedures.

There is a natural tendency to want to transcribe a medical document immediately rather than take a few moments to listen to the dictation in its entirety. As a beginning medical transcriptionist, listening to the entire document for any instructions, corrections, and comments will familiarize you with its content and alert you to potentially challenging sections of the report. It is helpful to stop and start the cassette as often as desired. In this way, you will familiarize yourself with the pronunciation and the meaning of the various words. Take time now to learn the fundamentals of medical transcription. The more time you spend previewing the dictated material, the more productive you will be and less time will be needed for transcribing the material.

The transcription process is to listen to a block of dictation, stop, and then accurately transcribe what you

BOX 4-2 Homonyms and Sound-Alike Medical Terms

Afferent (n)—moving toward the center

Efferent (n)—moving away from the center

Anuresis (n)—retention of urine in the bladder

Enuresis (n)—involuntary discharge of urine

Atopic (adj)—displaced

Atrophic (adj)—decrease in the size of a normally developed organ or tissue

Ectopic (adj)—located away from normal position

Aural (adj)—pertaining to the ear

Oral (adj)—pertaining to the mouth

Basal (adj)—basic, elemental, forming the base

Basil (n)—herb used in cooking

Chorda (n)—cord or sinew

Chordee (n)—downward deflection of the penis

Cirrhosis (n)—disease of the liver

Psoriasis (n)—chronic recurrent skin disease

Cite (v)—to quote

Site (n)—location in the body

Coarse (adj)—rough

Course (n)—duration of time

Colposcopy (n)—examination of the vagina and cervix with a colposcope

Culdoscopy (n)—direct visual examination of the female viscera through an endoscope

Dilation (n)—expansion of an organ or vessel

Dilution (n)—reduction of a concentration of active substance by adding a neutral agent

Discreet (adj)—cautious

Discrete (adj)—made up of separated parts

Dysphagia (n)—difficulty in swallowing

Dysphasia (n)—difficulty in speaking

Elicit (v)—to bring out

Illicit (n)—illegal

Eminent (adj)—prominent, famous

Imminent (adj)—about to occur

Facial (adj)—pertaining to the face

Fascial (adj)—pertaining to the fibrous connective tissue

Faucial (adj)—pertaining to the passage from the mouth to the pharynx

Fissure (n)—a narrow slit or groove on the surface of an organ

Fistula (n)—any abnormal tube-like passage within body tissue

Fundal (adj)—pertaining to a fundus

Fungal (adj)—pertaining to a condition caused by a fungus

Fundus (n)—general term for the bottom or base of an organ

Fungus (n)—general term for a group of eukaryotic organisms

Generic (adj)—nonspecific, nontrademark

Genetic (adj)—hereditary

Glands (n)—organs or groups of cells that produce or secrete substances

Glans (n)—small rounded mass

Hemostasis (n)—cessation of bleeding

Homeostasis (n)—maintain relative constant condition in the internal environment of the body

Ileum (n)—the last part of the small intestine between the jejunum and the large intestine

Ilium (n)—superior portion of the hipbone

In vitro (n)—in an artificial environment

In vivo (n)—within the living body

Malleolus (n)—rounded bone on either side of the ankle

Malleus (n)—largest of the three ossicles of the ear

Menorrhagia (n)—prolonged or heavy menses

Menorrhalgia (n)—pain during menstruation

Mucous (adj)—pertaining to or resembling mucus

Mucus (n)—sticky secretions of mucous membranes and glands

Palpation (n)—examination by touching

Palpitation (n)—rapid or fluttering heartbeat

Parental (adj)—pertaining to a parent

Parenteral (adj)—pertaining to treatment other than through the digestive system

Patience (n)—ability to suppress restlessness

Patients (n)—recipients of a healthcare services

Patient's (adj)—possessive form of the noun *patient*

Perianal (adj)—pertaining to the area around the anus

Perineal (adj)—pertaining to the area between the genitals and rectum

Peroneal (adj)—pertaining to the fibula

Perfuse (v)—to force blood or other fluid to flow

Profuse (adj)—abundant

Perfusion (n)—amount of blood reaching a tissue

Profusion (n)—abundance

Pericardial (adj)—pertaining to the area surrounding the heart

Precordial (adj)—pertaining to the area in front of the heart

Perineum (n)—pelvic floor

Peritoneum (n)—serous membrane lining the walls of the abdominal and pelvic cavities

Prostate (n)—male gland that surrounds the neck of the bladder and the urethra

Prostrate (adj)—lying face down

Radical (adj)—going to the root of the cause

Radicle (n)—one of the smallest branches of a vessel or nerve

Recession (n)—withdrawal of a part from its normal position

Continued

BOX 4-2 Homonyms and Sound-Alike Medical Terms—cont'd

Resection (n)—cutting out of a significant part of an organ or structure
Reflex (n)—involuntary reaction
Reflux (n)—abnormal backward or return flow of a fluid
Serious (adj)—not joking
Serous (adj)—pertaining to serum
Shoddy (adj)—tattered, worn
Shotty (adj)—resembling pellets used in shotgun cartridges

Tendinitis/tendonitis (n)—inflammation of a tendon
Tinnitus (n)—ringing in the ears
Ureteral (adj)—pertaining to the ureter
Urethral (adj)—pertaining to the urethra
Vesical (adj)—pertaining to the bladder
Vesicle (n)—blister
Viscous (adj)—sticky or glutinous
Viscus (n)—internal organ enclosed within a body cavity

have heard. Think about what you are transcribing. Concentration will avoid errors of wrong word choice and inconsistencies in text. When in doubt about a word, phonetically spell the word and either underscore or bold the word to remind you to verify its meaning. The dictator may repeat the words again, or you may receive a clue from the content of the report.

The final step in the transcription process is to proofread the document, correct your errors, and print the final document. Because medical transcriptionists are compensated based on speed and accuracy, it may be helpful to retranscribe (not retype) difficult reports to strengthen your skills.

PREPARING TO TRANSCRIBE

Before you begin to transcribe, gather together all necessary materials and equipment at your desk. If you organize your materials and plan your work, you should encounter less frustration and should be more productive. This textbook and its accompanying CD utilize new technology. In place of the traditional transcriber, you can now use your own personal computer, the CD, and a foot pedal that connects to your computer to transcribe dictation.

To utilize the traditional transcriber, audiocassettes, and personal computer, you will need the following:
1. A computer with a word processing software package installed. Word and WordPerfect are the two most common word processing packages.
2. Transcriber
3. Headset or earphones
4. Foot pedal
5. Reference materials
6. Printer and paper
7. Audiocassette with dictated material

If you are using the new technology, you will need the following:
1. A computer with MS Word package installed.
2. Headset or earphones
3. PC foot pedal adaptor and its software

4. Reference materials
5. Printer and paper
6. CD-ROM with dictated material

Connecting your earphones to the transcriber allows you to hear the dictation. The three parts of an earphone are the chin band, cord, and connection tip. If you are having trouble hearing with your earphones, check the earphone connection; the tip may not be in tight contact with the transcriber. Also, the cord itself could be worn or cracked and may need replacement. Remember that earphones collect debris and wax and should be cleaned with rubbing alcohol after every use.

Make sure your foot pedal is connected to the transcriber and the transcriber is turned on. The foot pedal allows you to keep your hands free for keyboarding. A foot pedal consists of two parts: the pedal and the cord. Pressing the foot pedal causes the transcriber to play. As soon as you release the pedal with your foot, the machine stops. If you press on the foot pedal and nothing happens, check the cord connection to make sure it is plugged firmly into the transcriber.

Foot pedals are available in a variety of styles. With most models, the center of the foot pedal is the position to press for play, fast forward is on the right, and rewind is on the left. Some foot pedals have only two options: right for play and left for rewind (there is no fast forward). Check the directions of the model that you are using before you begin to transcribe a document.

The Transcriber
The transcriber operates similar to a musical cassette player. Figure 4-1 shows the location of the usual features that appear on the base control board on most portable and desktop transcriber models.

On/Off or Power Button
This button is used to turn the transcriber on and off and is indicated by a power light.

Index Counters
Some transcribers have an index counter that measures the length of dictation on a cassette. This is a useful tool

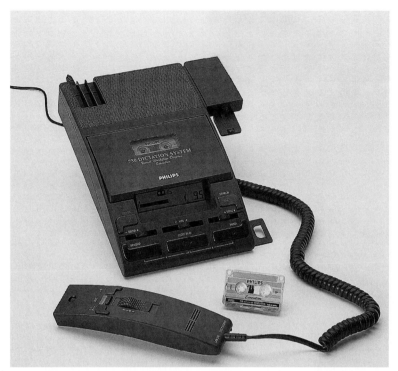

Figure 4-1 Features of the transcriber. *(Courtesy Phillips Speech Processing, Atlanta, Georgia.)*

for finding the correct dictation or scanning cassettes. As the tape is scanned, it is also rewound. At the end of every dictation series, you can hear a beep. At this point, the index counter lights up and marks where the dictation ends for each series on the control strip.

Auto Playback or Auto Rewind
The auto backspace button allows you to replay a word or a string of words. With a digital dictation system, this feature is adjusted by a computer system.

Speaker
Use the speaker button to listen aloud to dictation.

Eject
The eject button opens the cassette door. Press it to insert or remove a cassette.

Speed Control
You can increase or decrease the speed control knob while you are learning. Either extreme, whether too slow or too fast, will only distort the sound. Keep this in mind when you are trying to understand a garbled word. It sometimes helps to set the speed at a normal conversational level to understand the dictator more clearly.

Volume Control
You can increase or decrease the volume knob to compensate for a louder or softer voice.

Tone
The tone feature mutes or accentuates consonants (treble or bass) for nasal tones or a stuttering style of dictation.

Erase
This feature allows you to clear or erase tapes. Be careful with this button to make sure you do not erase dictation before it is transcribed.

Tapes
The most frequently used audiocassette transcriber, the standard cassette transcriber, uses $3^{15}/_{16} \times 2^{1}/_{2} \times 2^{1}/_{2}$–inch standard audiocassettes. These cassettes are sold everywhere.

The microcassette transcriber uses the smallest cassette tapes on the market today, the microsize audiocassette tapes ($2 \times 1^{1}/_{4}$ inches). These cassettes are frequently used in physician offices and clinics because of their size and convenience. The dictating machines that accommodate them are handheld, pocket-sized models. The cassettes are sold in supermarkets, department stores, and business supply stores.

The minicassette transcriber uses a cassette tape size whose use is almost exclusively limited to transcribing machines. These minisized audiotapes are $2^{3}/_{16} \times 1^{3}/_{8}$ inches. Minicassettes are frequently used in physician offices that have been in practice for many years because the minicassette preceded the microcassette. Many physicians still continue to use minicassette dictating machines. Minicassettes are generally sold in dictation specialty stores.

PRODUCTION FOR PAY SUMMARY

In medical transcription the transcriptionist's salary is often based on the amount of work produced rather than a regular monthly salary. The character is the preferred method of measuring productivity and has been supported by several national allied health organizations. A character is any letter, number, symbol, or function key necessary for the final appearance and content of a document, including the space bar, enter key, underscore, bold, and any character contained within a macro, header, or footer. Most employers pay on production determined by characters by line, primarily a 65-character line. Because many transcription environments have now transitioned to MS Word from Word Perfect, word-counting formulas are becoming obsolete. The Production for Pay calculations in the software program that accompanies this textbook uses word count of the document.

The Production for Pay summary in Table 4-1 is an example of how a transcriptionist's wage is determined for documents transcribed in this textbook. The summary includes the total number of words produced, total production time, and total number of errors to compute the net production pay. A rate of $0.15 per minute per net production word is used as an arbitrary amount to compute wages. For example: You have just completed a 260-word history and physical examination report in 13 minutes with two uncorrected errors,

as shown in Table 4-2. Completing the Production for Pay summary, you earned $2.70 for this report. If you transcribed at the same production rate for an hour, you would earn approximately $11.

WELCOME TO FEDDES WELLNESS CENTER

Beginning in Chapter 5, you will apply your knowledge of the transcription process as a medical transcriptionist employed at the fictitious medical office practice, FedDes Wellness Center. To make the process of learning transcription easier, the next sections provide you with specific formatting guidelines, a physician directory, and an audiocassette directory.

Document formats and dictation styles vary from office to office. Because of this diversity, each facility has its own format and guidelines for transcribing a physician's dictation. In large institutions, medical committees develop their own manual of style that is followed by all transcriptionists throughout the facility. Healthcare facilities owned by hospital organizations must adhere to Joint Commission on Accreditation of Healthcare Organizations (JCAHO) rules and regulations regarding formatting medical reports. In single or small practices, the transcriptionist is given more freedom in style usage, as long as it conforms to known standards. The *FedDes Wellness Center's Transcription Guidelines* should enable you to focus on developing your transcription skills without the confusion of conflicting technical guidelines. After you understand and have practiced this formatting style, it will be easier to grasp alternative styles as you progress in your career.

FedDes Wellness Center Transcription Guidelines

FedDes Wellness Center has its own format and guidelines for transcribing physician's dictation. All the rules and guidelines presented in Chapter 2 and Chapter 3, as well as those described in this section, apply to the medical documents that are transcribed at FedDes Wellness Center. To research extensive technical questions, FedDes Wellness Center complies with *The AAMT Book of Style for Medical Transcription*, 2nd edition.

Formatting Guidelines
1. All medical reports use the block style format with 1-inch margins. No tabulation appears in the document. Letters are formatted with a 2-inch first-page top margin to accommodate a letterhead and 1-inch second-page top margin.
2. Lowercase letters for both sets of initials, with a colon between them and no periods, are used for

TABLE 4-1 PRODUCTION FOR PAY SUMMARY	
Document No.	
Total Word Count	
Total Production Time	
Words per Minute (Total Word Count ÷ Total Production Time)	
Total Error Value (Error Analysis Chart)	
Net Production (Words per Minute − Total Error Value)	
Production for Pay ($0.15 × Net Production)	

TABLE 4-2. COMPLETED PRODUCTION FOR PAY SUMMARY	
Document No.	1
Total Word Count	260
Total Production Time	13 minutes
Words per Minute (Total Word Count ÷ Total Production Time)	20
Total Error Value (Error Analysis Chart)	2
Net Production (Words per Minute – Total Error Value)	18
Production for Pay ($0.15 × Net Production)	$2.70

the dictator and transcriptionist initials placed at the end of a medical report.

3. All medical letters use open punctuation. No punctuation marks follow the salutation and complimentary closing.

4. The complete headings, sections/topics, and subheadings are always used. These are keyed in all capital letters.

5. The dictated words *current date* must be transcribed as the actual month, day, and year. The dictated words *yesterday's date* should be transcribed as the day before the actual date the document is transcribed.

6. Identifying statistical data must be included on medical reports.

   Example
   CHART NOTE
   Patient Name: Felter, Michael
   Date of Birth: July 3, 1954
   Examination Date: *current date*

   Example
   HISTORY AND PHYSICAL EXAMINATION
      REPORT
   Patient Name: Doe, Jane
   File Number: 1235678
   Date of Birth: January 3, 1950
   Examination Date: *current date*
   Physician: Charles P. Davis, MD

   Example
   X-RAY REPORT
   Patient Name: Doe, Jane
   File Number: 1235678
   Date of Birth: January 3, 1950
   Examination Date: *current date*
   Ordering Physician: Izzy Sertoli, MD

   Example
   PROCEDURE REPORT
   Patient Name: Doe, Jane
   File Number: 1235678
   Date of Birth: January 3, 1950
   Examination Date: *current date*
   Ordering Physician: Izzy Sertoli, MD

   Example
   CONSULTATION REPORT
   Patient Name: Doe, Jane
   File Number: 1235678
   Date of Birth: January 3, 1950
   Examination Date: *current date*
   Requesting Physician: Izzy Sertoli, MD

7. All medical documents formatted as a letter should include a reference line above the salutation line.

   Example
   Re: Betty Williams
      Date of Birth: February 2, 1949
      Examination: RIGHT BREAST SONOGRAM

   Dear Dr. Davis

8. When a medical report is longer than one page, the name of the report, patient's name, file number, and page number are keyed in the header pane on each printed page.

   Example
   HISTORY AND PHYSICAL EXAMINATION
      REPORT
   Patient Name: Doe, Jane
   File Number: 1235678
   Page 2

9. For multiple-page letters, the header includes the patient's name, date, and page number beginning at the 1-inch top margin.

Example
Patient Name
Date
Page 2

10. When a medical report is longer than one page, the word *continued* is keyed in the footer pane on each printed page before the last page. Medical letters do not have a footer.

11. Do not carry a single line of a report or letter onto a continuation page.

12. Do not allow a continuation page to include only the signature block and the data following it.

13. The signature line includes the physician's or dictator's name and title entered four lines below the final line of text, flush left. The dictator and transcriptionist initials are placed at the end of each report. Enter the initials flush left and two lines below the physician's name. Use all lowercase letters for both sets of initials with a colon or diagonal between them, without the use of periods. The date of the dictation, indicated by the letter D, and date the document was transcribed, indicated by the letter T, are entered flush left below the initials of the dictator and transcriptionist.

Example

Potter T. Bucky, MD

ptb:cd
D: 11/20/xx (date the report was dictated)
T: 11/21/xx (date the report was transcribed)

14. Keep the numeral and unit of measure together at line breaks. This is important when transcribing a drug and its corresponding dosage.
Example: The specimen measured 3 cm in diameter.
Erythromycin 250 mg t.i.d. was prescribed.

Usage Guidelines

1. When the age of the patient is mentioned within the body of the transcript, the patient's year of birth is not provided, and the student will need to calculate this date.

2. All dates are spelled out in medical documents regardless of where the date appears on a report or letter.
Example: The patient was seen in this office on Monday, January 12, 20xx.

3. A comma separates each vital sign.
Example: BP 108/72, pulse 78 and regular, respirations 20/min.

4. Drug allergies are typed in all capitals.
Example
ALLERGIES: TETRACYCLINE.

5. Drug dosages are expressed in Latin abbreviations and transcribed in lowercase letters with periods and no internal spaces.
Example: The patient was started on Keflex, 250 mg q.i.d.

6. Measurements of tumors are expressed in metric terms.
Example: The tumor measured $12 \times 12 \times 6$ mm.

7. A zero is placed *before* a decimal that lacks a whole number.
Example: The lesion measured 0.75×1 cm.

8. Mixed numbers are transcribed in figures (Arabic numerals).
Example: The $5\frac{1}{2}$-year-old female was seen at 1 p.m.

9. Figures are used almost exclusively as opposed to spelled-out numbers to improve clarity and avoid potential mistakes. There are always exceptions, and judgment and discretion are needed when deciding whether to use numerals or to spell out numbers.
Examples
Mrs. Jones is widowed, but she resides with one of her three children.
Patient complains of right elbow pain for the past 3 weeks.
The patient smokes 2 packs per day and has done so for 24 years.

10. Figures are used in lists. MS Word autonumbering feature is used to create numbered lists.
Example
IMPRESSION
1. Acute appendicitis.
2. Rule out ureteral calculus.

11. Figures are used to indicate the patient's weight, height, blood pressure (BP), pulse, and respiration. Figures are used to indicate patient's age, except at the beginning of a sentence.
Examples
This is the second admission for this 2-year-old.
Two-year-old patient was admitted for the second time.
Her physical findings are: Weight 25 pounds, height 21 inches, BP 142/72, pulse 117, respirations 20/min.

12. Figures and the number sign are used for suture materials.
Example: The subcutaneous tissues were closed with interrupted #3-0 plain catgut.

13. Figures are used for ranges and ratios.
Example: She has vomited 4-5 times in the past 24 hours, and the vomit is mostly a bile-colored, watery liquid.

14. Figures are used to refer to grade, phase, and pregnancy and delivery.

    Examples

    She was diagnosed with grade 3/6 holosystolic murmur.

    The patient is gravida 1, para 1.

15. The plurals of single-digit numbers, letters, and symbols are formed by adding *s*.

16. The plurals of double-digit numbers and all-capital abbreviations are formed by adding the letter *s*.

    Example: The patient's blood pressure has been relatively well controlled, with systolic pressures running 140-150s.

17. Roman numerals are generally used to express stages and clotting factors.

    Examples

    She was diagnosed with stage IV decubitus ulcer.

    Prothrombin time is a test to measure the activity of factors I, II, V, VII, and X, which participate in the extrinsic pathway of coagulation.

18. Roman numerals are used for standard leads and intercostal space positions.

    Example: There is reciprocal depression in leads I and II.

19. Ordinal numbers are used to indicate order or position in a series rather than quantity. As with all numbers in medical reports, AAMT recommends using numerals (figures): 1st, 2nd, 3rd, etc.

    Example: On the 3rd day, the baby's temperature was normal.

20. Do not use superscripts and subscripts when expressing electrocardiographic leads, vertebral columns, chemical compounds, and so on.

    Examples

    The leads are V1 through V6.

    We used distilled H2O.

21. Do not use the degree symbol when expressing temperature. The word *degree* is included only if dictated. Fahrenheit or Celsius is included only if dictated and is expressed as a capital letter, *F* or *C*.

    Example: Her temperature was 98.6 F.

22. The letter × is used to abbreviate *by* and *times* when it precedes a number or another abbreviation.

    Examples

    The lesion on her leg is 1.5 × 1 cm.

    The patient was prescribed Augmentin, 500 mg p.o. t.i.d. × 2 weeks.

23. A hyphen is used between numbers and *year old*.

    Example: The patient was a 26-year-old female.

24. A hyphen is used between two "like" vowels.

    Example: We will plan to see the patient in 3 weeks for re-evaluation.

25. A hyphen is used to take the place of the word *to* or *through* to identify ranges.

    Example: The last time he vomited was 4-5 hours ago.

26. Hyphens are used to form compound adjectives.

    Example: Although the stated age of this patient is 45, his speech is child-like.

27. A diagonal or virgule (/) is used to indicate the word *per* in laboratory values and respirations or the word *over* in blood pressure.

    Example: BP 120/80, pulse 106 and regular, temperature 37.2° C, respirations 14/min.

28. The number or pound (#) symbol is used to abbreviate the word *number* when followed by a medical instrument or apparatus.

    Example: The small piece of metal was removed with a #25-gauge needle.

29. Do not use an abbreviation for common nonmetric units of measure to express weight, depth, distance, height, length, and width, except in tables.

    Example: The patient was 5 feet 3 inches and weighed 105 pounds.

30. One space follows end-of-sentence punctuation.

    Example: The patient is a 45-year-old computer programmer. He presents with a sinus headache.

31. One space follows commas, semicolons, and colons.

    Examples

    She denies associated fever, chills, or hematemesis.

    Pupils are constricted and midline; they react to light.

32. Space once after a period that ends an abbreviation.

    Example: Dr. Smith was called for the consultation.

33. No spaces are used after a period within an abbreviation.

    Example: Her medication was ordered t.i.d. by her doctor.

34. No spaces are used before or after a hyphen, apostrophe, or diagonal.

    Example: The patient was a well-developed, well-nourished 29-year-old in mild distress.

35. No spaces are used between symbol and referent.

    Example: Her temperature was 98.6°.

FedDes Wellness Center Approved Abbreviation List

AB	abortion
ABG	arterial blood gas
ACTH	adrenocorticotropic hormone
A&D	ascending and descending
ADL	activities of daily living
AP	anteroposterior
A&P	auscultation and percussion

ARD	acute respiratory distress	LLQ	left lower quadrant
ASAP	as soon as possible	LMP	last menstrual period
ASCVD	atherosclerotic cardiovascular disease	LUQ	left upper quadrant
AV	atrioventricular	MI	myocardial infarction
BCC	basal cell carcinoma	MM	mucous membrane
BE	barium enema	NKA	no known allergies
BLE	bilateral lower extremities	NOS	not otherwise specified
BLT	bilateral tubal ligation	NPH	no previous history
BM	bowel movement	NSAID	nonsteroidal anti-inflammatory drug
BP	blood pressure	NSR	normal sinus rhythm
BPH	benign prostatic hypertrophy	NTP	normal temperature and pressure
BS	blood sugar, bowel sounds	OB-GYN	obstetrics and gynecology
BUN	blood urea nitrogen	PA	posteroanterior
BUS	Bartholin, urethral, and Skene (glands)	P&A	percussion and auscultation
CABG	coronary artery bypass graft surgery	PERL	pupils equal and reactive to light
CAD	coronary artery disease	PERLA	pupils equal and reactive to light and accommodation
CBC	complete blood count		
CHF	congestive heart failure	PERRLA	pupils equal, round, reactive to light and accommodation
CNS	central nervous system		
COPD	chronic obstructive pulmonary disease	PID	pelvic inflammatory disease
CPR	cardiopulmonary resuscitation	PIP	proximal interphalangeal
CR	cardiorespiratory	PSA	prostate-specific antigen
C&S	culture and sensitivity	RBC	red blood cell (count)
CT	computerized tomography	RLQ	right lower quadrant
CVA	cerebrovascular accident	ROM	range of motion
D&C	dilation and curettage	RRR	regular rate and rhythm
DJD	degenerative joint disease	RUQ	right upper quadrant
DOE	dyspnea on exertion	SGOT	serum glutamic-oxaloacetic transaminase
DPT	diphtheria-pertussis-tetanus (vaccine)	SOB	shortness of breath
DTR	deep tendon reflexes	STD	sexually transmitted disease
DVT	deep vein thrombosis	T&A	tonsillectomy and adenoidectomy
EAC	external auditory canal	TAB	therapeutic abortion
ECG	electrocardiogram	TM	tympanic membrane
EGD	esophagogastroduodenoscopy	TPR	temperature, pulse, respirations
EKG	electrocardiogram	TUR	transurethral resection
EOM	extraocular movements	TURP	transurethral resection of the prostate
EOMI	extraocular movements intact	UA	urinalysis
ER	emergency room	URI	upper respiratory infection
ESR	erythrocyte sedimentation rate	UTI	urinary tract infection
FB	foreign body	UV	ultraviolet
FBS	fasting blood sugar	VPB	ventricular premature beat
FUO	fever of unknown origin	VS	vital signs
GB	gallbladder	V&T	volume and tension
GI	gastrointestinal	WBC	white blood cell (count)
GYN	gynecology/gynecologist	WF	white female
HCG	human chorionic gonadotropin	WM	white male
H&P	history and physical	WNL	within normal limits
HPI	history of present illness		
I&D	incision and drainage		
IM	intramuscular		
INR	International Normalized Ratio		
IV	intravenous		
IVP	intravenous pyelogram		
KUB	kidneys, ureters, bladder		
L&A	light and accommodation		

FedDes Wellness Center Physician Directory

The center is at 101 Wellness Way Drive, New York, NY 10036. Providers on site include 24 physicians, a physical therapist, and a certified nurse practitioner.

Family Practice Division, Suite 300

Charles P. Davis, MD

J. Thomas Geiger, MD
Matthew D. Sponch, MD
Izzy Sertoli, MD
P. H. Waters, MD
Melissa A. Anconeus, MS, PT
Pamela S. Barthonin, MA, RN, CRNP

Orthopedic Division, Suite 133
David Treppe, MD
James P. Osseous, MD
Harry A. Medulla, MD

Urology Division, Suite 237
Helen Loop, MD
Theodore Trigone, MD
Benjamin Keytone, MD

Pulmonary Medicine Division, Suite 451
Allan Bolus, MD
Neal Alveoli, MD
Douglas Sputum, MD

Gastroenterology Division, Suite 279

Gwenn Maltase, MD
Kate Cobalamin, MD
Anna Bolism, MD

Cardiology Division, Suite 413
Erica Purkinje, MD
Lucas Site, MD
A.B. Doner, MD
Adam Valence, MD

Diagnostic Imaging Division, Suite 157
William C. Roentgen, MD
Hounsfield T. Scanner, MD
Potter T. Bucky, MD
Scott E. Film, MD

Audiocassette Directory

Eight audiocassettes accompany *Essentials of Medical Transcription*, as listed in Table 4-3.

TABLE 4-3 AUDIOCASSETTES TO ACCOMPANY *ESSENTIALS OF MEDICAL TRANSCRIPTION*			
TAPE NUMBER	NUMBER OF DICTATIONS	CHAPTER NUMBER	CHAPTER TITLE
1	4T-1 through 4T-3, supplemental dictation	4	Transcription Process
1, 2	5T-1 through 5T-23, supplemental dictation	5	Office Medical Transcription from the Family Practice
2	6T-1 through 6T-19 supplemental dictation	6	Office Medical Transcription from the Orthopedic Practice
3	7T-1 through 7T-15, supplemental dictation	7	Office Medical Transcription from the Urology Practice
4	8T-1 through 8T-12, supplemental dictation	8	Office Medical Transcription from the Pulmonary Medicine Practice
5, 6	9T-1 through 9T-15, supplemental dictation	9	Office Medical Transcription from the Gastroenterology Practice
7, 8	10T-1 through 10T-12, supplemental dictation	10	Office Medical Transcription from the Cardiology Practice
8	11T-1 through 11T-19, supplemental dictation	11	Office Medical Transcription from the Diagnostic Imaging Practice

Understanding the contents of medical documents is the first step to becoming an accomplished transcriptionist. Assess your knowledge of medical document content by completing two worksheets.

TEXTBOOK USERS

Select the best answer for each question or statement concerning reference materials.

Refer to the answer key for immediate feedback (Appendix E).

SOFTWARE USERS

Click on *Chapter 4, Activity 4-1*, and follow the directions.

Follow the same process for *Chapter 4, Activity 4-2*.

ACTIVITY 4-1
Word Search Worksheets

Part I Directions: Which reference book would you select to find the word or phrase to verify spelling, capitalization, punctuation, or definition?

1. Parkinson's disease
   (a) eponym word book
   (b) English dictionary
   (c) manual of style
   (d) a and b

2. *Afferent* or *efferent*
   (a) standard English dictionary
   (b) eponym word book
   (c) manual of style
   (d) a and c

3. Penicillin
   (a) medical dictionary
   (b) anatomy and physiology textbook
   (c) drug book
   (d) all the above

4. CABG
   (a) English dictionary
   (b) cardiology word book
   (c) abbreviation book
   (d) b and c

5. Bypass graft
   (a) surgery word book
   (b) orthopedic word book
   (c) urology word book
   (d) none of the above

6. LDH
   (a) pathology and lab word book
   (b) physician's drug reference book
   (c) abbreviation word book
   (d) a and c

7. Percutaneous transluminal angioplasty
   (a) drug book
   (b) radiology word book
   (c) eponym book
   (d) all the above

8. *Check up* or *check-up*
   (a) manual of style
   (b) eponym book
   (c) neither a nor b
   (d) a and b

9. *Xanax* or *Zantac*
   (a) eponym book
   (b) surgical book
   (c) drug book
   (d) cardiology book

10. *Elicit* or *illicit*
    (a) homonym book
    (b) manual of style
    (c) standard English dictionary
    (d) all the above

11. Retin-A
    (a) dermatology book
    (b) drug book
    (c) neither a nor b
    (d) a and b

12. The plural form of *vertebra*
    (a) medical dictionary
    (b) surgical word book
    (c) eponym book
    (d) none of the above

13. Down syndrome
    (a) English dictionary
    (b) manual of style
    (c) eponym book
    (d) a and c

14. *DeBakey clamp* or *DeBakey's clamp*
    (a) eponym book
    (b) manual of style
    (c) medical dictionary
    (d) all the above

15. *H influenzae* or *h influenzae*
    (a) manual of style
    (b) orthopedic word book
    (c) surgical book
    (d) cardiology book

16. *V1 and V2* or *V_1 or V_2*
    (a) dermatology
    (b) eponym book
    (c) manual of style
    (d) none of the above

ACTIVITY 4-1 *(cont'd)*

17. McMurray's test
    (a) orthopedic word book
    (b) eponym book
    (c) a and b
    (d) none of the above

18. San Antonio, TX
    (a) English dictionary
    (b) eponym word book
    (c) manual of style
    (d) abbreviation word book

19. Extirpative surgery
    (a) medical dictionary
    (b) English dictionary
    (c) surgical word book
    (d) all the above

20. Mucous or mucus
    (a) medical dictionary
    (b) English dictionary
    (c) a and b
    (d) neither a nor b

Part II Directions: Select the best word that completes the meaning of the sentence.

21. The patient who had _____ went to the urologist.
    (a) psoriasis
    (b) cirrhosis
    (c) anuran
    (d) enuresis

22. His _____ was 20/40 uncorrected.
    (a) sight
    (b) cite
    (c) site
    (d) zite

23. The medical assistant tried to _____ the patient's complaints.
    (a) illicit
    (b) elicit
    (c) ilicit
    (d) ellicit

24. Mr. Thompson suffered from _____ as a result of a stroke, making eating solid foods difficult.
    (a) dysphagia
    (b) menorrhagia
    (c) dysphasia
    (d) menorrhalgia

25. The physician examined the patient's breast by _____.
    (a) recession
    (b) palpation
    (c) resection
    (d) palpitation

26. The physician used eye drops for _____ in order to examine her eyes.
    (a) colposcopy
    (b) culdoscopy
    (c) dilation
    (d) dilution

27. The _____ was found to be normal on endoscopic examination.
    (a) ileum
    (b) illeum
    (c) ilium
    (d) illium

28. The boy denied any use of an _____ drug.
    (a) afferent
    (b) illicit
    (c) efferent
    (d) elicit

29. The examination revealed the man's _____ to be normal in size.
    (a) porcine
    (b) Bartholin's gland
    (c) prostate
    (d) prostrate

30. The stroke caused his left _____ weakness.
    (a) facial
    (b) faucial
    (c) fascial
    (d) fasucial

ACTIVITY 4-1 *(cont'd)*

31. The patient underwent a _____ mastectomy because of cancer.
    (a) radicle
    (b) radical
    (c) vesical
    (d) visicle

32. The pharmacist asked if the _____ drug would be acceptable.
    (a) genic
    (b) genetic
    (c) generic
    (d) genetric

33. The little boy found his mother _____ on the kitchen floor.
    (a) perineum
    (b) peritoneum
    (c) prostate
    (d) prostrate

34. The pathology report concludes the lesion is a _____ cell carcinoma.
    (a) basal
    (b) chorda
    (c) basil
    (d) chordee

35. The _____ laboratory tests were normal.
    (a) patients
    (b) patience
    (c) patient's
    (d) patients'

ACTIVITY 4-2
Word Search Worksheet

Part I Directions: Which reference book would you select to find the word or phrase to verify spelling, capitalization, punctuation, or definition?

1. Hodgkin's disease
   (a) eponym word book
   (b) English dictionary
   (c) manual of style
   (d) all the above

2. *Aural* or *oral*
   (a) standard English dictionary
   (b) eponym word book
   (c) manual of style
   (d) a and c

3. *gr3* or *grade 3*
   (a) ophthalmology word book
   (b) anatomy and physiology textbook
   (c) drug book
   (d) all the above

4. HNP
   (a) English dictionary
   (b) orthopedic word book
   (c) abbreviation book
   (d) b and c

5. Cholecystectomy
   (a) surgery word book
   (b) orthopedic word book
   (c) cardiology word book
   (d) none of the above

6. BRAT
   (a) gastroenterology word book
   (b) urology word book
   (c) abbreviation word book
   (d) a and c

7. Cystoscopy
   (a) drug book
   (b) medical dictionary
   (c) eponym book
   (d) all the above

8. *3 year old* or *3-year-old*
   (a) manual of style
   (b) eponym book
   (c) neither a nor b
   (d) a and b

9. *Xanax* or *Zantac*
   (a) eponym book
   (b) surgical book
   (c) drug book
   (d) cardiology book

10. *Shoddy* or *shotty*
    (a) homonym book
    (b) manual of style
    (c) eponym book
    (d) a and b

11. Denorex
    (a) dermatology book
    (b) drug book
    (c) neither a nor b
    (d) a and b

12. The plural form of *diverticulum*
    (a) medical dictionary
    (b) surgical word book
    (c) eponym book
    (d) none of the above

13. Tinel's sign
    (a) English dictionary
    (b) manual of style
    (c) eponym book
    (d) none of the above

14. *Potts clamp* or *Potts' clamp*
    (a) eponym book
    (b) English dictionary
    (c) surgical word book
    (d) a and c

15. *S aureus* or *s aureus*
    (a) manual of style
    (b) orthopedic word book
    (c) surgical book
    (d) cardiology book

16. *L1 and L2* or L_1 *and* L_2
    (a) abbreviation book
    (b) eponym book
    (c) manual of style
    (d) none of the above

ACTIVITY 4-2 (cont'd)

Part II Directions: Select the best word that completes the meaning of the sentence.

17. The smallest branch of a nerve is called a _____.
    (a) radicle
    (b) radical
    (c) vesical
    (d) visicle

18. The cutting out of a significant part of an organ or structure is referred to as _____.
    (a) recession
    (b) resection
    (c) reflex
    (d) reflux

19. Both great toenails were deformed by _____.
    (a) fundus
    (b) fungus
    (c) fungel
    (d) fundal

20. The rash was diagnosed as _____ dermatitis.
    (a) atopic
    (b) ectopic
    (c) atropic
    (d) topic

21. The child's feet were covered with small _____ from red ant bites.
    (a) fauces
    (b) viscous
    (c) vesicles
    (d) viscus

22. The fracture site was tender to _____.
    (a) palpitation
    (b) palpation
    (c) perfusion
    (d) profusion

23. It was concluded that the _____ was caused by prostatic hypertrophy.
    (a) anuresis
    (b) dysphagia
    (c) anuran
    (d) dysphasia

24. The patient was diagnosed with _____ of the liver.
    (a) cirrhosis
    (b) psoriasis
    (c) tinnitus
    (d) tendinitis

25. The patient was diagnosed with severe gastroesophageal _____.
    (a) perfusion
    (b) reflex
    (c) profusion
    (d) reflux

26. The colonoscopy was performed all the way to the terminal _____.
    (a) ileum
    (b) illeum
    (c) ilium
    (d) illium

27. The patient was placed on _____ feedings after the gastrectomy.
    (a) perineal
    (b) parental
    (c) parenteral
    (d) peroneal

28. The _____ closure was accomplished with 0 silk after the hysterectomy.
    (a) parenteral
    (b) perineal
    (c) peroneal
    (d) parental

29. After the stroke, James had experienced _____ and was unable to communicate.
    (a) menorrhagia
    (b) dysphasia
    (c) menorrhalgia
    (d) dysphasis

30. The _____ lesions were found by examining the mouth.
    (a) oral
    (b) chorda
    (c) aural
    (d) chordee

ACTIVITY 4-2 *(cont'd)*

31. The _____ physician had an article published in the *Journal of the American Medical Association*.
    (a) imminent
    (b) iminent
    (c) eminent
    (d) emminent

32. The Tay-Sachs disease was found to be _____.
    (a) generic
    (b) genetic
    (c) discreet
    (d) discrete

33. The examination of the female viscera through an endoscope is _____.
    (a) culdoscopy
    (b) resection
    (c) colposopy
    (d) recession

34. Mr. James complained of _____ and pain in his ears.
    (a) tinnitus
    (b) tendenitis
    (c) tendinitis
    (d) tinitus

35. Her favorite recipe included _____.
    (a) glands
    (b) glans
    (c) basal
    (d) basil

Being able to format and transcribe medical documents is the second step to becoming an accomplished transcriptionist. If you have not already done so, create a template for a chart note, history and physical examination, and letter and then transcribe the documents *4T-1*, *4T-2*, and *4T-3* from your audiocassette.

TEXTBOOK USERS

Open your word processing package.

Transcribe and proofread dictation *4T-1*, referring to the FedDes Physician Directory and using the formatting guidelines established in Chapter 2.

Identify and correct all errors.

Save your work on your student disk.

Follow the same process for dictations *4T-2* and *4T-3*.

Manually complete the error analysis chart for each document.

Manually complete the Production for Pay summary for each report.

SOFTWARE USERS

Click on *Chapter 4, Activity 4-3*, and follow the directions.

Follow the same process for *Chapter 4, Activities 4-4 and 4-5*.

Let's pause a minute and see how well you have mastered the information in this chapter. This section allows you to evaluate your understanding of reference materials and how to use them.

TEXTBOOK USERS

Select the best answer for each question or statement concerning reference materials.
Refer to the answer key (Appendix E) for immediate feedback.

SOFTWARE USERS

Click on *Chapter 4, Check Your Progress*, and follow the directions.

CHECK YOUR PROGRESS

Directions: Select true (T) or false (F) for each statement on reference materials and the transcription process.

1. T or F   Ten characters are calculated to equal one word for production pay.

2. T or F   Hospital medical committees may develop their own manuals of style as long as they comply with accreditation standards.

3. T or F   Electronic medical spellers can be customized to include a transcriptionist's troublesome words.

4. T or F   A *macro* is a word processing file that contains recorded commands for a series of tasks.

5. T or F   Productivity tools increase speed and accuracy.

6. T or F   Resources found on the Internet are helpful to a transcriptionist.

7. T or F   Medical terms are sometimes formed by back formation.

8. T or F   It is acceptable practice to guess at dictated words when all efforts have been exhausted to find the terms.

9. T or F   When transcribing, it is realistic to keep pace with the dictating voice.

10. T or F   As a beginning student transcriptionist, you must be concerned with speed.

11. T or F   Before transcribing, it is important to have all materials available.

12. T or F   Fast forward is located on the right side of a foot pedal.

13. T or F   Very fast or very slow speed extremes will distort the sound.

14. T or F   The transcriptionist's salary is never based on a regular monthly salary.

15. T or F   The transcription process is the integration of listening, keyboarding, and understanding the dictation.

16. T or F   An awareness of the style and phrasing of medical dictation will make it easier to understand the dictation.

17. T or F   Word books are only available in certain specialties.

18. T or F   *Eponyms* are adjectives taken from a surname and used to describe a term.

19. T or F   All manuals of style offer the same guidelines.

20. T or F   Knowledge of how to effectively use reference materials will not increase productivity.

21. T or F   Medical words are not listed in the same manner as words found in an English dictionary.

22. T or F   Pronunciation guides are not included in word books.

23. T or F   Drug books are updated annually.

24. T or F   Electronic reference materials include dictionaries and spellers.

25. T or F   Document formats remain consistent between medical facilities.

CHECK YOUR PROGRESS *(cont'd)*

Directions: Which reference book would you select to find the word or phrase to verify spelling, capitalization, punctuation, or definition?

26. TUR
    (a) urology word book
    (b) surgical word book
    (c) abbreviation word book
    (d) all of the above

27. *5 year old* or *5-year-old*
    (a) manual of style
    (b) eponym word book
    (c) English dictionary
    (d) none of the above

28. Foley catheter
    (a) eponym word book
    (b) English dictionary
    (c) PDR
    (d) all the above

29. *Patient* or *patience*
    (a) standard English dictionary
    (b) eponym word book
    (c) manual of style
    (d) a and c

30. Keflex
    (a) English dictionary
    (b) anatomy and physiology textbook
    (c) drug word book
    (d) all the above

31. K wire
    (a) English dictionary
    (b) orthopedic word book
    (c) abbreviation book
    (d) b and c

32. Circumcision
    (a) surgery word book
    (b) orthopedic word book
    (c) cardiology word book
    (d) none of the above

33. D&C
    (a) drug book
    (b) cardiology word book
    (c) abbreviation word book
    (d) radiology word book

34. Diphenhydramine
    (a) drug book
    (b) laboratory word book
    (c) eponym book
    (d) all the above

35. *X ray* or *x-ray*
    (a) manual of style
    (b) eponym book
    (c) neither a nor b
    (d) a and b

36. *Xanax* or *Zantac*
    (a) eponym book
    (b) surgical book
    (c) drug book
    (d) cardiology book

37. *Basal* or *basil*
    (a) homonym book
    (b) drug word book
    (c) eponym book
    (d) all the above

38. Cortaid
    (a) dermatology book
    (b) drug book
    (c) neither a nor b
    (d) a and b

39. The plural form of *thorax*
    (a) medical dictionary
    (b) surgical word book
    (c) eponym book
    (d) none of the above

CHECK YOUR PROGRESS (cont'd)

Directions: Select the best word that completes the meaning of the sentence.

40. There was radiographic evidence of _____ esophagitis noted in the distal end of the patient's esophagus.
    (a) reflux
    (b) atopic
    (c) reflex
    (d) atropic

41. She denies the use of _____ drugs, including marijuana.
    (a) elicit
    (b) ellicit
    (c) illicit
    (d) ilicit

42. The physician diagnosed the patient with a distal left _____ obstruction due to calculi.
    (a) ureteral
    (b) urethral
    (c) atopic
    (d) atropic

43. The patient presented with pruritic red lesions on his face, leading the physician to a diagnosis of _____ dermatitis.
    (a) ureteral
    (b) urethral
    (c) atopic
    (d) atropic

44. The surgeon performed a deep _____ of the capsule throughout the bladder.
    (a) resection
    (b) dilation
    (c) recession
    (d) dilution

45. The radiologist's impression was that there was a soft tissue mass in the terminal _____ .
    (a) ilium
    (b) ileum
    (c) illium
    (d) illeum

46. The patient's chronic liver diseases include _____.
    (a) cirrhosis
    (b) hemostasis
    (c) psoriasis
    (d) homeostasis

47. The neurological examination showed the patient's _____ to be equal and active.
    (a) refluxes
    (b) atopic
    (c) reflexes
    (d) atropic

48. The patient experienced cardiac _____ after strenuous exercise.
    (a) palpitation
    (b) palptation
    (c) palpation
    (d) palpaition

49. Mary complained of a burning and itching sensation of the _____ following an episiotomy.
    (a) parineal
    (b) peroneal
    (c) peritoneum
    (d) perineum

50. The surgeon removed the placenta from the incision side superior to the anterior _____.
    (a) fundal
    (b) fundus
    (c) fungal
    (d) fungus

Skill Building and Simulation in Medical Transcription

Chapter 5

Office Medical Transcription from the Family Practice

OBJECTIVES

At the completion of Chapter 5, you should be able to do the following:
1. Match medical terms associated with the family practice specialty.
2. Spell medical terms associated with the family practice specialty.
3. Transcribe medical terms in sentence structure.
4. Proofread, edit, and correct medical documents associated with the family practice specialty that contain various errors.
5. Transcribe and proofread authentic medical documents associated with the family practice specialty.

INTRODUCTION TO THE FAMILY PRACTICE ROTATION

Terminology
Pretest
Activities
    5-1: Keyboarding Medical Terms and Definitions
    5-2: Spelling Medical Terms
    5-3: Transcribing Medical Sentences, *5T-1*
Check Your Progress

Proofreading
Pretest, *5T-2*
Activities
    5-4: Proofreading Worksheet
    5-5: Proofreading Worksheet
    5-6: Proofreading Transcription Exercise, *5T-3*
    5-7: Proofreading Transcription Exercise, *5T-4*
Check Your Progress, *5T-2*

Transcription
Pretest, *5T-5* and *5T-6*
Family Practice Transcription at FedDes Wellness Center
Index of Dictations and Associated Transcription Tips, *5T-7* through *5T-23*
Check Your Progress, *5T-5* and *5T-6*

Anatomical Illustrations and Medical Images

What's Ahead

The FedDes Wellness Center has five family practitioners, one physical therapist, one registered nurse, and one physician assistant on staff. The medical team treats the general health of the individual and the family. Pediatric patients are seen for well-baby care and infectious diseases, such as sore throats, gastroenteritis, and croup. Young adults are seen for infectious diseases and acute injuries, such as sprains, minor lacerations, and nondisplaced fractures. Older adults are seen for both acute and chronic illnesses, such as arthritis, hypertension, and diabetes mellitus. Patients requiring critical care are co-managed with the appropriate specialist. In addition, obstetrics and gynecology are incorporated into the practice, including pelvic examinations and Papanicolaou (Pap) smears.

The physicians in FedDes Family Practice Division perform and interpret routine x-rays in their offices. More sophisticated imaging, such as MRI, CT scans, and nuclear medicine studies, are referred to an outside facility and interpreted by a radiologist.

In this unit, you assume the role of a medical transcriptionist employed at FedDes Wellness Center. **Please follow the guidelines pertaining to capitalization, numbers, punctuation, abbreviations, measurements, symbols, and use of templates to create medical reports at FedDes Wellness Center.** This material is reviewed in Unit I. The transcription exercises list the type of report, patient's name, and physician(s) as well as the associated transcription tips.

You will work with the textbook and a CD-ROM or audiocassettes. Your mastery of family practice transcription is assessed through worksheets, timed transcription exercises, the error analysis chart, and the Production for Pay summary.

All answer keys are found in the textbook (Appendix E) and CD-ROM, providing immediate feedback. After transcribing a report, you will proofread your work and correct any errors. Then you will compare your proofread work against a master transcript, categorize all errors, and tabulate the errors on the error analysis chart. The Production for Pay summary correlates your production to the FedDes Wellness Center pay scale. The scale is also linked to your grade. This system allows you to assess your mastery of transcription skills in a real-world scenario.

Let's find out if you can define and spell selected terminology and drugs of the family practice specialty that are included in this chapter.

TEXTBOOK USERS

Select the correctly spelled term that matches its definition.
Refer to the answer key (Appendix E) for immediate feedback.

SOFTWARE USERS

Click on *Chapter 1, Terminology Pretest*, and follow the directions.

NAME _____   DATE _____

Directions: Select the correctly spelled term that matches its definition.

1. A benign tumor in which cells are derived from glandular epithelium:
   (a) adenoma
   (b) adnema
   (c) adnexa
   (d) adenxa

2. A body defense method to prevent movement of an injured part:
   (a) flank
   (b) garding
   (c) guarding
   (d) flenk

3. A generic name for a broad-spectrum antibiotic that is active against a wide range of gram-positive and gram-negative organisms:
   (a) doxycycline
   (b) pencillin
   (c) doxycyclene
   (d) penicillin

4. An abnormal sound heard on chest auscultation that is caused by an obstructed airway:
   (a) nystagmus
   (b) rhonchus
   (c) rhinchus
   (d) nystigmus

5. An abnormal rhythm of the heart:
   (a) distal
   (b) destal
   (c) galop
   (d) gallop

6. An enlargement of the thyroid gland:
   (a) hepatosplenomegaly
   (b) hepatosplenmegaly
   (c) thyromegaly
   (d) thyramegaly

7. A knot or knot-like mass:
   (a) ganglion
   (b) ganlion
   (c) fundus
   (d) fundes

8. A reversed response occurring on withdrawal of a stimulus:
   (a) reband
   (b) rebound
   (c) evert
   (d) revert

9. A small nodule, tumor, or growth:
   (a) buccal
   (b) bucca
   (c) granuloma
   (d) granduloma

10. A small, soft structure hanging from the free edge of the soft palate:
    (a) vulva
    (b) vuvla
    (c) ulvula
    (d) uvula

11. A small, tongue-shaped anatomic structure:
    (a) lingula
    (b) linula
    (c) lamina
    (d) lamena

12. A sound or murmur heard on auscultation:
    (a) bruit
    (b) palpitation
    (c) brut
    (d) palpation

13. A spasm of the orbicular muscle of the eyelid:
    (a) hyperlipidemia
    (b) blepharospasm
    (c) blefarospasm
    (d) hyprelipidemia

14. A thin, flat layer:
    (a) lingula
    (b) linula
    (c) lamina
    (d) lamena

15. A member of a widespread genus of gram-negative, nonmotile bacteria:
    (a) chlamydia
    (b) chlamidia
    (c) myalgia
    (d) mialgia

PRETEST *(cont'd)*

16. A generic name for an ophthalmic antibiotic:
    (a) sulfactamide
    (b) sulfacetamide
    (c) meclizine
    (d) meslicine

17. An antiemetic especially effective for control of nausea and vomiting of motion sickness:
    (a) sulfactamide
    (b) sulfacetamide
    (c) meclizine
    (d) meslicine

18. An endoscope for examining the peritoneal cavity:
    (a) laparoscope
    (b) sigmoidoscope
    (c) laproscopy
    (d) sigmoidscopy

19. An incision of the tympanic membrane:
    (a) adenopathy
    (b) adinopathy
    (c) myringomy
    (d) myringotomy

20. An opening, mouth, or bone:
    (a) oss
    (b) os
    (c) pruritus ani
    (d) puritus anis

21. An unusually rapid, strong, or irregular heartbeat:
    (a) bruit
    (b) palpitation
    (c) brut
    (d) palpation

22. Any of a large group of natural or semisynthetic antibacterial antibiotics:
    (a) doxycycline
    (b) pencillin
    (c) doxycyclene
    (d) penicillin

23. Around the rectum:
    (a) perrectal
    (b) prerectal
    (c) perirectal
    (d) parirectal

24. Coughing and spitting of blood:
    (a) sputum
    (b) sputim
    (c) hemoptysis
    (d) hemotysis

25. External genital organs in the female:
    (a) vulva
    (b) vuvla
    (c) ulvula
    (d) uvula

26. Accumulation of fluid and cellular debris in the tissues:
    (a) exdate
    (b) exudate
    (c) edema
    (d) exdema

27. Inflammation of the mucous membrane of the nose:
    (a) mucosa
    (b) mucos
    (c) rhinitis
    (d) rinitis

28. Intense chronic itching in the anal region:
    (a) pruritus ani
    (b) puritus ani
    (c) rhinitis
    (d) rinitis

29. Involuntary rapid rhythmic movement of the eyeball:
    (a) nystagmus
    (b) rhonchus
    (c) rhinchus
    (d) nystigmus

30. Labored or difficult breathing:
    (a) dysuria
    (b) dyspnia
    (c) dyspnea
    (d) dysurea

31. Muscular pain:
    (a) chlamydia
    (b) chlamidia
    (c) myalgia
    (d) mialgia

PRETEST *(cont'd)*

32. Painful menstruation:
    (a) amenorrhea
    (b) dysmenorrhea
    (c) amenorhea
    (d) dysmenorhea

33. Painful or difficult urination:
    (a) dysuria
    (b) dyspnia
    (c) dyspnea
    (d) dysurea

34. Pertaining to the cheek:
    (a) buccal
    (b) bucca
    (c) granuloma
    (d) granduloma

35. Redness of the skin:
    (a) orthopnea
    (b) erthema
    (c) orthopea
    (d) erythema

36. Resembling a polyp:
    (a) polypiod
    (b) polypod
    (c) polypoid
    (d) polypide

37. The ability to breathe easily only in an upright position:
    (a) orthopnea
    (b) erthema
    (c) orthopea
    (d) erythema

38. Absence of the menses:
    (a) amenorrhea
    (b) dysmenorrhea
    (c) amenorhea
    (d) dysmenorhea

39. Accumulation of excess fluid in the tissues of the body:
    (a) exdate
    (b) exadate
    (c) edema
    (d) exdema

40. The state of lying down:
    (a) fundus
    (b) fundes
    (c) decubitus
    (d) decubitis

41. Bluish discoloration of the skin and mucous membranes due to excessive concentration of reduced hemoglobin in the blood:
    (a) labyrinthitis
    (b) cayonsis
    (c) labrinthitis
    (d) cyanosis

42. The bottom or base of an organ:
    (a) fundus
    (b) fundes
    (c) decubitus
    (d) decubitis

43. Elevated concentration of any lipid or all the lipids in the plasma:
    (a) hyperlipidemia
    (b) blepharospasm
    (c) blefarospasm
    (d) hyprelipidemia

44. Enlargement of the glands, especially the lymph nodes:
    (a) hepatosplenomegaly
    (b) adenopathy
    (c) hepasplenomegaly
    (d) adenompathy

45. Enlargement of the liver and spleen:
    (a) hepatosplenomegaly
    (b) adenopathy
    (c) hepasplenomegaly
    (d) adenompathy

46. Escape of fluid from blood vessels because of rupture or seepage, usually into a body cavity:
    (a) aeration
    (b) effusion
    (c) eration
    (d) efusion

PRETEST *(cont'd)*

47. Examination of the interior of the sigmoid colon:
    (a) laparoscope
    (b) sigmoidscope
    (c) laproscopy
    (d) sigmoidoscopy

48. Exchange of carbon dioxide for oxygen by the blood in the lungs:
    (a) aeration
    (b) effusion
    (c) eration
    (d) efusion

49. Farther from any point of reference; remote:
    (a) disal
    (b) galop
    (c) distal
    (d) gallop

50. Increase in the severity of a disease or its symptoms:
    (a) exaceration
    (b) exacerbation
    (c) auscultation
    (d) auscutation

51. Inflammation of the internal ear; otitis interna:
    (a) labyrinthitis
    (b) rhinitis
    (c) labrinthitis
    (d) rinitis

52. The act of listening for sounds produced within the body with the unaided ear or with a stethoscope:
    (a) palpitation
    (b) palpation
    (c) auscultation
    (d) auscutation

53. The mucous membrane:
    (a) mucoso
    (b) mucosa
    (c) mucousa
    (d) mucus

54. The mucous secretion from the lungs, bronchi, and trachea that is ejected through the mouth:
    (a) sputum
    (b) sputim
    (c) hemoptysis
    (d) hemotysis

55. The side of the body between the ribs and ilium:
    (a) flank
    (b) fundus
    (c) flanke
    (d) fundes

56. Tissues or body parts that are near or next to one another:
    (a) adenoma
    (b) adnema
    (c) adnexa
    (d) adenxa

57. To turn inside out:
    (a) reband
    (b) rebound
    (c) evert
    (d) revert

58. Agent used as an expectorant:
    (a) terpin
    (b) trepin
    (c) meclizine
    (d) mecilizine

59. Using both hands:
    (a) bimanaul
    (b) bimanual
    (c) bymanaul
    (d) bymanual

60. A blister:
    (a) blib
    (b) bleb
    (c) bleib
    (d) beb

61. Generic name for a corticosteroid:
    (a) ortho tri-cyclen
    (b) ortho tri-cyclin
    (c) triamcinolone
    (d) triamcinoline

62. Trade name for a corticosteroid for bronchial asthma (pocket inhaler):
    (a) Vancenase
    (b) Vancinase
    (c) Phenergan
    (d) Phenergin

TERMINOLOGY

PRETEST *(cont'd)*

63. Trade name for a powder for extraocular muscle injection:
    (a) Botex
    (b) Botox
    (c) Skelaxin
    (d) Skelaxen

64. Trade name for a preparation of amoxicillin, an antibiotic:
    (a) Co-Polymer
    (b) Copolymer
    (c) Amoxil
    (d) Amosil

65. Trade name for a combination preparation of amoxicillin, an antibiotic:
    (a) Klonopin
    (b) Augmenten
    (c) Klonpin
    (d) Augmentin

66. Trade name for a selective estrogen receptor modulator used to prevent postmenopausal osteoporosis:
    (a) Paxil
    (b) Pasil
    (c) Evista
    (d) Evixta

67. Trade name for an antidepressant:
    (a) Paxil
    (b) Pasil
    (c) Evista
    (d) Evixta

68. Trade name for a skeletal muscle relaxant:
    (a) Botex
    (b) Botox
    (c) Skelaxin
    (d) Skelaxen

69. Trade name for a topical antibiotic:
    (a) Proctocreem HC
    (b) Proctocream HC
    (c) Neosporen
    (d) Neosporin

70. Trade name for a triphasic oral contraceptive:
    (a) Ortho Tri-Cyclen
    (b) Ortho Tri Cyclin
    (c) Triamcinolone
    (d) Triamcinoline

71. Trade name for an anticonvulsant:
    (a) Klonopin
    (b) Augmenten
    (c) Klonpin
    (d) Augmentin

72. Trade name for an antihistamine, antiemetic:
    (a) Vancenase
    (b) Vancinase
    (c) Phenergan
    (d) Phenergin

73. Trade name for an antihyperlipidemic that reduces cholesterol synthesis:
    (a) Lipitir
    (b) Lipitor
    (c) Lo-Ovral
    (d) Lo-Oral

74. Trade name for an oral contraceptive:
    (a) Lipitir
    (b) Lipitor
    (c) Lo-Ovral
    (d) Lo-Oral

75. Trade name for a combination analgesic and antipyretic:
    (a) Darvoset
    (b) Darvocet
    (c) Melantonox
    (d) Melantonex

76. Trade name for preparations of lidocaine; classified as an antiarrhythmic, anesthetic:
    (a) Xylocaine
    (b) Ophthetic
    (c) Xylociane
    (d) Ophetic

77. Trade name for proparacaine hydrochloride; eye drops:
    (a) Xylocaine
    (b) Ophthetic
    (c) Xylociane
    (d) Ophetic

78. Trade name for a topical corticosteroid anti-inflammatory used as anorectal cream:
    (a) Proctocreem HC
    (b) Proctocream HC
    (c) Neosporen
    (d) Neosporin

79. Trade name for one of the immune-modulating drugs:
    (a) Co-Polymer
    (b) Amoxil
    (c) Copolymer
    (d) Amosil

80. Trade name for a calcium channel blocker, antihypertensive:
    (a) Naprosyn
    (b) Naporsyn
    (c) Norvasc
    (d) Norvasic

81. Trade name for an antibiotic:
    (a) Claritin
    (b) Clariten
    (c) Baixin
    (d) Biaxin

82. Trade name for an antiplatelet agent:
    (a) Presantine
    (b) Persantine
    (c) Prilosec
    (d) Prelosec

83. Trade name for a drug used to prevent NSAID-induced gastric ulcers:
    (a) Cytotec
    (b) Cytotic
    (c) Ditropan
    (d) Ditropen

84. Trade name for a urinary antispasmodic:
    (a) Cytotec
    (b) Cytotic
    (c) Ditropan
    (d) Ditropen

85. Trade name for an antibiotic:
    (a) Indocen
    (b) Indocin
    (c) E.E.A.
    (d) E.E.S.

86. Trade name for a nonsteroidal anti-inflammatory drug (NSAID):
    (a) Indocen
    (b) Indocin
    (c) E.E.A.
    (d) E.E.S.

87. Trade name for a gastric acid–secretion inhibitor:
    (a) Presantine
    (b) Persantine
    (c) Prilosec
    (d) Prelosec

88. Trade name for a sleep aid:
    (a) Melatonex
    (b) Melatonix
    (c) Darvocet
    (d) Darvocit

89. Trade name for a nonsedating antihistamine:
    (a) Claritin
    (b) Clariten
    (c) Baixin
    (d) Biaxin

90. Trade name for an NSAID, antihypertensive:
    (a) Naprosyn
    (b) Naporsyn
    (c) Norvasc
    (d) Norvasic

Activity 5-1

Keyboarding Medical Terms and Definitions

Let's learn to spell and define selected terminology and drugs of the family practice specialty that are included in this chapter. Keyboarding these terms is an effective way to improve your skills.

Word Processing Users

Open your word processing package. Read and type each word and its definition as shown below.

Save your work on your student disk.

1. Adenoma (ad-ah-<u>no</u>-mah) is a benign tumor in which cells are derived from glandular epithelium.
2. Adenopathy (ad-ah-<u>nop</u>-ah-the) is the enlargement of the glands, especially the lymph nodes.
3. Adnexa (ad-<u>nek</u>-sa) are the tissues or body parts that are near or next to one another.
4. Aeration (aer-<u>a</u>-shun) is the exchange of carbon dioxide for oxygen by the blood in the lungs.
5. Amenorrhea (ah-men-o-<u>re</u>-ah) is the absence of the menses.
6. Auscultation (aw-skul-<u>ta</u>-shun) is the act of listening for sounds produced within the body with the unaided ear or with a stethoscope.
7. Bimanual (bi-<u>man</u>-u-al) means using both hands.
8. Bleb (bleb) is a bulla or blister.
9. Blepharospasm (<u>blef</u>-ah-ro-spazm) is a spasm of the orbicular muscle of the eyelid.
10. Bruit (<u>bru</u>-it) is a sound or murmur heard on auscultation.
11. Buccal (<u>buk</u>-al) pertains to the cheek.
12. *Chlamydia* (klah-<u>mid</u>-e-ah) is a member of a widespread genus of sexually transmitted gram-negative, nonmotile bacteria.
13. Cyanosis (si-ah-<u>no</u>-sis) is the bluish discoloration of the skin due to lack of oxygenated blood.
14. Decubitus (de-<u>ku</u>-bi-tus) pertains to lying down.
15. Distal (<u>dis</u>-tal) means farther from any point of reference; remote.
16. Doxycycline (dok-se-<u>si</u>-klen) is a generic name for a broad-spectrum antibiotic that is active against a wide range of gram-positive and gram-negative organisms.
17. Dysmenorrhea (dis-men-o-<u>re</u>-ah) is painful menstruation.
18. Dyspnea (<u>disp</u>-ne-ah) is labored or difficult breathing.
19. Dysuria (dis-<u>u</u>-re-ah) is painful or difficult urination.

20. Edema (ed-<u>e</u>-mah) is the accumulation of excess fluid in the tissues of the body.
21. Effusion (e-<u>fu</u>-zhun) is the escape of fluid from blood vessels because of rupture or seepage, usually into a body cavity.
22. Erythema (er-i-<u>the</u>-mah) is redness of the skin.
23. Evert (e-<u>vert</u>) is to turn inside out.
24. Exacerbation (eg-zas-er-<u>ba</u>-shun) is an increase in the severity of a disease or its symptoms.
25. Exudate (<u>eks</u>-u-date) is an accumulation of fluid and cellular debris in the tissues.
26. Flank is the side of the body between the ribs and ilium.
27. Fundus (<u>fun</u>-dus) is the bottom or base of an organ.
28. Gallop (<u>gal</u>-op) is an abnormal rhythm of the heart.
29. Ganglion (<u>gang</u>-gle-on) is a knot or knotlike mass.
30. Granuloma (gran-u-<u>lo</u>-mah) is a small nodule, tumor, or growth.
31. Guarding (<u>gahr</u>-ding) is a body defense method to prevent movement of an injured part.
32. Hemoptysis (he-<u>mop</u>-ti-sis) is the coughing and spitting of blood.
33. Hepatosplenomegaly (hep-a-to-sple-no-<u>meg</u>-ah-le) is the enlargement of the liver and spleen.
34. Hyperlipidemia (hi-per-lip-i-<u>de</u>-me-ah) is the elevated concentration of any or all lipids in the plasma.
35. Labyrinthitis (lab-i-rin-<u>thi</u>-tis) is the inflammation of the internal ear; otitis interna.
36. Lamina (<u>lam</u>-i-nah) is a thin, flat layer.
37. Laparoscope (lap-ah-ro-skop) is an endoscope for examining the peritoneal cavity.
38. Lingula (<u>ling</u>-gu-lah) is a small, tongue-shaped anatomic structure.
39. Meclizine (<u>mek</u>-li-zeen) is an antiemetic especially effective for control of nausea and vomiting of motion sickness.
40. Mucosa (mu-<u>ko</u>-sah) is the mucous membrane.
41. Myalgia (mi-<u>al</u>-je-ah) is muscular pain.
42. Myringotomy (mir-in-<u>got</u>-o-me) is an incision of the tympanic membrane.
43. Nystagmus (ni-<u>stag</u>-mus) is an involuntary rapid rhythmic movement of the eyeball.
44. Orthopnea (or-thop-<u>ne</u>-ah) is the ability to breathe easily only in an upright position.
45. Os (os) is an opening, mouth, or bone.
46. Palpitation (pal-pi-<u>ta</u>-shun) is an unusually rapid, strong, or irregular heartbeat.

47. Penicillin (pen-i-<u>sil</u>-in) is a natural or semisynthetic antibacterial antibiotic.
48. Perirectal (per-i-<u>rek</u>-tal) means around the rectum.
49. Polypoid (<u>pol</u>-y-poid) means resembling a polyp.
50. Pruritus ani (proo-<u>ri</u>-tus a-ni) is the intense chronic itching in the anal region.
51. Rebound (<u>re</u>-bownd) is a reversed response occurring on withdrawal of a stimulus.
52. Rhinitis (ri-<u>ni</u>-tis) is the inflammation of the mucous membrane of the nose.
53. Rhonchus (<u>rong</u>-kus) is an abnormal sound heard on chest auscultation that is caused by an obstructed airway.
54. Sigmoidoscopy (sig-moi-<u>dos</u>-ko-pe) is the examination of the interior of the sigmoid colon.
55. Sputum (<u>spu</u>-tum) is the mucous secretion from the lungs, bronchi, and trachea that is ejected through the mouth.
56. Sulfacetamide (sul-fah-<u>set</u>-ah-mid) is a generic name for an ophthalmic antibiotic.
57. Terpin (<u>ter</u>-pin) is used as an expectorant.
58. Thyromegaly (thi-ro-<u>meg</u>-ah-le) is enlargement of the thyroid gland.
59. Uvula (<u>u</u>-vu-lah) is a small, soft structure hanging from the free edge of the soft palate.
60. Vulva (<u>vul</u>-vah) is the external genital organs in the female.
61. Amoxil (ah-<u>moks</u>-il) is the trade name for a preparation of amoxicillin, an antibiotic.
62. Augmentin (awg-men-tin) is the trade name for a combination preparation of amoxicillin, an antibiotic.
63. Biaxin (bi-<u>ak</u>-sin) is the trade name for an antibiotic.
64. Botox (bo-toks) is the trade name for a powder for extraocular muscle injection.
65. Claritin (<u>klar</u>-i-tin) is the trade name for a nonsedating antihistamine.
66. Copolymer (ko-<u>pol</u>-i-mer) is the trade name for any of the group of immune-modulating drugs.
67. Cytotec (<u>si</u>-to-tek) is the trade name for a drug used for the prevention of NSAID-induced gastric ulcers.
68. Darvocet (<u>dar</u>-vo-set) is the trade name for a combination analgesic and antipyretic.
69. Ditropan (<u>di</u>-tro-pan) is the trade name for a urinary antispasmodic.
70. E.E.S. (e-e-s) is the trade name for an antibiotic.
71. Evista (e-<u>vis</u>-ta) is the trade name for a selective estrogen receptor modulator used to prevent postmenopausal osteoporosis.
72. Indocin (<u>in</u>-do-sin) is the trade name for a nonsteroidal anti-inflammatory drug (NSAID).
73. Klonopin (<u>klon</u>-o-pin) is the trade name for an anticonvulsant and antianxiety drug.
74. Lipitor (<u>lip</u>-i-tor) is the trade name for an antihyperlipidemic that reduces cholesterol synthesis.
75. Lo-Ovral (lo-<u>ov</u>-ral) is the trade name for an oral contraceptive.
76. Melatonex (mel-a-<u>to</u>-neks) is the trade name for a sleep aid.
77. Naprosyn (<u>na</u>-pro-sin) is the trade name for an NSAID.
78. Neosporin (ne-o-<u>spor</u>-in) is the trade name for a topical antibiotic.
79. Norvasc (<u>nor</u>-vask) is the trade name for a calcium channel blocker and antihypertensive.
80. Ophthetic (op-<u>the</u>-tik) is the trade name for proparacaine hydrochloride eye drops.
81. Ortho Tri-Cyclen (<u>or</u>-tho tri-<u>si</u>-klen) is the trade name for a triphasic oral contraceptive.
82. Paxil (<u>paks</u>-il) is the trade name for an antidepressant.
83. Persantine (<u>per</u>-san-tine) is the trade name for an antiplatelet agent.
84. Phenergan (<u>fen</u>-er-gan) is the trade name for an antihistamine and antiemetic.
85. Prilosec (<u>pril</u>-o-sek) is the trade name for a gastric acid–secretion inhibitor.
86. Proctocream HC (<u>prok</u>-to-kreem) is the trade name for a topical corticosteroid anti-inflammatory used as anorectal cream.
87. Skelaxin (skel-aks-in) is the trade name for a skeletal muscle relaxant.
88. Triamcinolone (tri-am-<u>sin</u>-o-lon) is the generic name for a corticosteroid.
89. Vancenase (van-san-az) is the trade name for a corticosteroid for bronchial asthma and pocket inhaler.
90. Xylocaine (<u>zi</u>-lo-cane) is the trade name for preparations of lidocaine and is classified as an antiarrhythmic and anesthetic.

Do you remember back in school when you had to write each spelling word 10 times? Because you had to physically write each word, your mind and body were focused on the assignment, and the method worked. Let's follow this successful method by reinforcing the spelling of selected terms and drugs found in the family practice specialty through keyboarding drills.

WORD PROCESSING USERS

Open your word processing package. Read, mentally spell, and type each word in its sequence.
Save your work on your student disk.

1. adenoma adenopathy adnexa adenoma adenopathy adnexa adenoma adenopathy adnexa
2. aeration amenorrhea auscultation aeration amenorrhea auscultation aeration amenorrhea
3. bimanual blepharospasm bruit bleb blepharospasm bruit bimanual blepharospasm bleb
4. buccal chlamydia buccal chlamydia buccal chlamydia buccal chlamydia buccal chlamydia
5. cyanosis decubitus distal cyanosis decubitus distal cyanosis decubitus distal cyanosis decubitus distal
6. dysmenorrhea dyspnea dysuria dysmenorrhea dyspnea dysuria dysmenorrhea dyspnea
7. edema effusion erythema edema effusion erythema edema effusion erythema edema effusion
8. evert exacerbation exudate evert exacerbation exudate evert exacerbation exudate evert
9. flank fundus gallop flank fundus gallop flank fundus gallop flank fundus gallop flank fundus
10. ganglion granuloma guarding ganglion granuloma guarding ganglion granuloma guarding
11. hemoptysis hepatosplenomegaly hemoptysis hepatosplenomegaly hemoptysis
12. hyperlipidemia labyrinthitis hyperlipidemia labyrinthitis hyperlipidemia labyrinthitis

13. lamina laparoscope lingula lamina laparoscope lingula lamina laparoscope lingula lamina
14. mucosa myalgia myringotomy mucosa myalgia myringotomy mucosa myalgia myringotomy
15. nystagmus orthopnea os nystagmus orthopnea os nystagmus orthopnea os nystagmus os
16. palpitation penicillin perirectal palpitation penicillin perirectal palpitation penicillin perirectal
17. polypoid pruritus ani rebound polypoid pruritus ani rebound polypoid pruritus ani rebound
18. rhinitis rhonchus sigmoidoscopy rhinitis rhonchus sigmoidoscopy rhinitis rhonchus rhinitis
19. sputum terpin thyromegaly sputum terpin thyromegaly sputum terpin thyromegaly sputum
20. doxycycline uvula vulva doxycycline uvula vulva doxycycline uvula vulva doxycycline
21. doxycycline meclizine doxycycline meclizine doxycycline meclizine doxycycline meclizine
22. Amoxil Augmentin Botox Amoxil Augmentin Botox Amoxil Augmentin Botox Amoxil
23. Biaxin Claritin Copolymer Biaxin Claritin Copolymer Biaxin Claritin Copolymer Biaxin
24. Cytotec Ditropan E.E.S. Cytotec Ditropan E.E.S. Cytotec Ditropan E.E.S. Cytotec Ditropan
25. Darvocet Evista Klonopin Darvocet Evista Klonopin Darvocet Evista Klonopin Darvocet
26. Indocin Melatonex Naprosyn Indocin Melatonex Naprosyn Indocin Melatonex Naprosyn
27. Lipitor Lo-Ovral Neosporin Lipitor Lo-Ovral Neosporin Lipitor Lo-Ovral Neosporin Lipitor
28. Norvasc Persantine Prilosec Norvasc Persantine Prilosec Norvasc Persantine Prilosec
29. Ophthetic Ortho Tri-Cyclen Paxil Ophthetic Ortho Tri-Cyclen Paxil Ophthetic Ortho Tri-Cyclen
30. Phenergan Proctocream HC Skelaxin Phenergan Proctocream HC Skelaxin Phenergan
31. triamcinolone Vancenase Xylocaine triamcinolone Vancenase Xylocaine triamcinolone

Transcribing Medical Sentences

Now you are ready to make the transition from keyboarding medical terms, a visual process, to transcribing medical terms, an aural process. You are going to use audio-cassette tapes or your CD-ROM rather than printed material. Sentences 71 and 74 contain dangerous abbreviations and need to be transcribed according to the guidelines established in this textbook and the recommendations of *The AAMT Book of Style,* Appendix B.

WORD PROCESSING USERS

Open your word processing package. Insert the appropriate audiocassette in your transcribing machine and find dictation *5T-1.*

You will be transcribing spelling words in sentence structure.

Listen carefully to each sentence on the audiocassette before transcribing.

Rewind and type (transcribe) the sentences.

Save your work on your student disk.

Refer to the answer key (Appendix E) for immediate feedback.

SOFTWARE USERS

Click on *Chapter 5, Terminology Activity 5-3 (5T-1),* and follow the directions.

TERMINOLOGY

Let's pause a minute and see how well you are doing. This section allows you to evaluate your mastery of keyboarding and spelling of selected terms and drugs found in the family practice specialty.

TEXTBOOK USERS

Select the correctly spelled term that matches its definition.
Refer to the answer key (Appendix E) for immediate feedback.

SOFTWARE USERS

Click on *Chapter 5, Terminology Check Your Progress*, and follow the directions.

NAME _____   DATE _____

CHECK YOUR PROGRESS

Directions: Select the correctly spelled term that matches its definition.

1. Intense chronic itching in the anal region:
   (a) pruritus ani
   (b) puritus ani
   (c) rhinitis
   (d) rinitis

2. An abnormal sound heard on chest auscultation due to an obstructed airway:
   (a) nystagmus
   (b) rhonchus
   (c) rhinchus
   (d) nystigmus

3. A generic name for a broad-spectrum antibiotic that is active against a wide range of gram-positive and gram-negative organisms:
   (a) doxycycline
   (b) pencillin
   (c) doxycyclene
   (d) penicillin

4. A disorder in the rhythm of the heart:
   (a) distal
   (b) destal
   (c) galop
   (d) gallop

5. An enlargement of the thyroid gland:
   (a) hepatosplenomegaly
   (b) hepatosplenmegaly
   (c) thyromegaly
   (d) thyramegaly

6. A body defense method to prevent movement of an injured part:
   (a) flank
   (b) garding
   (c) guarding
   (d) flenk

7. A reversed response occurring on withdrawal of a stimulus:
   (a) reband
   (b) rebound
   (c) evert
   (d) revert

8. A small nodule, tumor, or growth:
   (a) buccal
   (b) bucca
   (c) granuloma
   (d) granduloma

9. A knot or knotlike mass:
   (a) ganglion
   (b) ganlion
   (c) fundus
   (d) fundes

10. A small, tongue-shaped anatomic structure:
    (a) lingula
    (b) linula
    (c) lamina
    (d) lamena

11. A sound or murmur heard on auscultation:
    (a) bruit
    (b) palpitation
    (c) brut
    (d) palpation

12. A spasm of the orbicular muscle of the eyelid:
    (a) hyperlipidemia
    (b) blepharospasm
    (c) blefarospasm
    (d) hyprelipidemia

13. A small, soft structure hanging from the free edge of the soft palate:
    (a) vulva
    (b) vuvla
    (c) ulvula
    (d) uvula

14. A member of a widespread genus of gram-negative, nonmotile bacteria:
    (a) chlamydia
    (b) chlamidia
    (c) myalgia
    (d) mialgia

15. A generic name for an ophthalmic antibiotic:
    (a) sulfactamide
    (b) sulfacetamide
    (c) meclizine
    (d) meslicine

CHECK YOUR PROGRESS *(cont'd)*

16. Coughing and spitting of blood:
    (a) sputum
    (b) sputim
    (c) hemoptysis
    (d) hemotysis

17. A thin, flat layer:
    (a) lingula
    (b) linula
    (c) lamina
    (d) lamena

18. An incision of the tympanic membrane:
    (a) adenopathy
    (b) adinopathy
    (c) myringomy
    (d) myringotomy

19. A benign tumor in which cells are derived from glandular epithelium:
    (a) adenoma
    (b) adnema
    (c) adnexa
    (d) adenxa

20. An unusually rapid, strong, or irregular heartbeat:
    (a) bruit
    (b) palpitation
    (c) brut
    (d) palpation

21. An endoscope for examining the peritoneal cavity:
    (a) laparoscope
    (b) sigmoidoscope
    (c) laproscopy
    (d) sigmoidscopy

22. Around the rectum:
    (a) perrectal
    (b) prerectal
    (c) perirectal
    (d) parirectal

23. An opening, mouth, or bone:
    (a) oss
    (b) os
    (c) pruritus ani
    (d) puritus anis

24. A generic name for any of a large group of natural or semisynthetic antibacterial antibiotics:
    (a) doxycycline
    (b) pencillin
    (c) doxycyclene
    (d) penicillin

25. Accumulation of fluid and cellular debris in the tissues:
    (a) exdate
    (b) exudate
    (c) edoma
    (d) exdem

26. Inflammation of the mucous membrane of the nose:
    (a) mucosa
    (b) mucos
    (c) rhinitis
    (d) rinitis

27. An antiemetic especially effective for control of nausea and vomiting of motion sickness:
    (a) sulfactamide
    (b) sulfacetamide
    (c) meclizine
    (d) meslicine

28. Involuntary rapid rhythmic movement of the eyeball:
    (a) nystagmus
    (b) rhonchus
    (c) rhinchus
    (d) nystigmus

29. Bluish discoloration of the skin and mucous membranes due to excessive concentration of reduced hemoglobin in the blood:
    (a) labyrinthitis
    (b) cayonsis
    (c) labrinthitis
    (d) cyanosis

30. Muscular pain:
    (a) chlamydia
    (b) chlamidia
    (c) myalgia
    (d) mialgia

CHECK YOUR PROGRESS (cont'd)

31. External genital organs in the female:
    (a) vulva
    (b) vuvla
    (c) ulvula
    (d) uvula

32. Painful or difficult urination:
    (a) dysuria
    (b) dyspnia
    (c) dyspnea
    (d) dysurea

33. Pertaining to the cheek:
    (a) buccal
    (b) bucca
    (c) granuloma
    (d) granduloma

34. Redness of the skin:
    (a) orthopnea
    (b) erthema
    (c) orthopea
    (d) erythema

35. Painful menstruation:
    (a) amenorrhea
    (b) dysmenorrhea
    (c) amenorhea
    (d) dysmenorhea

36. The ability to breathe easily only in an upright position:
    (a) orthopnea
    (b) erthema
    (c) orthopea
    (d) erythema

37. Absence of the menses:
    (a) amenorrhea
    (b) dysmenorrhea
    (c) amenorhea
    (d) dysmenorhea

38. Labored or difficult breathing:
    (a) dysuria
    (b) dyspnia
    (c) dyspnea
    (d) dysurea

39. The state of lying down:
    (a) fundus
    (b) fundes
    (c) decubitus
    (d) decubitis

40. Resembling a polyp:
    (a) polypiod
    (b) polypod
    (c) polypoid
    (d) polypide

41. The bottom or base of an organ:
    (a) fundus
    (b) fundes
    (c) decubitus
    (d) decubitis

42. Elevated concentration of any lipid or all lipids in the plasma:
    (a) hyperlipidemia
    (b) blepharospasm
    (c) blefarospasm
    (d) hyprelipidemia

43. Accumulation of excess fluid in a fluid compartment:
    (a) exdate
    (b) exadate
    (c) edema
    (d) exdema

44. Enlargement of the liver and spleen:
    (a) hepatosplenomegaly
    (b) adenopathy
    (c) hepasplenomegaly
    (d) adenompathy

45. Escape of fluid from blood vessels because of rupture or seepage, usually into a body cavity:
    (a) aeration
    (b) effusion
    (c) eration
    (d) efusion

46. Examination of the interior of the sigmoid colon:
    (a) laparoscope
    (b) sigmoidscope
    (c) laproscopy
    (d) sigmoidoscopy

CHECK YOUR PROGRESS (cont'd)

TERMINOLOGY

47. Enlargement of the glands, especially the lymph nodes:
    (a) hepatosplenomegaly
    (b) adenopathy
    (c) hepasplenomegaly
    (d) adenompathy

48. Farther from any point of reference; remote:
    (a) disal
    (b) galop
    (c) distal
    (d) gallop

49. Increase in the severity of a disease or its symptoms:
    (a) exaceration
    (b) exacerbation
    (c) auscultation
    (d) auscutation

50. Inflammation of the internal ear; otitis interna:
    (a) labyrinthitis
    (b) rhinitis
    (c) labrinthitis
    (d) rinitis

51. The act of listening for sounds produced within the body with the unaided ear or with a stethoscope:
    (a) palpitation
    (b) palpation
    (c) auscultation
    (d) auscutation

52. Exchange of carbon dioxide for oxygen by the blood in the lungs:
    (a) aeration
    (b) effusion
    (c) eration
    (d) efusion

53. The mucous secretion from the lungs, bronchi, and trachea that is ejected through the mouth:
    (a) sputum
    (b) sputim
    (c) hemoptysis
    (d) hemotysis

54. The side of the body between the ribs and ilium:
    (a) flank
    (b) fundus
    (c) flanke
    (d) fundes

55. Tissues or body parts that are near or next to one another:
    (a) adenoma
    (b) adnema
    (c) adnexa
    (d) adenxa

56. The mucous membrane:
    (a) mucoso
    (b) mucosa
    (c) mucousa
    (d) mucus

57. Agent used as an expectorant:
    (a) terpin
    (b) trepin
    (c) meclizine
    (d) mecilizine

58. Using both hands:
    (a) bimanaul
    (b) bimanual
    (c) bymanaul
    (d) bymanual

59. To turn inside out:
    (a) reband
    (b) rebound
    (c) evert
    (d) revert

60. A blister:
    (a) blib
    (b) bleb
    (c) bleib
    (d) beb

61. Trade name for a corticosteroid for bronchial asthma; pocket inhaler:
    (a) Vancenase
    (b) Vancinase
    (c) Phenergan
    (d) Phenergin

CHECK YOUR PROGRESS *(cont'd)*

62. Trade name for a powder for extraocular muscle injection:
    (a) Botex
    (b) Botox
    (c) Skelaxin
    (d) Skelaxen

63. Generic name for a corticosteroid:
    (a) ortho tri-cyclen
    (b) ortho tricyclin
    (c) triamcinolone
    (d) triamcinoline

64. Trade name for a preparation of amoxicillin, an antibiotic:
    (a) Klonopin
    (b) Augmenten
    (c) Klonpin
    (d) Augmentin

65. Trade name for a selective estrogen receptor modulator used to prevent postmenopausal osteoporosis:
    (a) Paxil
    (b) Pasil
    (c) Evista
    (d) Evixta

66. Trade name for a preparation of amoxicillin, an antimicrobial:
    (a) Co-Polymer
    (b) Copolymer
    (c) Amoxil
    (d) Amosil

67. Trade name for a skeletal muscle relaxant:
    (a) Botex
    (b) Botox
    (c) Skelaxin
    (d) Skelaxen

68. Trade name for a topical antibiotic:
    (a) Proctocreem HC
    (b) Proctocream HC
    (c) Neosporen
    (d) Neosporin

69. Trade name for an antidepressant:
    (a) Paxil
    (b) Pasil
    (c) Evista
    (d) Evixta

70. Trade name for an anticonvulsant:
    (a) Klonopin
    (b) Augmenten
    (c) Klonpin
    (d) Augmentin

71. Trade name for preparations of lidocaine; classified as an antiarrhythmic, anesthetic:
    (a) Xylocaine
    (b) Ophthetic
    (c) Xylociane
    (d) Ophetic

72. Trade name for a triphasic oral contraceptive:
    (a) Ortho Tri-Cyclen
    (b) Ortho-Tricyclin
    (c) Triamcinolone
    (d) Triamcinoline

73. Trade name for an oral contraceptive:
    (a) Lipitir
    (b) Lipitor
    (c) Lo-Ovral
    (d) Lo-Oral

74. Trade name for a combination analgesic and antipyretic:
    (a) Darvoset
    (b) Darvocet
    (c) Melantonox
    (d) Melantonex

75. Trade name for an antihyperlipidemic that reduces cholesterol synthesis:
    (a) Lipitir
    (b) Lipitor
    (c) Lo-Ovral
    (d) Lo-Oral

76. Trade name for proparacaine hydrochloride; eye drops:
    (a) Xylocaine
    (b) Ophthetic
    (c) Xylociane
    (d) Ophetic

TERMINOLOGY

CHECK YOUR PROGRESS (cont'd)

77. Trade name for a topical corticosteroid anti-inflammatory used as anorectal cream:
    (a) Proctocreem HC
    (b) Proctocream HC
    (c) Neosporen
    (d) Neosporin

78. Trade name for an antihistamine, antiemetic:
    (a) Vancenase
    (b) Vancinase
    (c) Phenergan
    (d) Phenergin

79. Trade name for an immune modulator:
    (a) Co-Polymer
    (b) Amoxil
    (c) Copolymer
    (d) Amosil

80. Trade name for a nonsteroidal anti-inflammatory drug (NSAID):
    (a) Naprosyn
    (b) Naporsyn
    (c) Norvasc
    (d) Norvasic

81. Trade name for an antibiotic:
    (a) Claritin
    (b) Clariten
    (c) Baixin
    (d) Biaxin

82. Trade name for an antiplatelet agent:
    (a) Presantine
    (b) Persantine
    (c) Prilosec
    (d) Prelosec

83. Trade name for a drug used to prevent NSAID-induced gastric ulcers:
    (a) Cytotec
    (b) Cytotic
    (c) Ditropan
    (d) Ditropen

84. Trade name for an analgesic:
    (a) Melatonex
    (b) Melatonix
    (c) Darvocet
    (d) Darvocit

85. Trade name for a urinary antispasmodic:
    (a) Cytotec
    (b) Cytotic
    (c) Ditropan
    (d) Ditropen

86. Trade name for an antibiotic:
    (a) Indocen
    (b) Indocin
    (c) E.E.A.
    (d) E.E.S.

87. Trade name for an NSAID:
    (a) Indocen
    (b) Indocin
    (c) E.E.A.
    (d) E.E.S.

88. Trade name for a gastric acid–secretion inhibitor:
    (a) Presantine
    (b) Persantine
    (c) Prilosec
    (d) Prelosec

89. Trade name for a sleep aid:
    (a) Melatonex
    (b) Melatonix
    (c) Darvocet
    (d) Darvocit

90. Trade name for a nonsedating antihistamine
    (a) Claritin
    (b) Clariten
    (c) Baixin
    (d) Biaxin

Professional transcriptionists proofread their own work. Can you?

WORD PROCESSING USERS

Open your word processing package.

Insert the appropriate audiocassette in your transcribing machine and find dictation *5T-2*.

Transcribe and proofread dictation *5T-2*, using formatting guidelines established in Chapter 2.

Identify and correct all errors.

Save your work on your student disk.

After completing the transcription, refer to the answer key.

Manually complete the error analysis chart.

Manually complete the Production for Pay summary.

SOFTWARE USERS

Click on *Chapter 5, Proofreading Pretest (5T-2)*, and follow the directions.

Finding your own errors and correcting them is not easy, but it is an essential skill for your success as a medical transcriptionist. The two worksheets in this activity will help you develop your proofreading skills.

TEXTBOOK USERS

Proofread and correct errors in the medical documents shown in *Activities 5-4 and 5-5*.
Refer to the answer key (Appendix E) for immediate feedback.
Manually complete the error analysis chart for each document.

SOFTWARE USERS

Click on *Chapter 5, Activity 5-4*, and follow the directions.
Follow the same process for *Chapter 5, Activity 5-5*.

PROOFREADING

ACTIVITY 5-4
Proofreading Worksheet

Directions: Proofread this medical document, which contains multiple errors. Use open punctuation and all other formatting guidelines established in this textbook.

CHART NOTE

Harris, Donna

Date of Birth: 10/21/50

Examination Date: *Current date*

SUBJECT
Donna comes in today for follow-up. Her weight have fortunately stayed the same. She still feels weak. Her blood word looks good. X-ray demonstrates prominent markings in the R middle lobe and a questionable nodular density in the R apex.

Her appetite remains about the same. Her living situation is unchanged and despite our best efforts we have really not been able to help her significantly with this.

OBJECTIVE
Weight 92 lbs BP 120/68. She has no cervical adenapathy. Lungs show decreased breathe sounds. Cardiac exam REGULAR IN RATE AND RHYTHM without murmurs, rubs or gallops appreciated. She has normal chest well excursion. Abdomen is soft. She has some tenderness in the right rib cage.

ASSESMENT
Copd
Weight loss which at this point has stabilized.

PLAN
I am planning to check apical lordotic views of this abnormality in her lung and have them compared with previous films. I will continue to follow her weight loss. I doubt that she has lung cancer , but, just to make sure, I will reevaluate that right upper lobe a little better. At this point I plan to follow her rib pain as well. I really wasn't able to elicit much information today.

Charles P. Davis, MD

D: *current date*
T: *current date*

ACTIVITY 5-5
Proofreading Worksheet

Directions: Proofread this medical document, which contains multiple errors. Use open punctuation and all other formatting guidelines established in this textbook.

Current date

J. Thomas Geiger, MD
Family Practice Division, Suite 300
101 Wellness Way Drive
New York, NY 10036
RE: Charlotte Mekola
         Date of birth: 10/19/58
         Examination: CHEST

Dear Dr. Gieger

There is a substantial area of alvelar infiltrate that involves the superior segment of the right lower lobe. I do not identify a mass or any definite hilar adenapathy. The lungs are otherwise clear. There is probably an element of Copd. The heart is mildly inlarged but the pulmonary vessels do not appear prominent. There is no efussion. The visualized bony thorax and soft tissues are remarkable for an acentuated kyphosis and probable osteoporosis.

IMPRESSION: Alveolar infiltrate in the superior segment of the left lower lobe. Simple pneumonia is the most likely diagnosis. A follow-up until clearing is reccommended.

Thank you for refering this patient to us.

Yours Truly,

Potter Bucky, MD/x

Now you are ready to make the transition from simply proofreading printed material to both transcribing and proofreading dictated material. This is the time to concentrate on building your medical vocabulary, which ultimately will improve your speed and accuracy. There are two activities in this section.

WORD PROCESSING USERS

Open your word processing package.

Insert the appropriate audiocassette in your transcribing machine and find dictation 5T-3.

Step 1: Listen to the entire dictation to gain an understanding of the medical concepts and terms involved in the report. Rewind the tape to the beginning of the dictation and transcribe what you hear. Do not worry about formatting, style, or speed. Simply type what you hear being dictated, using correct punctuation, capitalization, and spelling. Stop as needed to look up words you do not understand or cannot spell. Adjust the speed control of the transcriber to a comfortable level, starting slowly to ensure that no dictated words are missed, and then increase the speed as your accuracy improves.

Step 2: Rewind the tape and transcribe dictation *5T-3* again, including correct spacing and formatting. Proofread the report. Identify and correct all errors. Save your work on your student disk. Refer to the answer key, and manually complete the error analysis chart and Production for Pay summary.

Follow the same process for dictation *5T-4*.

SOFTWARE USERS

Click on *Chapter 5, Activity 5-6 (5T-3), Step 1,* and follow the directions. When you feel comfortable with the dictation, click on *Chapter 5, Activity 5-6 (5T-3), Step 2,* and follow the directions.

Follow the same process for *Chapter 5, Activity 5-7 (5T-4), Step 1* and *Chapter 5, Activity 5-7 (5T-4), Step 2*.

WORD PROCESSING USERS

Open your word processing package.

Insert the appropriate audiocassette in your transcribing machine and find dictation *5T-2*.

Transcribe and proofread dictation *5T-2*, using the formatting guidelines established in Chapter 2.

Identify and correct all errors.

Save your work on your student disk.

After completing the transcription, refer to the answer key.

Manually complete the error analysis chart.

Manually complete the Production for Pay summary.

SOFTWARE USERS

Click on *Chapter 5, Proofreading Check Your Progress (5T-2)*, and follow the directions.

Professional transcriptionists can transcribe and proofread their own work. Can you?

WORD PROCESSING USERS

Open your word processing package.

Insert the appropriate audiocassette in your transcribing machine and find dictation 5T-5.

Transcribe and proofread dictation 5T-5, using the formatting guidelines established in Chapter 2.

Save your work on your student disk.

Identify and correct all errors.

After completing the transcription, refer to the answer key.

Manually complete the error analysis chart.

Manually complete the Production for Pay summary.

Follow the same process for dictation 5T-6.

SOFTWARE USERS

Click on *Chapter 5, Transcription Pretest (5T-5)*, and follow the directions.

Follow the same process for *Chapter 5, Transcription Pretest (5T-6)*.

You have been hired as a transcriptionist at FedDes Wellness Center in the family practice division. Your supervisor has asked you to transcribe today's dictation.

WORD PROCESSING USERS

Open your word processing package.

Insert the appropriate audiocassette in your transcribing machine and find dictation *5T-7*.

Create or use your existing templates as necessary for the six types of reports (chart note, chart note using history and physical format, history and physical examination report, x-ray report, procedure report, consultation letter).

Transcribe and proofread dictation *5T-7*, using the formatting guidelines established in Chapter 2.

Identify and correct all errors.

Save your work on your student disk.

After completing the transcription, refer to the answer key.

Manually complete the error analysis chart.

Manually complete the Production for Pay summary.

Follow the same process for dictations *5T-8* through *5T-23*.

SOFTWARE USERS

Click on *Chapter 5, Transcription at FedDes Wellness Center, Dictation 5T-7*, and follow the directions.

Follow the same process for each of the remaining dictations (*5T-8* through *5T-23*).

TRANSCRIPTION

Remember to follow the guidelines pertaining to capitalization, numbers, punctuation, abbreviations, measurements, symbols, and use of templates to create medical reports at FedDes Wellness Center. This material is reviewed in Unit I.

5T-7

Chart Note Using SOAP Format
Patient's Name: Clark, Bertram
Physician: Charles P. Davis, MD

Transcription Tips

- The expression *o'clock* is used to refer to points on a circular surface.
  You hear the dictator say: Three o'clock position.
  You transcribe as: 3 o'clock position.
- The # symbol is used to abbreviate the word *number* followed by medical instrument or apparatus.
  You hear the dictator say: Number twenty-five gauge needle.
  You transcribe as: #25-gauge needle.
- Figures are used for measurements and with Latin abbreviations.
  You hear the dictator say: Place in eye two drops every two hours.
  You transcribe as: Place in eye 2 drops q.2h.
- A hyphen is used to join two or more words when used as an adjective that precedes a noun.
  The following word pair is dictated in this report: metallic-looking.
  The word *follow-up* is also hyphenated because it is a noun implying an appointment. You hear the dictator say: He will return tomorrow for a follow-up.
- The following medication is dictated in this report:
  Ophthetic: trade name for proparacaine hydrochloride eye drops.

5T-8

Chart Note Using SOAP Format
Patient's Name: Meckonni, James
Physician: Charles P. Davis, MD

Transcription Tips

- Vital signs are separated by commas and are transcribed as one sentence.
  You hear the dictator say: Temperature ninety-eight point four weight one hundred forty four pounds blood pressure one hundred twenty eight over seventy four pulse fifty six.
  You transcribe as: Temperature 98.4, weight 144 pounds, BP 128/74, pulse 56.
- Words beginning with *pre, re, post*, and *non* are generally not hyphenated: postnasal.
- The following medications are dictated in this report:
  Augmentin: trade name for a preparation of amoxicillin, an antibiotic.
  Vancenase: trade name for a corticosteroid for bronchial asthma; pocket inhaler.
- The letter *x* is used to abbreviate the word *times* when it precedes a number.
  You hear the dictator say: Augmentin five hundred milligrams by mouth three times a day times two weeks.
  You transcribe as:
  Augmentin 500 mg p.o. t.i.d. × 2 weeks.

5T-9

Chart Note Using SOAP Format
Patient's Name: Chesterfield, Fredrick
Physician: Charles P. Davis, MD

Transcription Tips

- Words beginning with *pre, re, post*, and *non* are generally not hyphenated: nonstop.
- A hyphen is used to join two or more words when used as an adjective that precedes a noun. The following word pair dictated in this report is hyphenated: over-the-counter.
- The following abbreviation is dictated in this report. The plurals of all-capital abbreviations are formed by adding the letter *s*.
  TM: tympanic membrane; TMs
- Capitalize trade names and brand names of drugs, not generic drugs. The following medications are dictated in this report:
  NyQuil: trade name for an antitussive, decongestant, antihistamine
  E.E.S.: trade name for an antibiotic
  Terpin hydrate with codeine: generic name for an expectorant

TRANSCRIPTION

Robitussin: trade name for an antitussive
- Figures are used in ranges.
  You hear the dictator say: four to five times during the day.
  You transcribe as: 4-5 times during the day.

5T-10

Chart Note Using SOAP Format
Patient's Name: Trepidor, Rodrigues
Physician: Charles P. Davis, MD

Transcription Tips
- A hyphen is used between numbers and *year old*.
  You hear the dictator say: A thirty two year old white male.
  You transcribe as: A 32-year-old white male.
- Words beginning with *pre, re, post*, and *non* are generally not hyphenated: nonproductive, nontoxic.
- The following abbreviation is dictated in this report:
  A&P: auscultation and percussion
- The following medication is dictated in this report:
  Amoxil: trade name for a preparation of amoxicillin, an antibiotic

5T-11

Chart Note Using SOAP Format
Patient's Name: Aswart, Sabine
Physician: Charles P. Davis, MD

Transcription Tips
- The following eponym is dictated:
  Romberg's sign: swaying or falling when standing with feet close together and eyes closed. If positive, the patient will sway and fall.
- Capitalize trade names and brand names of drugs, not generic drugs. The following medications are dictated in this report:
  meclizine: generic name for an antiemetic especially effective for control of nausea and vomiting of motion sickness
  Paxil: trade name for an antidepressant
  Klonopin: trade name for an anticonvulsant
- A hyphen is used when joining numbers or letters to form a word, phrase, or abbreviation.
  You hear the dictator say: B twelve injections.
  You transcribe as: B-12 injections.
- Words beginning with *pre, re, post*, and *non* are generally not hyphenated: nontender.

5T-12

Procedure Report, FLEXIBLE SIGMOIDOSCOPY WITH BIOPSY
Patient's Name: Inshetski, Ann
Physician: Charles P. Davis, MD

5T-13

History and Physical Examination Report
Patient's Name: Stephano, Jennifer
Physician: Charles P. Davis, MD

Transcription Tips
- The following abbreviations are dictated in this report:
  SOB: shortness of breath
  PERRLA: pupils equal, round, reactive to light and accommodation
  EOMs: extraocular movements
  P&A: percussion and auscultation
  DTRs: deep tendon reflexes
- The diagonal (/) is used to separate the indicators of visual acuity.
  You hear the dictator say: Visual acuity is twenty over thirty both in the left and right eye, but corrected twenty over twenty five.
  You transcribe as: Visual acuity is 20/30 both in the left and right eye, but corrected 20/25.
- A hyphen joins two or more words when used as an adjective that precedes a noun. The following word pair is not hyphenated because it is a verb: follow up.
- A hyphen is used when two or more words are viewed as a single word: well-child.

5T-14

Chart Note Using History and Physical Format
Patient's Name: Smythers, Jane
Physician: P. H. Waters, MD

Transcription Tips
- The following abbreviations are dictated in this report:
  EACs: external auditory canals
  SOB: shortness of breath
  P&A: percussion and auscultation
  TMs: tympanic membranes
- A hyphen is used to join two or more words when used as an adjective that precedes a noun. The following word pairs are dictated in this report: over-the-counter, follow-up.

- The following laboratory test is dictated in this report:
  Rapid Strep test: a throat culture for a sore
  throat caused by a streptococcus

5T-15

Chart Note Using History and Physical Format
Patient's Name: Mermain, Devon
Physician: Izzy Sertoli, MD

Transcription Tips
- The following words are not hyphenated because they end a sentence: checkup, up to date.
- The hyphen is used to take the place of the word *to* or *through* to identify ranges.
  You hear the dictator say: We should see him again in two to three years at his school.
  You transcribe as: We should see him again in 2-3 years at his school.

5T-16

X-ray Report, PA AND LATERAL CHEST X-RAY
Patient's Name: Holtzworth, Max
Physician: P. H. Waters, MD

Transcription Tips
- The following abbreviation is dictated in this report:
  COPD: chronic obstructive pulmonary disease

5T-17

Chart Note Using History and Physical Format
Patient's Name: Margolis, Davy
Physician: P. H. Waters, MD

Transcription Tips
- A dangerous abbreviation is dictated within this transcript.
  You will hear the dictator say: three cc of yellow serous fluid.
  You should transcribe as: 3 mL of yellow serous fluid.
- The following abbreviations are dictated in this report:
  ASO: antistreptolysin O. ASO is an antibody that inhibits streptolysin. Streptolysin is an oxygen-labile and antigenic hemolysin produced by most group A streptococci that lyse red blood cells.

ANA: antinuclear antibody. The ANA test is used as a screen to detect autoimmune disease and systemic lupus erythematosus. It cannot identify the specifics of the disease; it only identifies the presence of antibodies of autoimmune disease.
CBC: complete blood count
- The following medications are dictated in this report:
  Cytotec: trade name for a drug used for the prevention of NSAID-induced gastric ulcers
  Indocin: trade name for a nonsteroidal anti-inflammatory drug (NSAID)
  Naprosyn: trade name for an NSAID
  lidocaine: generic name for a topical local anesthetic
- Words beginning with *pre, re, post*, and *non* are generally not hyphenated: recheck.
- The # symbol is used to abbreviate the word *number* followed by medical instrument or apparatus.
  You hear the dictator say: number twenty two gauge needle.
  You transcribe as: #22-gauge needle.

5T-18

Chart Note Using History and Physical Format
Patient's Name: Duke, Marge
Physician: Gwenn Maltase, MD

Transcription Tips
- A hyphen is used to join two or more words when used as an adjective that precedes a noun. The following word pairs are dictated in this report: over-the-counter, follow-up.

5T-19

Chart Note Using History and Physical Format
Patient's Name: Levy, Susan
Physician: Gwenn Maltase, MD

Transcription Tips
- Generic drugs are not capitalized.
  You will hear the dictator say: Will just treat with ibuprofen, rest, and fluids.
  You should transcribe as: Will just treat with ibuprofen, rest, and fluids.
- A hyphen is used to take the place of the word *to* or *through* to identify ranges.
  You hear the dictator say: She will call if she is not improving over the next twenty four to forty eight hours.

You transcribe as: She will call if she is not improving over the next 24-48 hours.

5T-20

Consultation Letter
  Inside address: Mr. Ben Over, Customer Services, Simon Seez Managed Care, Inc., 911 Dividend Drive, Cashflow, NY 10039
  Reference line: Samuel Franklin, File Number 69024, Date of Birth January 1, 1986
  Physician: J. Thomas Geiger, MD

Transcription Tips
- The following abbreviation is dictated in this report: HMO: health maintenance organization
- A hyphen is used to join two or more words when used as an adjective that precedes a noun. The following word pair is dictated in this report: follow-up.
- The apostrophe is used to form the possessive of singular and plural nouns.
    You hear the dictator say: Thank you for your timely assistance in Mr. Franklin's treatment plan.
- The following medication is dictated:
    Copolymer: trade name for one of the immune-modulating drugs

5T-21

Physical Therapy Referral Letter
  Inside address: David Treppe, MD, Orthopedic Division, Suite 133, FedDes Wellness Center, New York, NY 10036
  Reference line: Betty Ross, File Number 51490, Date of Birth September 15, 19xx
  Physical Therapist: Melissa A. Anconeus, MS, PT

Transcription Tips
- A hyphen is used to join two or more words when used as an adjective that precedes a noun. The following word pairs are dictated in this report:
    30-foot
    right-sided
    left-sided
    pain-free
    part-time
    self-employed
    long-term
- A hyphen is used between two "like" vowels: anti-inflammatory, pre-existing.
- The percent sign (%) is used with words and figures.

You hear the dictator say: Cervical range of motion is restricted at seventy five percent of normal rotation.
  You transcribe as: Cervical range of motion is restricted at 75% of normal rotation.
  You hear the dictator say: treated with a one percent Xylocaine injection.
  You transcribe as: treated with a 1% Xylocaine injection.
- Figures with capital letters are used to refer to the vertebral column and spinal nerves.
    The hyphen is used to take the place of the word *through* to identify ranges.
    You hear the dictator say: There is left-sided point tenderness over the C five through C six paraspinal areas.
    You transcribe as: There is left-sided point tenderness over the C5-C6 paraspinal areas.
- The words *palpation* and *palpitation* are often confused in dictation. Listen carefully!
    Palpation is an examination by touching.
    Palpitation is a rapid or fluttering heartbeat.
    There is tenderness to palpation of the anterior glenohumeral capsule.
    No chest pain, edema, palpitations, orthopnea, leg cramps, or exertional dyspnea was noted.

5T-22

Chart Note Using SOAP Format
Patient's Name: Lee, My
Physician: Izzy Sertoli, MD

Transcription Tips
- The following abbreviation is dictated in this report: Pap: Papanicolaou test
- Figures are used to express pregnancy and delivery. For example: gravida 1, para 1
- The following laboratory tests are dictated in this report:
    Fasting Astra IV: a panel of four blood chemistry tests that require the patient to fast. The name of this test is linked to the manufacturer of the chemical analyzer, Astra.
    TSH: thyroid-stimulating hormone. The test measures the TSH level.
    Erythrocyte sedimentation rate (ESR) test is helpful in identifying and monitoring disease activity in infectious, inflammatory, and neoplastic conditions.
- The following medication is dictated in this report:
    Skelaxin: trade name for a skeletal muscle relaxant

TRANSCRIPTION

History and Physical Examination Report
Patient's Name: Feiffer, Madeline
Physician: Matthew Sponch, MD

Transcription Tips

- A hyphen is used to join two or more words when used as an adjective that precedes a noun. The following word pairs are dictated in this report: well-developed, well-nourished, 12-week.
- Figures are used almost exclusively as opposed to spelled-out numbers to improve clarity and avoid potential mistakes.

  You hear the dictator say: She is twelve weeks amenorrheic with complaints of vaginal spotting for the past three days.

  You transcribe as: She is 12 weeks amenorrheic with complaints of vaginal spotting for the past 3 days.

- The following abbreviation is dictated in this report: HPI: history of present illness
- The hyphen is used to take the place of the word *to* or *through* to identify ranges.

  You hear the dictator say: The cervix is open one to two centimeters.

  You transcribe as: The cervix is open 1-2 cm.

- Words beginning with *pre, re, post*, and *non* are generally not hyphenated: noncontributory, nontender.

  Professional transcriptionists can transcribe and proofread their own work with speed and accuracy. Have you mastered the family practice transcription rotation at FedDes Wellness Center?

Professional transcriptionists can transcribe and proofread their own work with speed and accuracy. Have you mastered the family practice transcription rotation at FedDes Wellness Center?

WORD PROCESSING USERS

Open your word processing package.

Insert the appropriate audiocassette in your transcribing machine and find dictation *5T-5*.

Transcribe and proofread dictation *5T-5*, using the formatting guidelines established in Chapter 2.

Save your work on your student disk.

Identify and correct all errors.

After completing the transcription, refer to the answer key.

Manually complete the error analysis chart.

Manually complete the Production for Pay summary.

Follow the same process for dictation *5T-6*.

SOFTWARE USERS

Click on *Chapter 5, Transcription Check Your Progress (5T-5)*, and follow the directions.

Follow the same process for *Chapter 5, Transcription Check Your Progress (5T-6)*.

Anatomical Illustrations and Medical Images

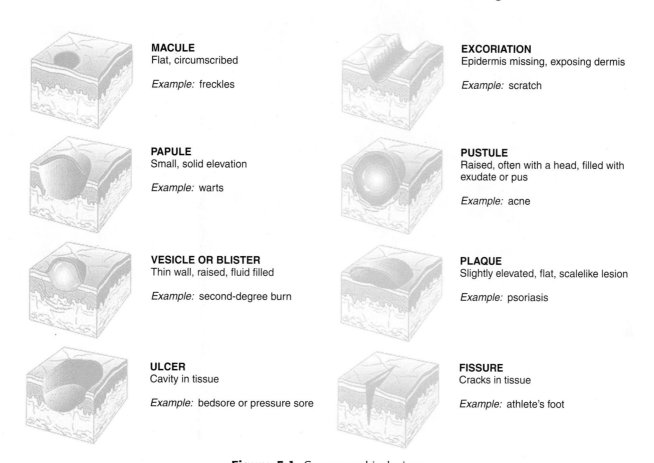

MACULE
Flat, circumscribed

Example: freckles

PAPULE
Small, solid elevation

Example: warts

VESICLE OR BLISTER
Thin wall, raised, fluid filled

Example: second-degree burn

ULCER
Cavity in tissue

Example: bedsore or pressure sore

EXCORIATION
Epidermis missing, exposing dermis

Example: scratch

PUSTULE
Raised, often with a head, filled with exudate or pus

Example: acne

PLAQUE
Slightly elevated, flat, scalelike lesion

Example: psoriasis

FISSURE
Cracks in tissue

Example: athlete's foot

Figure 5-1 Common skin lesions.

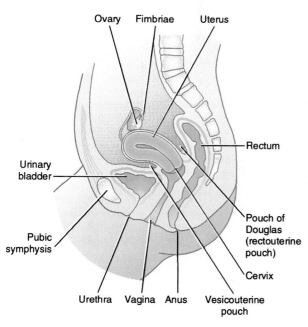

Figure 5-2 Sagittal view of female reproductive system.

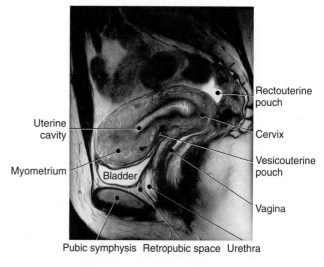

Figure 5-3 Sagittal magnetic resonance (MR) scan of female reproductive system. *(From Kelley LL, Petersen CM: Sectional anatomy for imaging professionals, St Louis, 1996, Mosby.)*

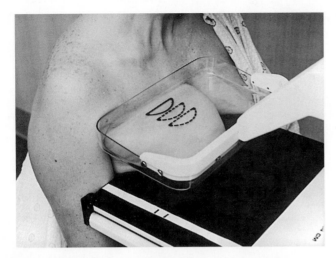

Figure 5-4 Patient positioned for craniocaudal projection of breast. *(From Ballinger PW, Frank ED: Merrill's atlas of radiographic positions and radiologic procedures, ed 10, St Louis, 2003, Mosby.)*

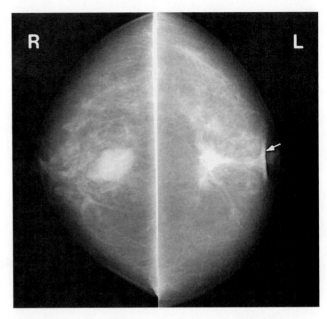

Figure 5-5 Craniocaudal projection of bilateral breast masses. *(From Ballinger PW, Frank ED: Merrill's atlas of radiographic positions and radiologic procedures, ed 10, St Louis, 2003, Mosby.)*

Chapter 6

Office Medical Transcription from the Orthopedic Practice

OBJECTIVES

At the completion of Chapter 6, you should be able to do the following:
1. Match medical terms associated with the orthopedic specialty with their definitions.
2. Spell medical terms associated with the orthopedic specialty.
3. Transcribe medical terms in sentence structure.
4. Proofread, edit, and correct medical documents associated with the orthopedic specialty that contain various errors.
5. Transcribe and proofread authentic medical documents associated with the orthopedic specialty.

INTRODUCTION TO THE ORTHOPEDIC ROTATION

What's Ahead

INTRODUCTION TO THE ORTHOPEDIC ROTATION

The FedDes Wellness Center has three *orthopedists*, or specialists in orthopedic medicine, on staff. *Orthopedics* is the field of medicine concerned with the diseases, injuries, and deformities of the musculoskeletal system. Patients who see an orthopedist may be suffering from a fracture, acute or chronic pain, inflammatory joint or stress injuries, osteoporosis, herniated intervertebral discs, or carpal tunnel syndrome.

During a physical examination by an orthopedist, the patient is first observed standing and walking. Posture, movement of the extremities, and any signs of pain are included in the observation. The examination includes full range of motion activities and strength assessment for each muscle group.

The physicians in FedDes Orthopedic Division perform and interpret routine x-rays in their offices. More sophisticated imaging, such as MRI, CT scans, and nuclear medicine studies, are referred to an outside facility and interpreted by a radiologist.

In this unit, you assume the role of a medical transcriptionist employed at FedDes Wellness Center. **Please remember to follow the guidelines pertaining to capitalization, numbers, punctuation, abbreviations, measurements, symbols, and use of templates to create medical reports at FedDes Wellness Center.** This material is reviewed in Unit I. The transcription exercises list the type of report, patient's name, and physician(s) as well as the associated transcription tips.

You will work with the textbook and a CD-ROM or audiocassettes. Your mastery of orthopedic transcription is assessed through worksheets, timed transcription exercises, the error analysis chart, and the Production for Pay summary.

All the answer keys are found in the textbook and CD-ROM, providing immediate feedback. After transcribing a report, you will proofread your work and correct any errors. Then you will compare your proofread work against a master transcript, categorize all errors, and tabulate the errors on the error analysis chart. The Production for Pay summary correlates your production to the FedDes Wellness Center pay scale. The scale is also linked to your grade. This system allows you to assess your mastery of transcription skills in a real-world scenario.

Let's find out if you can define and spell selected terminology and drugs of the orthopedic specialty that are included in this chapter.

WORD PROCESSING USERS

Select the correctly spelled term that matches its definition.
Refer to the answer key (Appendix E) for immediate feedback.

SOFTWARE USERS

Click on *Chapter 6, Terminology Pretest*, and follow the directions.

NAME _____   DATE _____

PRETEST

Directions: Select the correctly spelled term that matches its definition.

1. A finger or toe:
   (a) digit
   (b) falanx
   (c) fusiform
   (d) degit

2. A fracture of the distal end of the radius with displacement of the hand backward and upward:
   (a) Coles fracture
   (b) Colles fracture
   (c) Smith fracture
   (d) Smythe fracture

3. A fracture of the lower end of the radius with forward displacement of the lower fragment:
   (a) Coles fracture
   (b) Colles fracture
   (c) Smith fracture
   (d) Smythe fracture

4. Frequent cause of shoulder pain thought to be caused by pressure on the tendons of the shoulder:
   (a) radiculitis
   (b) rotator cuff tendenitis
   (c) radeculitis
   (d) rotator cuff tendinitis

5. Lubricating fluid of joints:
   (a) apophysis
   (b) apophyis
   (c) synova
   (d) synovia

6. The tearing away or ripping of a part or structure:
   (a) avulsion
   (b) crepitus
   (c) avolsion
   (d) creitus

7. Abnormal contact or pressure between two structures:
   (a) impingement
   (b) impingment
   (c) debredment
   (d) debridement

8. Abnormal, benign growth on the surface of a bone; also called *hyperostosis*:
   (a) ecchymosis
   (b) exostisis
   (c) echymosis
   (d) exostosis

9. Benign tumor composed mostly of fat cells:
   (a) lymphedema
   (b) lipoma
   (c) lipima
   (d) lymphodema

10. Affecting or relating to two sides:
    (a) bilateril
    (b) genu varum
    (c) bilateral
    (d) ganu varum

11. An attempt to exhale forcibly with the glottis, nose, and mouth closed:
    (a) Valsalva maneuver
    (b) Fabrey test
    (c) Fabre test
    (d) Valsava maneuver

12. An outgrowth of bone that is usually found around a joint:
    (a) apophysis
    (b) ostophyte
    (c) osteophyte
    (d) appophysis

13. Any outgrowth or swelling; a process or projection of a bone:
    (a) apophysis
    (b) ostophyte
    (c) osteophyte
    (d) appophysis

14. Between two joints:
    (a) bilateral
    (b) bilateril
    (c) intrarticuler
    (d) interarticular

15. Bowleg:
    (a) genu varum
    (b) gluteus medius
    (c) ganu varum
    (d) glutus medius

16. Commonly called a *bruise*, with trauma to the body part but no break in the skin surface:
    (a) contusion
    (b) volar
    (c) contrusion
    (d) volor

17. Condition of containing pus:
    (a) pisiform
    (b) pesiform
    (c) purulence
    (d) prulence

18. Describes the pathway of the x-ray beam as it passes through anteriorly and exits posteriorly; anteroposterior x-ray:
    (a) NKA x-ray
    (b) PA x-ray
    (c) AP x-ray
    (d) KAN x-ray

19. Directional term, from posterior to medial:
    (a) postmedial
    (b) posteromedial
    (c) peripheral
    (d) peripharel

20. Black and blue appearance of the skin:
    (a) ecchymosis
    (b) exostisis
    (c) echymosis
    (d) exostosis

21. Draw in or out by suction:
    (a) turgor
    (b) asporate
    (c) turger
    (d) aspirate

22. Swelling due to obstruction of lymph vessels:
    (a) lymphedema
    (b) lipoma
    (c) lipima
    (d) lymphodema

23. Escape of fluid from blood vessels because of rupture or seepage, usually into a body cavity:
    (a) crepitus
    (b) effussion
    (c) effusion
    (d) creptus

24. Examination of the interior of a joint with an arthroscope:
    (a) arthroscopy
    (b) hypertrophy
    (c) arthriscopy
    (d) hyprotrophy

25. General term for any bone of a finger or toe:
    (a) fusiform
    (b) falanx
    (c) phalanx
    (d) degit

26. Grating sound of bone fragments rubbing together:
    (a) crepitus
    (b) effussion
    (c) effusion
    (d) creptus

27. Increase in the size of an organ or structure:
    (a) greater trochanter
    (b) hypertrophy
    (c) greater trichanter
    (d) hyprotrophy

28. Inflammation of a tendon:
    (a) tendinitis
    (b) radiculitis
    (c) tendenitus
    (d) radeculitis

29. Large projection at the proximal end of the femur:
    (a) greater trochanter
    (b) hypertrophy
    (c) greater trichanter
    (d) hyprotrophy

30. Movement by a joint that decreases the angle between the two adjoining bones; the bending of a joint:
    (a) abduction
    (b) flixion
    (c) flexion
    (d) abuction

31. Movement of an extremity away from midline:
    (a) abuction
    (b) aduction
    (c) abduction
    (d) adduction

32. Movement of an extremity toward the midline:
    (a) abuction
    (b) aduction
    (c) abduction
    (d) adduction

33. New growth of bony tissue surrounding the bone ends in a fracture; part of the repair process of a fractured bone:
    (a) plantar
    (b) callus
    (c) planter
    (d) calus

34. Normal resiliency of the skin:
    (a) turgor
    (b) trugor
    (c) volar
    (d) volor

35. Occurring away from the center:
    (a) postmedial
    (b) posteromedial
    (c) peripheral
    (d) peripharel

36. One of the three muscles that form the buttocks; acts to abduct and rotate the thigh:
    (a) genu varum
    (b) gluteus medius
    (c) ganu varum
    (d) glutus medius

37. Pea-shaped, smallest carpal bone:
    (a) pisiform
    (b) pesiform
    (c) purulence
    (d) prulence

38. Performed with patient supine, thigh and knee flexed; the ankle is placed over the patella of the opposite leg, then the knee is depressed.
    (a) Valsalva maneuver
    (b) Fabrey test
    (c) Fabre test
    (d) Valsava maneuver

39. A spinous projection off the scapula:
    (a) acromon
    (b) faciculations
    (c) acromion
    (d) fasciculations

40. Pertaining to the palm of the hand or sole of the foot:
    (a) turgor
    (b) trugor
    (c) volar
    (d) volor

41. Reconstructive surgery to repair or reshape a diseased joint:
    (a) arthroscopy
    (b) arthriscropy
    (c) arthroplasty
    (d) arthroplasy

42. Relating to the sole of the foot:
    (a) plantar
    (b) callus
    (c) planter
    (d) calus

43. Removal of dead or damaged tissue:
    (a) impingement
    (b) impingment
    (c) debredment
    (d) debridement

44. Situated or occurring between bone:
    (a) calcaneus
    (b) interosseous
    (c) clacaneus
    (d) intreosseous

45. Spindle-shaped structure that is tapered at both ends:
    (a) fusiform
    (b) fusform
    (c) pisiform
    (d) pesiform

46. Supporting one's own weight without assistance:
    (a) weightbearing
    (b) weightbaring
    (c) trapezius
    (d) trapeius

47. Surgical removal of a meniscus:
    (a) menisectomy
    (b) mellelus
    (c) melleolus
    (d) meniscectomy

48. Symptoms of a specific disease:
    (a) asympmatic
    (b) symptomatology
    (c) symptomology
    (d) asymptomatic

49. Movement of a finger temporarily stopping in the extension or flexion position, then beginning again with a jerk:
    (a) jerking finger
    (b) trigger finger
    (c) jerk finger
    (d) trig finger

50. Divergence of pain from the site of injury to other areas of the body:
    (a) radiculitis
    (b) radaition
    (c) radiation
    (d) radiculation

51. Therapy program using simulated or real work tasks to improve strength and endurance gradually in anticipation of completing a full day's work:
    (a) workhardening
    (b) work hardening
    (c) workbearing
    (d) work bearing

52. Bending of a joint toward the posterior aspect of the body:
    (a) dorsiflexion
    (b) flixion
    (c) abduction
    (d) dorsflexion

53. Uncontrolled twitching of a group of muscle fibers:
    (a) acromon
    (b) faciculations
    (c) acromion
    (d) fasciculations

54. Without symptoms:
    (a) asympmatic
    (b) symptomatology
    (c) symptomology
    (d) asymptomatic

55. Triangular muscle of each side of the upper back:
    (a) metatarsus
    (b) trapezius
    (c) trapezsus
    (d) metatarus

56. Disease of the lymph nodes:
    (a) lymphadenopathy
    (b) lymphenopathy
    (c) lymphedema
    (d) lymphodema

57. Crescent-shaped fibrocartilage in the knee joint:
    (a) meniscus
    (b) malelus
    (c) menscus
    (d) malleolus

58. The long, medial bone of the forearm:
    (a) radius
    (b) radious
    (c) ulna
    (d) unla

59. Any of the five long bones of the foot between the ankle and toes:
    (a) metatarsus
    (b) trapezius
    (c) trapezsus
    (d) metatarus

60. Either of the two rounded projections on either side of the ankle joint:
    (a) meniscus
    (b) malelus
    (c) menscus
    (d) malleolus

61. The heel bone or os calcis:
    (a) colcaneus
    (b) calcaneus
    (c) ulna
    (d) unla

62. Inflammation of a spinal nerve root:
    (a) radiculitis
    (b) radaition
    (c) radiation
    (d) radiculation

NAME _____   DATE _____

PRETEST *(cont'd)*

63. Inflammation involving the folds of tissue surrounding the nail:
    (a) synovia
    (b) synomvia
    (c) parychia
    (d) paronychia

64. Trade name for a beta-adrenergic blocker:
    (a) Lopressor
    (b) Percocet
    (c) Lopresser
    (d) Percoset

65. Generic name for an antibiotic:
    (a) tetrasysline
    (b) spironolactone
    (c) spironlactone
    (d) tetracycline

66. Trade name for an opioid analgesic:
    (a) Lopressor
    (b) Percocet
    (c) Lopressar
    (d) Percoset

67. Trade name for an antihyperlipidemic:
    (a) Linoxin
    (b) Lipitor
    (c) Lanoxin
    (d) Lippitor

68. Trade name for an antiarrhythmic, cardiotonic:
    (a) Linoxin
    (b) Lipitor
    (c) Lanoxin
    (d) Lippitor

69. Generic name for a corticosteroid:
    (a) codeine
    (b) cortisone
    (c) codenine
    (d) cortisome

70. Generic name for an opioid analgesic:
    (a) codeine
    (b) cortisone
    (c) codenine
    (d) cortisome

71. Trade name for an antiarrhythmic, local anesthetic:
    (a) Xylocaine
    (b) Biaxin
    (c) Baixin
    (d) Xylacane

72. Generic name for a diuretic:
    (a) tetrasysline
    (b) spironolactone
    (c) spironlactone
    (d) tetracycline

73. Trade name for an antibiotic:
    (a) Xylocaine
    (b) Biaxin
    (c) Baixin
    (d) Xylacane

74. Trade name for a narcotic analgesic:
    (a) Keflex
    (b) Keplex
    (c) Vicoprofen
    (d) Vicoprophen

75. Trade name for an antibiotic:
    (a) Keflex
    (b) Keplex
    (c) Vicoprofen
    (d) Vicoprophen

76. Trade name for an anti-inflammatory:
    (a) Dolibid
    (b) Dolobid
    (c) Vicodin
    (d) Vicidin

77. Trade name for a narcotic analgesic:
    (a) Dolibid
    (b) Dolobid
    (c) Vicodin
    (d) Vicidin

78. Generic name for any of a large group of antibacterial antibiotics derived from strains of fungi:
    (a) pencilin
    (b) pennicilin
    (c) penicilin
    (d) penicillin

Let's learn to spell and define some orthopedic terms. Keyboarding these terms is an effective way to improve your skills.

WORD PROCESSING USERS

Open your word processing package.
Read and type each word and its definition as shown below.
Save your work on your student disk.

1. Abduction (ab-<u>duk</u>-shun) is the movement of an extremity away from the midline.
2. Acromion (ah-<u>kro</u>-me-on) is a spinous projection off the scapula.
3. Adduction (ad-<u>duk</u>-shun) is the movement of an extremity toward the midline.
4. Apophysis (ah-<u>pofi</u>-sis) is any outgrowth or swelling; a process or projection of a bone.
5. Arthroplasty (ar-<u>thro</u>-plas-te) is the reconstructive surgery to repair or reshape a diseased joint.
6. Arthroscopy (ar-<u>thros</u>-ko-pe) is the examination of the interior of a joint with an arthroscope.
7. Aspirate (<u>as</u>-pi-rate) is to draw in or out by suction.
8. Asymptomatic (a-<u>simp</u>-to-mat-ik) means without symptoms.
9. Avulsion (ah-<u>vul</u>-shun) is the tearing away or ripping of a part or structure.
10. Bilateral (bi-<u>lat</u>-er-al) means affecting or relating to two sides.
11. Calcaneus (kal-<u>kay</u>-nee-us) is the heel bone or os calcis.
12. Callus (<u>kal</u>-us) is the new growth of bony tissue surrounding the bone ends in a fracture; part of the repair process of a fractured bone.
13. Codeine (<u>ko</u>-deen or <u>ko</u>-dean) is the generic name for an opioid analgesic.
14. Colles fracture (<u>kol</u>-ez) is a fracture of the distal end of the radius with displacement of the hand backward and upward.
15. Contusion (kon-<u>to</u>-shun) is commonly called a *bruise*, with trauma to the body part but no break in the skin surface.
16. Cortisone (<u>cor</u>-ti-sone) is the generic name for a corticosteroid used to treat inflammations.
17. Crepitus (<u>krep</u>-i-tus) is a grating sound of bone fragments rubbing together.
18. Debridement (da-<u>breed</u>-ment) is the removal of dead or damaged tissue.
19. Digit (<u>dij</u>-it) is a finger or toe.
20. Dorsiflexion (dor-si-<u>flek</u>-shun) is the bending of a joint toward the posterior aspect of the body.
21. Ecchymosis (eki-<u>mo</u>-sis) is the black and blue appearance of the skin.
22. Effusion (e-<u>fu</u>-zhun) is the escape of fluid from blood vessels because of rupture or seepage, usually into a body cavity.
23. Exostosis (ek-sos-<u>to</u>-sis) is an abnormal, benign growth on the surface of a bone, also called *hyperostosis*.
24. Fasciculations (fa-sik-u-<u>la</u>-shun) are the uncontrolled twitching of a group of muscle fibers.
25. Flexion (<u>flek</u>-shun) is the movement by a joint that decreases the angle between the two adjoining bones; the bending of a joint.
26. Fusiform (<u>fu</u>-zi-form) is a spindle-shaped structure that is tapered at both ends.
27. Genu varum (<u>je</u>-nu va-rum) is bowleg.
28. Gluteus medius (<u>gloo</u>-te-us me-de-us) is one of the three muscles that form the buttocks; acts to abduct and rotate the thigh.
29. Greater trochanter (tro-<u>kan</u>-ter) is the large projection at the proximal end of the femur.
30. Hypertrophy (hi-<u>per</u>-tro-fe) is an increase in the size of an organ or structure.
31. Interarticular (in-ter-ar-<u>tik</u>-u-lar) is between two joints.
32. Interosseous (in-ter-<u>os</u>-e-us) is situated or occurring between bone.
33. Lipoma (li-<u>po</u>-mah) is a benign tumor composed mostly of fat cells.
34. Lymphadenopathy (lim-fad-e-<u>nop</u>-ah-the) is the disease of the lymph nodes.
35. Lymphedema (<u>lim</u>-fi-de-ma) is edema due to obstruction of lymph vessels.
36. Malleolus (mah-<u>lee</u>-o-lus) is either of the two rounded projections on either side of the ankle joint.
37. Meniscectomy (me-ni-<u>sek</u>-to-me) is the surgical removal of a meniscus.
38. Meniscus (me-<u>nis</u>-kus) is the crescent-shaped fibrocartilage in the knee joint.
39. Metatarsus (met-a-<u>tar</u>-sus) is any of the five long bones of the foot between the ankle and the toes.
40. Osteophyte (<u>os</u>-te-o-fight) is an outgrowth of bone that is usually found around a joint.
41. Paronychia (par-o-<u>nik</u>-e-ah) is the inflammation involving the folds of tissue surrounding the nail.

42. Penicillin (pen-i-<u>sil</u>-in) is the generic name for any of a large group of antibacterial antibiotics derived from strains of fungi of the genus *Penicillium*.

43. Peripheral (pe-<u>rif</u>-er-al) is occurring away from the center.

44. Phalanx (<u>fa</u>-langks) is the general term for any bone of a finger or toe.

45. Pisiform (<u>pi</u>-si-form) is the pea-shaped, smallest carpal bone.

46. Plantar (<u>plan</u>-tar) is relating to the sole of the foot.

47. Purulence (<u>pu</u>-roo-lens) is the condition of containing pus.

48. Radiculitis (rah-dik-u-<u>li</u>-tis) is the inflammation of a spinal nerve root.

49. Smith fracture is a fracture of the lower end of the radius with forward displacement of the lower fragment.

50. Spironolactone (spir-o-no-<u>lak</u>-tone) is the generic name for a diuretic.

51. Symptomatology (simp-to-mah-<u>tol</u>-o-je) is the symptoms of a specific disease.

52. Synovia (si-<u>no</u>-ve-ah) is the lubricating fluid of joints.

53. Tendinitis (ten-di-<u>ni</u>-tis) is the inflammation of a tendon; tendonitis.

54. Tetracycline (te-trah-<u>si</u>-klen) is the generic name for an antibiotic.

55. Trapezius (trah-<u>pee</u>-zee-us) is the triangular muscle on each side of the upper back.

56. Turgor (<u>tur</u>-gor) is the normal resiliency of the skin.

57. Ulna (<u>ul</u>-nah) is the long, medial bone of the forearm.

58. Volar (<u>vo</u>-lar) pertains to the palm of the hand or sole of the foot.

59. Biaxin (bi-<u>ak</u>-sin) is the trade name for an antibiotic.

60. Dolobid (<u>do</u>-lo-bid) is the trade name for an analgesic and anti-inflammatory.

61. Keflex (<u>kef</u>-leks) is the trade name for an antibiotic.

62. Lanoxin (lah-<u>nok</u>-sin) is the trade name for an antiarrhythmic and cardiotonic.

63. Lipitor (<u>lip</u>-i-tor) is the trade name for an antihyperlipidemic.

64. Lopressor (lo-<u>pres</u>-or) is the trade name for a beta-adrenergic blocker.

65. Percocet (<u>per</u>-ko-set) is the trade name for an opioid analgesic (Schedule II).

66. Vicodin (<u>vi</u>-co-din) is the trade name for a narcotic analgesic.

67. Vicoprofen (vik-o-<u>pro</u>-fen) is the trade name for a narcotic analgesic.

68. Xylocaine (<u>zi</u>-lo-cane) is the trade name for an antiarrhythmic and local anesthetic.

Spelling Medical Terms

Do you remember back in school when you had to write each spelling word ten times? Because you had to physically write each word, your mind and body were focused on the assignment, and the method worked. Let's follow this successful method by reinforcing the spelling of some orthopedic terms through keyboarding drills.

WORD PROCESSING USERS

Open your word processing package.
Read, mentally spell, and type each word in its sequence.
Save your work on your student disk.

1. abduction acromial adduction abduction acromial adduction abduction acromial adduction
2. apophysis arthroplasty aspirate apophysis arthroplasty aspirate apophysis arthroplasty
3. arthroscopy asymptomatic avulsion arthroscopy asymptomatic avulsion arthroscopy avulsion
4. bilateral codeine cortisone bilateral codeine cortisone bilateral codeine cortisone codeine
5. calcaneus contusion crepitus calcaneus contusion crepitus calcaneus contusion crepitus
6. debridement digit dorsiflexion debridement digit dorsiflexion debridement digit dorsiflexion
7. ecchymosis effusion exostosis ecchymosis effusion exostosis ecchymosis effusion exostosis
8. fasciculations flexion fusiform fasciculations flexion fusiform fasciculations flexion fusiform
9. genu varum gluteus medius greater trochanter genu varum gluteus medius greater trochanter
10. hypertrophy interarticular interosseous hypertrophy interarticular interosseous hypertrophy
11. lipoma lymphadenopathy lymphedema lipoma lymphadenopathy lymphedema lipoma
12. malleolus meniscectomy meniscus malleolus meniscectomy meniscus malleolus meniscectomy
13. metatarsus osteophyte paronychia metatarsus osteophyte paronychia metatarsus osteophyte
14. peripheral phalanx pisiform peripheral phalanx pisiform peripheral phalanx pisiform phalanx
15. plantar purulence radiculitis plantar purulence radiculitis plantar purulence radiculitis plantar
16. symptomatology synovia tendinitis symptomatology synovia tendinitis symptomatology
17. trapezius turgor ulna volar trapezius turgor ulna volar trapezius turgor ulna volar trapezius
18. penicillin spironolactone tetracycline penicillin spironolactone tetracycline penicillin
19. Lanoxin Lipitor Lopressor Lanoxin Lipitor Lopressor Lanoxin Lipitor Lopressor Lanoxin
20. Biaxin Dolobid Keflex Biaxin Dolobid Keflex Biaxin Dolobid Keflex Biaxin Dolobid Keflex
21. Percocet Vicodin Vicoprofen Xylocaine Percocet Vicodin Vicoprofen Xylocaine Percocet

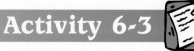
Now you are ready to make the transition from keyboarding medical terms, which is a visual process, to transcribing medical terms, an aural process. You are going to use audiocassette tapes or your CD-ROM rather than printed material.

WORD PROCESSING USERS

Open your word processing package.

Insert the appropriate audiocassette in your transcribing machine and find dictation *6T-1*.

You will be transcribing spelling words in sentence structure.

Listen carefully to each sentence on the audiocassette before transcribing.

Rewind and type (transcribe) the sentences.

Save your work on your student disk.

Refer to the answer key (Appendix E) for immediate feedback.

SOFTWARE USERS

Click on *Chapter 6, Terminology Activity 6-3 (6T-1)*, and follow the directions.

Let's pause a minute and see how well you are doing. This section allows you to evaluate your mastery of keyboarding and spelling selected terms and drugs found in the orthopedic specialty.

TEXTBOOK USERS

Select the correctly spelled term that matches its definition.
Refer to the answer key (Appendix E) for immediate feedback.

SOFTWARE USERS

Click on *Chapter 6, Terminology Check Your Progress*, and follow the directions.

TERMINOLOGY

CHECK YOUR PROGRESS

Directions: Select the correctly spelled term that matches its definition.

1. A finger or toe:
   (a) digit
   (b) falanx
   (c) fusiform
   (d) degit

2. Lubricating fluid of joints:
   (a) apophysis
   (b) apophyis
   (c) synova
   (d) synovia

3. A tearing away or ripping of a part or structure:
   (a) avulsion
   (b) crepitus
   (c) avolsion
   (d) creitus

4. Abnormal, benign growth on the surface of a bone; also called *hyperostosis*:
   (a) ecchymosis
   (b) exostisis
   (c) echymosis
   (d) exostosis

5. Benign tumor composed mostly of fat cells:
   (a) lymphedema
   (b) lipoma
   (c) lipima
   (d) lymphodema

6. Affecting or relating to two sides:
   (a) bilateril
   (b) genu varum
   (c) bilateral
   (d) ganu varum

7. An outgrowth of bone that is usually found around a joint:
   (a) apophysis
   (b) ostophyte
   (c) osteophyte
   (d) appophysis

8. Any outgrowth or swelling; a process or projection of a bone:
   (a) apophysis
   (b) ostophyte
   (c) osteophyte
   (d) appophysis

9. Between two joints:
   (a) bilateral
   (b) bilateril
   (c) interarticuler
   (d) interarticular

10. Bowleg:
    (a) genu varum
    (b) gluteus medius
    (c) ganu varum
    (d) glutus medius

11. Commonly called a *bruise*, with trauma to the body part but no break in the skin surface:
    (a) contusion
    (b) volar
    (c) contrusion
    (d) volor

12. Condition of containing pus:
    (a) pisiform
    (b) pesiform
    (c) purulence
    (d) prulence

13. Black and blue appearance of the skin:
    (a) ecchymosis
    (b) exostisis
    (c) echymosis
    (d) exostosis

14. Draw in or out by suction:
    (a) turgor
    (b) asporate
    (c) turger
    (d) aspirate

15. Swelling due to obstruction of lymph vessels:
    (a) lymphedema
    (b) lipoma
    (c) lipima
    (d) lymphodema

16. Escape of fluid from rupture or seepage of blood vessels, usually into a body cavity:
    (a) crepitus
    (b) effussion
    (c) effusion
    (d) creptus

CHECK YOUR PROGRESS *(cont'd)*

17. Examination of the interior of a joint with an arthroscope:
    (a) arthroscopy
    (b) hypertrophy
    (c) arthriscopy
    (d) hyprotrophy

18. General term for any bone of a finger or toe:
    (a) digit
    (b) falanx
    (c) phalanx
    (d) degit

19. Grating sound of bone fragments rubbing together:
    (a) crepitus
    (b) effussion
    (c) effusion
    (d) creptus

20. Increase in the size of an organ or structure:
    (a) greater trochanter
    (b) hypertrophy
    (c) greater trichanter
    (d) hyprotrophy

21. Large projection at the proximal end of the femur:
    (a) greater trochanter
    (b) hypertrophy
    (c) greater trichanter
    (d) hyprotrophy

22. Movement by a joint that decreases the angle between the two adjoining bones; the bending of a joint:
    (a) abduction
    (b) flixion
    (c) flexion
    (d) abuction

23. Movement of an extremity away from midline:
    (a) abuction
    (b) aduction
    (c) abduction
    (d) adduction

24. Movement of an extremity toward the midline:
    (a) abuction
    (b) aduction
    (c) abduction
    (d) adduction

25. New growth of bony tissue surrounding the bone ends in a fracture; part of the repair process of a fractured bone:
    (a) plantar
    (b) callus
    (c) planter
    (d) calus

26. Normal resiliency of the skin:
    (a) turgor
    (b) trugor
    (c) volar
    (d) volor

27. One of the three muscles that form the buttocks; acts to abduct and rotate the thigh:
    (a) genu varum
    (b) gluteus medius
    (c) ganu varum
    (d) glutus medius

28. Pea-shaped, smallest carpal bone:
    (a) pisiform
    (b) pesiform
    (c) purulence
    (d) prulence

29. A spinous projection off the scapula:
    (a) acromon
    (b) faciculations
    (c) acromion
    (d) fasciculations

30. Pertaining to the palm of the hand or sole of the foot:
    (a) turgor
    (b) trugor
    (c) volar
    (d) volor

31. Reconstructive surgery to repair or reshape a diseased joint:
    (a) arthroscopy
    (b) arthriscropy
    (c) arthroplasty
    (d) arthroplasy

32. Relating to the sole of the foot:
    (a) plantar
    (b) callus
    (c) planter
    (d) calus

NAME _____   DATE _____

CHECK YOUR PROGRESS *(cont'd)*

33. Situated or occurring between bone:
    (a) calcaneus
    (b) interosseous
    (c) clacaneus
    (d) introosseous

34. Spindle-shaped structure that is tapered at both ends:
    (a) fusiform
    (b) fusform
    (c) pisiform
    (d) pesiform

35. Surgical removal of a meniscus:
    (a) menisectomy
    (b) mellelus
    (c) melleolus
    (d) meniscectomy

36. Symptoms of a specific disease:
    (a) asympmatic
    (b) symptomatology
    (c) symptomology
    (d) asymptomatic

37. Bending of a joint toward the posterior aspect of the body:
    (a) dorsiflexion
    (b) flixion
    (c) abduction
    (d) dorsflexion

38. Uncontrolled twitchings of a group of muscle fibers:
    (a) acromon
    (b) faciculations
    (c) acromion
    (d) fasciculations

39. Without symptoms:
    (a) asympmatic
    (b) symptomatology
    (c) symptomology
    (d) asymptomatic

40. Triangular muscle of each side of the upper back:
    (a) metatarsus
    (b) trapezius
    (c) trapezsus
    (d) metatarus

41. Disease of the lymph nodes:
    (a) lymphadenopathy
    (b) lymphenopathy
    (c) lymphedema
    (d) lymphodema

42. Crescent-shaped fibrocartilage in the knee joint:
    (a) meniscus
    (b) malelus
    (c) menscus
    (d) malleolus

43. Long, medial bone of the forearm:
    (a) radius
    (b) radious
    (c) ulna
    (d) unla

44. Any of the five long bones of the foot between the ankle and toes:
    (a) metatarsus
    (b) trapezius
    (c) trapezsus
    (d) metatarus

45. Either of the two rounded projections on either side of the ankle joint:
    (a) meniscus
    (b) malelus
    (c) menscus
    (d) malleolus

46. The heel bone or os calcis:
    (a) colcaneus
    (b) calcaneus
    (c) ulna
    (d) unla

47. Inflammation involving the folds of tissue surrounding the nail:
    (a) synovia
    (b) synomvia
    (c) parychia
    (d) paronychia

48. Trade name for a beta-adrenergic blocker:
    (a) Lopressor
    (b) Percocet
    (c) Lopressar
    (d) Percoset

CHECK YOUR PROGRESS *(cont'd)*

49. Generic name for an antibiotic:
    (a) tetrasysline
    (b) spironolactone
    (c) spironlactone
    (d) tetracycline

50. Trade name for an opioid analgesic:
    (a) Lopressor
    (b) Percocet
    (c) Lopresor
    (d) Percoset

51. Trade name for an antihyperlipidemic:
    (a) Linoxin
    (b) Lipitor
    (c) Lanoxin
    (d) Lippitor

52. Trade name for an antiarrhythmic, cardiotonic:
    (a) Linoxin
    (b) Lipitor
    (c) Lanoxin
    (d) Lippitor

53. Generic name for a corticosteroid:
    (a) codeine
    (b) cortisone
    (c) codenine
    (d) cortisome

54. Generic name for an opioid analgesic:
    (a) codeine
    (b) cortisone
    (c) codenine
    (d) cortisome

55. Trade name for an antiarrhythmic, local anesthetic:
    (a) Xylocaine
    (b) Biaxin
    (c) Baixin
    (d) Xylacane

56. Generic name for a diuretic:
    (a) tetrasysline
    (b) spironolactone
    (c) spironlactone
    (d) tetracycline

57. Trade name for an antibiotic:
    (a) Xylocaine
    (b) Biaxin
    (c) Baixin
    (d) Xylacane

58. Trade name for a narcotic analgesic:
    (a) Keflex
    (b) Keplex
    (c) Vicoprofen
    (d) Vicoprophen

59. Trade name for an antibiotic:
    (a) Keflex
    (b) Keplex
    (c) Vicoprofen
    (d) Vicoprophen

60. Trade name for an anti-inflammatory:
    (a) Dolibid
    (b) Dolobid
    (c) Vicodin
    (d) Vicidin

61. Trade name for a narcotic analgesic:
    (a) Dolibid
    (b) Dolobid
    (c) Vicodin
    (d) Vicidin

62. Generic name for any of a large group of antibacterial antibiotics derived from strains of fungi:
    (a) pencilin
    (b) pennicilin
    (c) penicilin
    (d) penicillin

WORD PROCESSING USERS

Open your word processing package.

Insert the appropriate audiocassette in your transcribing machine and find dictation *6T-2*.

Transcribe and proofread dictation *6T-2*, using the formatting guidelines established in Chapter 2.

Identify and correct all errors.

Save your work on your student disk.

After completing the transcription, refer to the answer key.

Manually complete the error analysis chart.

Manually complete the Production for Pay summary.

SOFTWARE USERS

Click on *Chapter 6, Proofreading Pretest (6T-2)*, and follow the directions.

PROOFREADING

TEXTBOOK USERS

Proofread and correct errors in the medical documents shown in *Activities 6-4 and 6–5*.

Refer to the answer key (Appendix E) for immediate feedback.

Manually complete the error analysis chart for each document.

SOFTWARE USERS

Click on *Chapter 6, Activity 6-4*, and follow the directions.

Follow the same process for *Chapter 6, Activity 6-5*.

ACTIVITY 6-4
Proofreading Worksheet

Directions: Proofread this medical document, which contains multiple errors. Use open punctuation and all other formatting guidelines established in this textbook.

HITORY AND PHYSICAL EXAMINATION REPORT
Winster, Penny
File Number: 41390
Date of birth: March 16, 19xx
Examination Date: *current date*
James P. Osseous, MD
HISTORY:
HISTORY OF PRESENT ILLNESS
I had the pleasure of seeing Penny in the office today. This is a 43 year old right hand dominant woman who saw Dr.Zart for left rotator cuff tendinitis. She has impingment. A MRI shown acromial spur, no sign of a rotator cuff tear. He has an early syst formation. She has undergone two injections. The first did not help. The second seemed to help her for a few days. She has had physical therapy for three months.
PAST MEDICAL HISTORY
Significant for cardiac arhythmia.
MEDICATIONS
She is intermittently on Lopressar. She hasn't always been real compliant with that if she is not having any problems. Allergies: Codine.
REVIEW OF SYMPTOMS
She denies liver or kidney disease. She has had an ulcer in the remote past. She has not had any problems with it recently.
FAMILY HISTORY
$^1/_2$ pack per day smoker for fifteen years.
PHYSICAL EXAMINATION
On examination, this is a welldeveloped woman in no a cute distress. She has full pain less range of motion of her neck. Has has pain in the Neer and Hawkins impingments tests. Active adduction is 135 degrees. Forward flexion is 125 degrees. Passively, I could take her the rest of the way. Her strength is mildly diminished in external rotation, good in internal and abduction. She has a negative lift-off test. She is missing about two levels internal rotation up her back. She has pain with cross chest adduction. There is no pain at the sternoclavicular or AC joint. No clavicular tenderness is noted. Neurovascularly, she is intact.

DIAGNOSTIC TESTS
I reviewed the MRI as above. We got an AP and outlet x-ray which shows a type III acronion.

continued

PROOFREADING

ACTIVITY 6-4 *(cont'd)*
Proofreading Worksheet

HISTORY AND PHYSICAL EXAMINATION REPORT
Winster, Penny
File Number: 41390
Page 2

PLAN
Penny has chronic impingment. We discussed the options. We are going to procede with arthoscopic subacromial decompresion. We discussed the surgery and the risks involved which she understands. All questions were answered and an instruction booklet given. We will schedule this in a timely fashion after appropriate postoperative testing.

James P. Osseous, MD/xx D: 6/28/xx

PROOFREADING

PROOFREADING

Directions: Proofread this medical document, which contains multiple errors. Use open punctuation and all other formatting guidelines established in this textbook.

CHART NOTE
Lucy Smith
DOB: February 28, 19xx
Examination Date: *current date*

SUBJECTIVE
Lucy is an 84 year old female who falled directly onto her right hand yesterday.

OBJECTIVE
She suffered a wrist fracture. She is right hand dominant. He can move his fingers okay and has good perpheral circulation and sensation. T here is considerable echymosis and a little bit of deformity of the wrist. X rays show a reversed Coles or Smith fracture.

ASSESSMENT
Reversed Coles fracture, left wrist.

PLAN
I have proceeded with reduction of the fracture with 1 % Xylocane local anesthesia and have placed her in a sugar tong splint. Post reduction x-rays shows essentially an anatomic reduction. I am going to plan to keep her immobilized for six weeks. I will have her return to the office in one wk for an x-ray throught the cast.

James P. Osseous, M.D

Now you are ready to make the transition from simply proofreading printed material to both transcribing and proofreading dictated material. This is the time to concentrate on building your medical vocabulary, which ultimately will improve your speed and accuracy. There are two activities in this section.

WORD PROCESSING USERS

Open your word processing package.

Insert the appropriate audiocassette in your transcribing machine and find dictation *6T-3*.

Step 1: Listen to the entire dictation to gain an understanding of the medical concepts and terms involved in the report. Rewind the tape to the beginning of the dictation and transcribe what you hear. Do not worry about formatting, style, or speed. Simply type what you hear being dictated, using correct punctuation, capitalization, and spelling. Stop as needed to look up words you do not understand or cannot spell. Adjust the speed control of the transcriber to a comfortable level, starting slowly to ensure no dictated words are missed, and then increase the speed as your accuracy improves.

Step 2: Rewind the tape and transcribe document *6T-3* again, including correct spacing and formatting. Proofread the report. Identify and correct all errors. Save your work on your student disk. Refer to the answer key, and manually complete the error analysis chart and Production for Pay summary.

Follow the same process for dictation *6T-4*.

SOFTWARE USERS

Click on *Chapter 6, Activity 6-6 (6T-3), Step 1,* and follow the directions. When you feel comfortable with the dictation, click on *Chapter 6, Activity 6-6 (6T-3), Step 2,* and follow the directions.

Follow the same process for *Chapter 6, Activity 6-7 (6T-4), Step 1* and *Chapter 6, Activity 6-7 (6T-4), Step 2.*

Let's pause a minute and see how well you are doing. This section allows you to evaluate your success at transcribing and proofreading orthopedic reports.

WORD PROCESSING USERS

Open your word processing package.

Insert the appropriate audiocassette in your transcribing machine and find dictation *6T-2*.

Transcribe and proofread dictation *6T-2*, using the formatting guidelines established in Chapter 2.

Identify and correct all errors.

Save your work on your student disk.

After completing the transcription, refer to the answer key.

Manually complete the error analysis chart.

Manually complete the Production for Pay summary.

SOFTWARE USERS

Click on *Chapter 6, Proofreading Check Your Progress (6T-2)*, and follow the directions.

PROOFREADING

Professional transcriptionists can transcribe and proofread their own work. Can you?

WORD PROCESSING USERS

Open your word processing package.

Insert the appropriate audiocassette in your transcribing machine and find dictation 6T-5.

Transcribe and proofread dictation 6T-5, using the formatting guidelines established in Chapter 2.

Save your work on your student disk.

Identify and correct all errors.

After completing the transcription, refer to the answer key.

Manually complete the error analysis chart.

Manually complete the Production for Pay summary.

Follow the same process for dictation 6T-6.

SOFTWARE USERS

Click on *Chapter 6, Transcription Pretest (6T-5)* and follow the directions.

Follow the same process for *Chapter 6, Transcription Pretest (6T-6)*.

You have been hired as a transcriptionist at FedDes Wellness Center in the orthopedic division. Your supervisor has asked you to transcribe today's dictation.

WORD PROCESSING USERS

Open your word processing package.

Insert the appropriate audiocassette in your transcribing machine and find dictation 6T-7.

Create or use an existing template as necessary for the six types of reports (chart note, chart note using history and physical format, history and physical examination report, x-ray report, procedure report, consultation letter).

Transcribe and proofread dictation 6T-7, using the formatting guidelines established in Chapter 2.

Identify and correct all errors.

Save your work on your student disk.

After completing the transcriptions, refer to the answer key.

Manually complete the error analysis chart.

Manually complete the Production for Pay summary.

Follow the same process for dictations 6T-8 through 6T-19.

SOFTWARE USERS

Click on *Chapter 6, Transcription at FedDes Wellness Center, Dictation 6T-7*, and follow the directions.

Follow the same process for each of the remaining dictations (*6T-8* through *6T-19*).

INDEX OF DICTATIONS AND ASSOCIATED TRANSCRIPTION TIPS

Remember to follow the guidelines pertaining to capitalization, numbers, punctuation, abbreviations, measurements, symbols, and use of templates to create medical reports at FedDes Wellness Center. This material is reviewed in Unit I.

6T-7

X-ray Report
Patient's Name: Mary Ann Dubroy
Ordering Physician: Izzy Sertoli, MD
Physician: Harry A. Medulla, MD

Transcription Tips

- A hyphen is used between numbers and *year old*.
  You hear the dictator say: twenty one old female.
    You transcribe as: 21-year-old female.
- Ordinal numbers are used to indicate order or position in a series rather than quantity. As with all numbers in medical reports, AAMT recommends using numerals (figures): 1st, 2nd, 3rd, etc. This report mentions 5th metacarpal.

6T-8

Chart Note Using History and Physical Format
Patient's Name: Peter Hammer
Physician: James P. Osseous, MD

Transcription Tips

- A hyphen is used when two or more words are viewed as a single word.
    You hear the dictator say: Steri strips were removed.
    You transcribe as: Steri-Strips were removed.
- The hyphenated form, follow-up, is used for the noun and adjective forms. For the verb, the two-word form, follow up, is used.
    Peter returned for follow-up today.
- A hyphen is used between two "like" vowels: re-evaluation.
- Numerals or figures should be used almost exclusively as opposed to spelled-out numbers.
    You hear the dictator say: He started weightbearing approximately nine days ago and felt his cast was very loose.
    You transcribe this sentence as: He started weightbearing approximately 9 days ago and felt his cast was very loose.

6T-9

X-ray Report
Patient's Name: Rachel Winterman
Ordering Physician: Charles P. Davis, MD
Physician: David Treppe, MD

Transcription Tips

- A hyphen is used between numbers and *year old*.
    You hear the dictator say: This is a fifty four year old female
    You transcribe this phrase as: This is a 54-year-old female
- The following new term is dictated in this report:
    Calcaneal (kal-ka-ne-al): pertaining to the irregular quadrangular bone at the back of the tarsus; also called the heel bone and os calcis.

6T-10

X-ray Report
Patient's Name: Lance Newhouse
Ordering Physician: P. H. Waters, MD
Physician: Harry A. Medulla, MD

Transcription Tips

- Ordinal numbers are used to indicate order or position in a series rather than quantity. As with all numbers in medical reports, AAMT recommends using numerals (figures): 4th middle phalanx.
- The following abbreviation is dictated in this report:
    PIP joint: proximal interphalangeal joint, articulation between proximal and middle phalanx
- Words beginning with *pre, re, post*, and *non* are generally not hyphenated: nondisplaced.

6T-11

Chart Note Using History and Physical Format
Patient's Name: Tommy Butger
Physician: David Treppe, MD

Transcription Tips

- Ordinal numbers are used to indicate order or position in a series rather than quantity. As with all numbers in medical reports, AAMT recommends using numerals (figures): 5th metatarsal.
- Words beginning with *pre, re, post*, and *non* are generally not hyphenated: nontender.
- The following term is transcribed as one word: weightbearing (supporting one's own weight).

6T-12

Chart Note Using History and Physical Format
Patient's Name: James Harris
Physician: David Treppe, MD

Transcription Tips

- A hyphen is used to join two or more words when it is used within an adjective clause that precedes a noun. The following word pair is dictated in this report: 8-week.
- Figures are used for measurements and Latin terms.
- Figures are used in ranges and ratios.
- A hyphen is used to take the place of the word *to* or *through* to identify ranges.
- Remember that the figure and the word *degree* must remain on the same line of the chart note.

> You hear the dictator say: Dorsiflexion is ten to fifteen degrees with plantar flexion to twenty-five degrees.
>
> You transcribe as: Dorsiflexion is 10-15 degrees with plantar flexion to 25 degrees.

6T-13

Chart Note Using History and Physical Format
Patient's Name: Patricia Willis
Physician: James P. Osseous, MD

Transcription Tips

- Ordinal numbers are used to indicate order or position in a series rather than quantity. As with all numbers in medical reports, AAMT recommends using numerals (figures): 1st dorsal interosseous, 2nd metacarpal.
- A hyphen is used with words beginning with *ex* and *self*: self-referred.
- The following new term is dictated in this report:
  > lipomatous (li-<u>po</u>-mah-tus): affected with or of the nature of lipoma
- The following acronym is dictated in this report. Remember that acronyms are typed in all capital letters.
  > MRI: magnetic resonance imaging

6T-14

History and Physical Examination in Letter Format
Patient's Name: Juan Rodriquez
Physician: Harry A. Medulla, MD
Inside Address: John Mastersetti, MD, Pleasantville Family Health, 792 West Walnut Street, Westerville, OH 78910

Transcription Tips

- In order for this letter to fit on one page, leave only 2 blank lines between the dateline and the inside address and 2 blank lines separating the last line of text and the signature block.
- The following abbreviations are dictated in this report and are keyed in all capital letters:
  > I&D: incision and drainage
  > ER: emergency room
  > DIP joint: distal interphalangeal joint, articulation between middle and distal phalanx
- A hyphen is used to join two or more words when they are used within an adjective clause that precedes a noun. The following word pair is dictated in this report: right-hand.
- Latin abbreviations are expressed in lowercase letters with periods: p.o. (per os, by mouth).
- Capitalize the name of specific departments or sections in a hospital or institution.
  > You hear the dictator say: He was seen in the county hospital emergency room.
  > You transcribe this sentence as: He was seen in the County Hospital Emergency Room.

6T-15

Chart Note Using History and Physical Format
Patient's Name: William Grant
Physician: Harry A. Medulla, MD

Transcription Tips

- The following term is transcribed as two words: a lot.
- The following is a troublesome spelling term: posteromedial.
- The term *status post* means *after the condition* and may be abbreviated as *S/P*.
- The following abbreviation is dictated in this report: MCL: medial collateral ligament
- A hyphen is used between two "like" vowels: re-evaluation.

6T-16

Chart Note Using History and Physical Format
Patient's Name: John Phillips
Physician: Harry A. Medulla, MD

Transcription Tips

- The following medication is dictated in this report:
  > Vicodin: trade name for an opioid analgesic
- The following acronym is dictated in this report. Remember that acronyms are typed in all capital letters.

MRI: magnetic resonance imaging
- The following abbreviation is dictated in this report:
  AP: directional term for anterior to posterior
- A hyphen is used between two "like" vowels: re-evaluation.

6T-17

History and Physical Examination Report
Patient's Name: Sam Evertson
Physician: Harry A. Medulla, MD

Transcription Tips

- The following are new terms:
  Radiation (ra-de-<u>a</u>-shun) is the divergence of pain from the site of injury to other areas of the body.
  Impingement is an abnormal contact or pressure between two structures.
- Figures are used for age, weight, height, blood pressure, pulse, and respiration.
  You hear the dictator say: Blood pressure one hundred twelve over seventy-four pulse sixty-four and regular respirations sixteen per minute.
  You transcribe as: BP 112/74, pulse 64 and regular, respirations 16/min.
- The following abbreviation is dictated in this report.
  AC joint: acromioclavicular joint, articulation between acromion and clavicle
- A hyphen is used to join two or more words when used as an adjective that precedes a noun: 3-month.
- The following drug is dictated in this report:
  penicillin: the generic name for any of the large group of natural or semisynthetic antibacterial antibiotics

6T-18

History and Physical Examination Report
Patient's Name: Jerry Madison
Physicians: James P. Osseous, MD; Enrique Hernandez, MD

Transcription Tips

- A hyphen is used to join two or more words when used as an adjective that precedes a noun: light-duty, 2-week, follow-up.
- Capitalize eponyms. Eponyms are surnames teamed with a disease, instrument, or surgical procedure. The following eponym is dictated in this report: Achilles reflexes.

- An apostrophe is used to form the possessive of singular and plural nouns.
  You hear the dictator say: I reviewed the patients x rays.
  You transcribe as: I reviewed the patient's x-rays.
- The following drugs are dictated in this report:
  Vicoprofen: trade name for an opioid analgesic
  Dolobid: trade name for an NSAID, a nonsteroidal anti-inflammatory drug
- Latin abbreviations are expressed in lowercase letters with periods: b.i.d. (bis in die, twice a day).
- Figures are used for measurements and Latin terms. No period follows metric abbreviations unless the abbreviation ends a sentence.
  You hear the dictator say: I have changed his prescription to Dolobid five hundred milligrams to be taken on a b eye d basis.
  You transcribe as: I have changed his prescription to Dolobid 500 mg to be taken on a b.i.d. basis.
- The following procedure is dictated in this report:
  Valsalva (val-<u>sal</u>-vah) maneuver is an attempt to exhale forcibly with the glottis, nose, and mouth closed.
- Figures are used with the + or − symbols.
- Reflexes are usually graded on a scale from zero to four plus as follows: 4+ is very brisk and may indicate disease; 3+ is brisker than average but not necessarily indicative of disease; 2+ is normal; 1+ is low normal; and 0 is no response and may indicate neuropathy.
  You hear the dictator say: He had two plus and symmetric patella as well as Achilles reflexes.
  You transcribe as: He had 2+ and symmetric patella as well as Achilles reflexes.
- Figures and capital letters are used to refer to the vertebral column and spinal nerves.
  You hear the dictator say: There is evidence of discogenic abnormality at L four through five.
  You transcribe as: There is evidence of discogenic abnormality at L4-5.
- Figures are used almost exclusively as opposed to spelled-out numbers to improve clarity and avoid potential mistakes.
  You hear the dictator say: The patient smokes two packs per day and has done so for twenty-four years.
  You transcribe as: The patient smokes 2 packs per day and has done so for 24 years.

TRANSCRIPTION

History and Physical Examination Using Letter Format

Patient's Name: Clara B. Jackson

Physician: James P. Osseous, MD

Inside Address: Peter R. Desman, MD, Orange Hill Family Practice, 214 Orchard Road, Brooklyn, NY 11245

Transcription Tips

- Figures are used for measurements and Latin terms. No period follows metric abbreviations unless the abbreviation ends a sentence: p.r.n. (pro re nata, as circumstances may require).
- A hyphen is used to join two or more words when used as an adjective that precedes a noun: follow-up.
- The following procedure is dictated in this report:
  lupus test: used to determine lupus vulgaris or lupus erythematosus

Professional transcriptionists can transcribe and proofread their own work with speed and accuracy. Have you mastered the orthopedic transcription rotation at FedDes Wellness Center?

WORD PROCESSING USERS

Open your word processing package.

Insert the appropriate audiocassette in your transcribing machine and find dictation *6T-5*.

Transcribe and proofread dictation *6T-5*, using the formatting guidelines established in Chapter 2.

Save your work on your student disk.

Identify and correct all errors.

After completing the transcriptions, refer to the answer key.

Manually complete the error analysis chart for each document.

Manually complete the Production for Pay summary for each document.

Follow the same process for dictation *6T-6*.

SOFTWARE USERS

Click on *Chapter 6, Transcription Check Your Progress (6T-5)*, and follow the directions.

Follow the same process for *Chapter 6, Transcription Check Your Progress (6T-6)*.

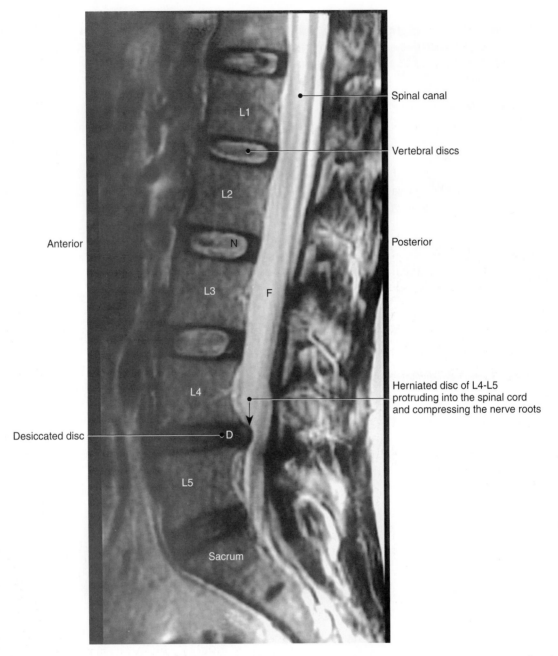

Figure 6-1 Lumbar spine. *(From Ballinger PW, Frank ED:* Merrill's atlas of radiographic positions and radiologic procedures, *ed 10, St Louis, 2003, Mosby.)*

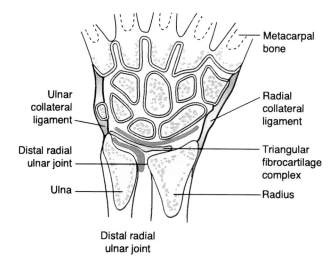

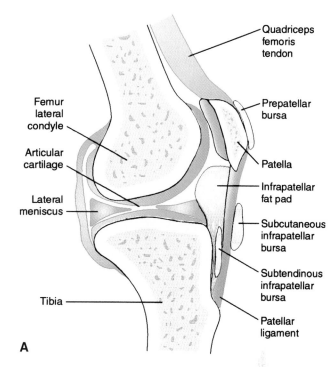

Figure 6-2 Coronal view of wrist with ligaments.

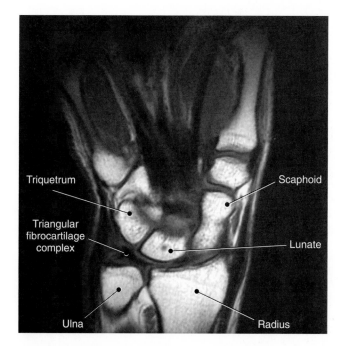

Figure 6-3 Coronal magnetic resonance (MR) scan of wrist. *(From Kelley LL, Peterson CM: Sectional anatomy for imaging professionals, St Louis, 1966, ed 9, Mosby.)*

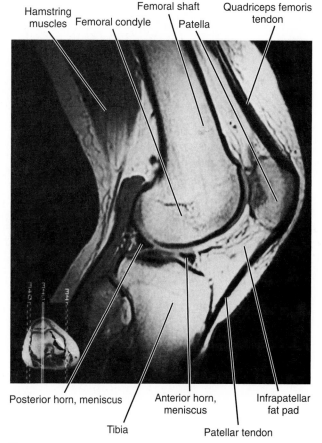

Figure 6-4 A, Sagittal view of knee. **B**, Sagittal magnetic resonance (MR) scan of knee. *(B from Kelley LL, Petersen CM: Sectional anatomy for imaging professionals, St Louis, 1996, Mosby.)*

Chapter 7

Office Medical Transcription from the Urology Practice

OBJECTIVES

At the completion of Chapter 7, you should be able to do the following:
1. Match medical terms associated with the urology specialty with their definitions.
2. Spell medical terms associated with the urology specialty.
3. Transcribe medical terms in sentence structure.
4. Proofread, edit, and correct medical documents associated with the urology specialty that contain various errors.
5. Transcribe and proofread authentic medical documents associated with the urology specialty.

INTRODUCTION TO THE UROLOGY ROTATION

What's Ahead

The FedDes Wellness Center has three urologists (specialists in urology) on staff. *Urology* is the study of the urinary tract in both women and men. The urologist treats male patients for problems with the urogenital system, which includes the male sexual organs.

In this unit, you assume the role of a medical transcriptionist employed at FedDes Wellness Center. **Please remember to follow the guidelines pertaining to capitalization, numbers, punctuation, abbreviations, measurements, symbols, and use of templates to create medical reports at FedDes Wellness Center.** This material is reviewed in Unit I. The transcription exercises list the type of report, patient's name, and physician(s) as well as the associated transcription tips.

You will work with the textbook and CD-ROM or accompanying audiocassettes. Your mastery of urology transcription is assessed through worksheets, timed transcription exercises, the error analysis chart, and the Production for Pay summary.

All answer keys are found in the textbook (Appendix E) and CD-ROM, providing immediate feedback. After transcribing a report, you will proofread your work and correct any errors. Then you will compare your proofread work against a master transcript, categorize all errors, and tabulate the errors on the error analysis chart. The Production for Pay summary correlates your production to the FedDes Wellness Center pay scale. The scale is also linked to your grade. This system allows you to assess your mastery of transcription skills in a real-world scenario.

Let's find out if you can define and spell selected terminology and drugs of the urology specialty that are included in this chapter.

TEXTBOOK USERS

Select the correctly spelled term that matches its definition.
Refer to the answer key (Appendix E) for immediate feedback.

SOFTWARE USERS

Click on *Chapter 7, Terminology Pretest*, and follow the directions.

NAME _____   DATE _____

PRETEST

Directions: Select the correctly spelled term that matches its definition.

1. Generic name for a bactericidal antibiotic:
   (a) bacitracin
   (b) bactracine
   (c) meclizine
   (d) mecizine

2. A colorless blood corpuscle:
   (a) occlude
   (b) oclude
   (c) leukocyte
   (d) leuocyte

3. A cystoscope that gives a wide-angle view of the bladder:
   (a) syncope
   (b) synscope
   (c) pandoscope
   (d) panendoscope

4. A discharge or escape of fluid from a vessel into the tissues:
   (a) extravasation
   (b) extrevasation
   (c) fulguration
   (d) fulgeration

5. Generic name for a diuretic, antihypertensive agent:
   (a) hydrochlorozide
   (b) hydrochlorothiazide
   (c) hydrocele
   (d) hydrosele

6. A diagnostic x-ray study of kidneys, ureter, and bladder:
   (a) nephrogram
   (b) nepherogram
   (c) urogram
   (d) urologram

7. A herniation of part of the rectum into the vagina:
   (a) cystocele
   (b) cystosele
   (c) rectosele
   (d) rectocele

8. A hollow or depressed area:
   (a) fossa
   (b) fosa
   (c) meatus
   (d) metus

9. A normal alkaline constituent of urine and blood:
   (a) creatinine
   (b) creatine
   (c) incontinence
   (d) incontinance

10. An accumulation of fluid in a sac-like cavity:
    (a) hydrosele
    (b) hydrocele
    (c) urethrosele
    (d) urethrocele

11. A radiograph of an artery:
    (a) arterogram
    (b) arterigram
    (c) arteriogram
    (d) arteiogram

12. A sac or pouch in the walls of a canal or organ:
    (a) verumontanum
    (b) verumonum
    (c) diverticulum
    (d) diverticum

13. A seam or ridge noting the line of junction of halves of a part:
    (a) coapte
    (b) coapt
    (c) rafe
    (d) raphe

14. A skin discoloration caused by a hemorrhage:
    (a) hydronephrosis
    (b) hydronphrosis
    (c) ecchymosis
    (d) echymosis

15. A small beam or supporting structure:
    (a) trabeculation
    (b) traculation
    (c) concomitant
    (d) concommitant

16. A triangular area:
    (a) staghorn
    (b) staghorne
    (c) trigon
    (d) trigone

17. Above the pubis:
    (a) periumbilical
    (b) supraumbilical
    (c) suprapubic
    (d) peripubic

18. An abnormal concretion, stone:
    (a) calculus
    (b) calcus
    (c) coudé
    (d) coudus'

19. Generic name for an angiotensin-converting enzyme inhibitor:
    (a) captopril
    (b) amoxicillin
    (c) catopril
    (d) amoxcillin

20. Generic name for an antibiotic:
    (a) captopril
    (b) amoxicillin
    (c) catopril
    (d) amoxcillin

21. Generic name for an antiemetic, antihistamine, motion sickness relief:
    (a) bacitracin
    (b) bactracine
    (c) meclizine
    (d) mecizine

22. An endoscope especially designed for passing through the urethra into the bladder:
    (a) cystoscope
    (b) cystourethroscope
    (c) cystscope
    (d) cystourescope

23. An incision of a duct or organ for the removal of calculi:
    (a) laminectomy
    (b) laminotomy
    (c) lithotomy
    (d) lithectomy

24. An instrument for examining the posterior urethra and bladder:
    (a) cystoscope
    (b) cystourethroscope
    (c) cystscope
    (d) cystourescope

25. An instrument placed in the vagina to support the uterus or rectum:
    (a) pessary
    (b) pesary
    (c) pissary
    (d) pisary

26. An opening:
    (a) fossa
    (b) fosa
    (c) meatus
    (d) metus

27. Around the umbilicus:
    (a) periumbilical
    (b) supraumbilical
    (c) suprapubic
    (d) peripubic

28. Bent or elbowed:
    (a) calculus
    (b) calcus
    (c) coudé
    (d) coudus'

29. Labored or difficult breathing:
    (a) dispnea
    (b) dyspnea
    (c) diuresis
    (d) dyuresis

30. Pertaining to the atrium and ventricle of the heart:
    (a) vas deferens
    (b) atriventricular
    (c) vas defens
    (d) atrioventricular

TERMINOLOGY

PRETEST *(cont'd)*

31. Pertaining to the genitalia and urinary organs:
    (a) genitorinary
    (b) genitourinary
    (c) pyruia
    (d) pyuria

32. Pus in the urine:
    (a) genitorinary
    (b) genitourinary
    (c) pyruia
    (d) pyuria

33. Taking place at the same time:
    (a) trabeculation
    (b) traculation
    (c) concomitant
    (d) concommitant

34. A calculus of the renal pelvis usually extending into multiple calices:
    (a) staghorn
    (b) staghorne
    (c) trigon
    (d) trigone

35. Removal of the gallbladder:
    (a) cholecystectomy
    (b) cystometrography
    (c) chocystectomy
    (d) cystorography

36. Destruction of living tissue by electric sparks generated by a high-frequency current:
    (a) extravasation
    (b) extrevasation
    (c) fulguration
    (d) fulgeration

37. Discharge of blood in the urine:
    (a) heme
    (b) hematuria
    (c) heman
    (d) hemeturia

38. Distention of the renal pelvis and calices with urine:
    (a) hydronephrosis
    (b) hydronphrosis
    (c) ecchymosis
    (d) echymosis

39. Elevation on the floor of the prostatic portion of the urethra where the seminal ducts enter:
    (a) verumontanum
    (b) verumonum
    (c) diverticulum
    (d) diverticum

40. The essential elements of an organ:
    (a) perenchyma
    (b) parenchyma
    (c) bardycardia
    (d) bradycardia

41. To cut a portion of a tissue or organ:
    (a) flank
    (b) flanke
    (c) desect
    (d) resect

42. Excision of one or both ovaries:
    (a) oophorectomy
    (b) colporrhaphy
    (c) ophorectomy
    (d) colporhaphy

43. The excretory duct of the testis:
    (a) vas deferens
    (b) atriventricular
    (c) vas defens
    (d) atrioventricular

44. X-ray study of the renal pelvis and ureters:
    (a) pyelogram
    (b) pylegram
    (c) cystorograph
    (d) cystumetrogram

45. The graphic record of the pressure in the bladder at varying stages of filling:
    (a) cholecystectomy
    (b) cystometrography
    (c) chocystectomy
    (d) urogram

46. Herniation of the urinary bladder into the vagina:
    (a) cystocele
    (b) cystosele
    (c) rectosele
    (d) rectocele

PRETEST *(cont'd)*

47. The inability to control excretory functions:
    (a) creatinine
    (b) creatine
    (c) incontinence
    (d) incontinance

48. Increased excretion of urine:
    (a) dispneic
    (b) dyspneic
    (c) diuresis
    (d) dyuresis

49. Inflammation of the gallbladder:
    (a) cystitis
    (b) cystisis
    (c) cholcystitis
    (d) cholecystitis

50. Inflammation of the kidney and renal pelvis:
    (a) urethrogonitis
    (b) urethrotrigonitis
    (c) pyelonephritis
    (d) pyelonphritis

51. Inflammation of the urethra and trigone of the bladder:
    (a) urethrogonitis
    (b) urethrotrigonitis
    (c) pyelonephritis
    (d) pyelonphritis

52. Inflammation of the urinary bladder:
    (a) cystitis
    (b) cystisis
    (c) cholcystitis
    (d) cholecystitis

53. The nonprotein, insoluble, iron constituent of hemoglobin:
    (a) heme
    (b) hematuria
    (c) heman
    (d) hemeturia

54. The penis:
    (a) fallus
    (b) fallis
    (c) phalus
    (d) phallus

55. Poisoning from retained and absorbed urinary substances:
    (a) urosepsis
    (b) urethrocele
    (c) urethepsis
    (d) urothcele

56. Prolapse of the female urethra through the urinary meatus:
    (a) urosepsis
    (b) urethrocele
    (c) urethepsis
    (d) urothcele

57. The side of the body between the ribs and ilium:
    (a) flank
    (b) flanke
    (c) desect
    (d) resect

58. Slowness of the heartbeat:
    (a) perenchyma
    (b) parenchyma
    (c) bardycardia
    (d) bradycardia

59. The supply of vessels to a specific region:
    (a) vasculature
    (b) vaculature
    (c) nephrectomy
    (d) neprectomy

60. Surgical excision of the lamina:
    (a) laminectomy
    (b) laminotomy
    (c) lithotomy
    (d) lithectomy

61. Surgical removal of the kidney:
    (a) vasculature
    (b) vaculature
    (c) nephrectomy
    (d) neprectomy

62. Suturing of the vagina:
    (a) oophorectomy
    (b) colporrhaphy
    (c) ophorectomy
    (d) colporhaphy

TERMINOLOGY

PRETEST *(cont'd)*

63. Temporary suspension of consciousness; fainting:
    (a) syncope
    (b) synscope
    (c) pandoscope
    (d) panendoscope

64. To bring together, as in suturing a laceration:
    (a) coapte
    (b) coapt
    (c) rafe
    (d) raphe

65. To close tight:
    (a) occlude
    (b) oclude
    (c) leukocyte
    (d) leuocyte

66. Trade name for a diuretic:
    (a) Calen
    (b) Calan
    (c) Aldatone
    (d) Aldactone

67. Trade name for a diuretic, antiglaucoma agent:
    (a) Neptazane
    (b) Netazane
    (c) Noroxin
    (d) Norxin

68. Trade name for an antibacterial, urinary tract anti-infective:
    (a) Neptazane
    (b) Netazane
    (c) Noroxin
    (d) Norxin

69. Trade name for an antibacterial, antibiotic:
    (a) Maxquine
    (b) Maxaquin
    (c) Lopressor
    (d) Lopressar

70. Trade name for an antibacterial, antibiotic:
    (a) Ciprro
    (b) Cipro
    (c) Cardura
    (d) Carduro

71. Trade name for an antiarrhythmic, anesthetic:
    (a) Xylocine
    (b) Perpine
    (c) Propine
    (d) Xylocaine

72. Trade name for a nonsteroidal anti-inflammatory drug; analgesic for acute, moderately severe pain:
    (a) Toradol
    (b) Torodol
    (c) Tolinase
    (d) Tolenase

73. Trade name for a topical antiglaucoma agent:
    (a) Timoptic
    (b) Timptic
    (c) Trimpix
    (d) Trimpex

74. Trade name for an antianginal, antiarrhythmic, antihypertensive:
    (a) Calen
    (b) Calan
    (c) Aldatone
    (d) Aldactone

75. Trade name for an antianginal, antihypertensive:
    (a) Maxquine
    (b) Maxaquin
    (c) Lopressor
    (d) Lopressar

76. Trade name for an antidiarrheal:
    (a) Imadium
    (b) Imodium
    (c) Emadium
    (d) Emodium

77. Trade name for an antiglaucoma agent; eye drops:
    (a) Xylocine
    (b) Perpine
    (c) Propine
    (d) Xylocaine

78. Trade name for an antihypertensive, antiadrenergic:
    (a) Ciprro
    (b) Cipro
    (c) Cardura
    (d) Carduro

PRETEST *(cont'd)*

79. Trade name for an antibacterial, antibiotic:
    (a) Timoptic
    (b) Timptic
    (c) Trimpix
    (d) Trimpex

80. Trade name for an antibiotic:
    (a) Bactrim
    (b) Betadine
    (c) Backrim
    (d) Betdine

81. Trade name for a topical antibacterial, antiseptic:
    (a) Bactrim
    (b) Betadine
    (c) Backrim
    (d) Betdine

82. Trade name for an antidiabetic agent:
    (a) Toradol
    (b) Torodol
    (c) Tolinase
    (d) Tolenase

Let's learn to spell and define selected terminology and drugs of the urology specialty that are included in this chapter. Keyboarding these terms is an effective way to improve your skills.

WORD PROCESSING USERS

Open your word processing package.
Read and type each word and its definition as shown below.
Save your work on your student disk.

1. Amoxicillin (ah-moks-i-<u>sil</u>-in) is a generic name for an antibiotic.
2. Arteriogram (ar-<u>te</u>-re-o-gram) is a radiograph of an artery.
3. Atrioventricular (a-tre-o-ven-<u>trik</u>-u-lar) pertains to the atrium and the ventricle of the heart.
4. Bacitracin (bas-i-<u>tra</u>-sin) is a generic name for an antibacterial.
5. Bradycardia (brad-e-<u>kar</u>-de-ah) is the slowness of the heartbeat.
6. Calculus (<u>kal</u>-ku-lus) is an abnormal concretion, stone.
7. Captopril (<u>kap</u>-to-pril) is a generic name for an angiotensin-converting enzyme inhibitor.
8. Cholecystectomy (ko-le-sis-<u>tec</u>-to-me) is the removal of the gallbladder.
9. Cholecystitis (ko-le-sis-<u>ti</u>-tis) is inflammation of the gallbladder.
10. Coapt (ko-<u>apt</u>) is to bring together, as in suturing a laceration.
11. Colporrhaphy (kol-<u>por</u>-ah-fe) is the suturing of the vagina.
12. Concomitant (kon-<u>kom</u>-I-tant) means taking place at the same time.
13. Coudé (<u>koo</u>-dae) is bent or elbowed.
14. Creatinine (kre-<u>at</u>-i-nin) is a normal alkaline constituent of urine and blood.
15. Cystitis (sis-<u>ti</u>-tis) is inflammation of the urinary bladder.
16. Cystocele (<u>sis</u>-to-sel) is herniation of the urinary bladder into the vagina.
17. Cystometrography (sis-to-me-<u>trog</u>-ra-fe) is the graphic record of the pressure in the bladder at varying stages of filling.
18. Cystoscope (<u>sis</u>-to-skop) is an endoscope especially designed to permit visual inspection of the interior of the bladder.

19. Cystourethroscope (sis-to-u-<u>re</u>-thro-skop) is an instrument for examining the posterior urethra and bladder.
20. Diuresis (di-u-<u>re</u>-sis) is an increased excretion of urine.
21. Diverticulum (di-ver-<u>tik</u>-u-lum) is a sac or pouch in the walls of a canal or organ.
22. Dyspneic (disp-<u>ne</u>-ic) pertains to labored or difficult breathing.
23. Ecchymosis (ek-i-<u>mo</u>-sis) is a skin discoloration caused by a hemorrhage.
24. Extravasation (eks-trav-ah-<u>za</u>-shun) is a discharge or escape of fluid from a vessel into the tissues.
25. Flank is the side of the body between the ribs and ilium.
26. Fossa (<u>fos</u>-ah) is a hollow or depressed area.
27. Fulguration (ful-gu-<u>ra</u>-shun) is the destruction of living tissue by electric sparks generated by a high-frequency current.
28. Genitourinary (<u>jen</u>-i-to-<u>u</u>-ri-ner-e) pertains to the genitalia and urinary organs.
29. Hematuria (hem-ah-<u>tu</u>-re-ah) is the discharge of blood in the urine.
30. Heme (hem) is the nonprotein, insoluble, iron constituent of hemoglobin.
31. Hydrocele (<u>hi</u>-dro-sel) is the accumulation of fluid in a sac-like cavity.
32. Hydrochlorothiazide (hi-dro-klor-o-<u>thi</u>-ah-zid) is a generic name for a diuretic and antihypertensive agent.
33. Hydronephrosis (hi-dro-ne-<u>fro</u>-sis) is the distention of the renal pelvis and calices with urine.
34. Incontinence (in-<u>kon</u>-ti-nens) is the inability to control excretory functions.
35. Laminectomy (lam-i-<u>nek</u>-to-me) is the surgical excision of the lamina.
36. Leukocyte (<u>loo</u>-ko-site) is a colorless blood corpuscle.
37. Lithotomy (li-<u>thot</u>-o-me) is an incision of a duct or organ for the removal of calculi.
38. Meatus (me-<u>a</u>-tus) is an opening.
39. Meclizine (<u>mek</u>-li-zen) is a generic name for an antiemetic, antihistamine, and agent for motion sickness relief.
40. Nephrectomy (ne-<u>frek</u>-to-me) is the surgical removal of the kidney.
41. Occlude (o-<u>klood</u>) is to close tight.
42. Oophorectomy (o-of-o-<u>rek</u>-to-me) is the excision of one or both ovaries.

43. Panendoscope (pan-en-do-skop) is a cystoscope that gives a wide-angle view of the bladder.
44. Parenchyma (pah-reng-ki-mah) are the essential elements of an organ.
45. Periumbilical (per-e-um-bil-i-kal) is around the umbilicus.
46. Pessary (pes-ah-re) is an instrument placed in the vagina to support the uterus or rectum.
47. Phallus (fal-us) is the penis.
48. Pyelogram (pi-e-lo-gram) is an x-ray study of the renal pelvis and ureters.
49. Pyelonephritis (pi-e-lo-ne-fri-tis) is inflammation of the kidney and renal pelvis.
50. Pyuria (pi-u-re-ah) is pus in the urine.
51. Raphe (ra-fe) is a seam or ridge noting the line of junction of halves of a part.
52. Rectocele (rek-to-sel) is a hernia protrusion of part of the rectum into the vagina.
53. Resect (re-sekt) is to cut off or cut out a portion of a tissue or organ.
54. Staghorn (stag-horn) is the calculus of the renal pelvis usually extending into multiple calices.
55. Suprapubic (soo-prah-pu-bik) is above the pubis.
56. Syncope (sing-ko-pe) is the temporary suspension of consciousness; fainting.
57. Trabeculation (trah-bek-u-la-shun) is a small beam or supporting structure.
58. Trigone (tri-gon) is a triangular area.
59. Urethrocele (u-re-thro-sel) is the prolapse of the female urethra through the urinary meatus.
60. Urethrotrigonitis (u-re-thro-tri-go-ni-tis) is the inflammation of the urethra and trigone of the bladder.
61. Urogram (u-ro-gram) is a diagnostic x-ray study of the kidneys, ureters, and bladder.
62. Urosepsis (u-ro-sep-sis) is the poisoning from retained and absorbed urinary substances.
63. Vas deferens (vas def-er-ens) is the excretory duct of the testis.
64. Vasculature (vas-ku-lah-tur) is the supply of vessels to a specific region.

65. Verumontanum (ver-oo-mon-ta-num) is the elevation on the floor of the prostatic portion of the urethra where the seminal ducts enter.
66. Aldactone (al-dak-ton) is the trade name for a diuretic.
67. Bactrim (bak-trim) is the trade name for an antibiotic.
68. Betadine (bat-ah-dine) is the trade name for a topical antibacterial and antiseptic.
69. Calan (kal-an) is the trade name for an antianginal, antiarrhythmic, and antihypertensive.
70. Cardura (kar-du-rah) is the trade name for an antihypertensive and antiadrenergic.
71. Cipro (si-pro) is the trade name for a fluoroquinolone antibiotic and antibacterial.
72. Imodium (i-mo-de-um) is the trade name for an antidiarrheal.
73. Lopressor (lo-pres-or) is the trade name for an antianginal and antihypertensive.
74. Maxaquin (mak-sa-kwin) is the trade name for a fluoroquinolone antibiotic and antibacterial.
75. Neptazane (nep-ta-zan) is the trade name for a diuretic and antiglaucoma agent.
76. Noroxin (nor-ok-sin) is the trade name for an antibacterial and urinary tract anti-infective.
77. Propine (pro-pine) is the trade name for an antiglaucoma agent; eye drops.
78. Timoptic (tim-op-tik) is the trade name for a topical antiglaucoma agent.
79. Tolinase (tol-i-nas) is the trade name for an antidiabetic agent.
80. Toradol (tor-a-dol) is the trade name for a nonsteroidal anti-inflammatory drug and analgesic for acute, moderately severe pain.
81. Trimpex (trimp-eks) is the trade name for an antibacterial and antibiotic.
82. Xylocaine (zi-lo-kan) is the trade name for an anesthetic and antiarrhythmic.
83. Guaiac (gwi-ak) is a reagent used in tests for occult blood.

TERMINOLOGY

Do you remember back in school when you had to write each spelling word ten times? Because you had to physically write each word, your mind and body were focused on the assignment, and the method worked. Let's follow this successful method by reinforcing the spelling of selected terms and drugs found in the urology specialty through keyboarding drills.

WORD PROCESSING USERS

Open your word processing package.
Read, mentally spell, and type each word in its sequence.
Save your work on your student disk.

1. amoxicillin arteriogram atrioventricular amoxicillin arteriogram atrioventricular
2. bacitracin bradycardia calculus bacitracin bradycardia calculus bacitracin bradycardia
3. captopril cholecystectomy cholecystitis captopril cholecystectomy cholecystitis
4. coapt colporrhaphy concomitant coapt colporrhaphy concomitant coapt colporrhaphy
5. coudé creatinine cystitis coudé creatinine cystitis coudé creatinine cystitis coudé
6. cystocele cystometrography cystoscope cystocele cystometrography cystoscope
7. cystourethroscope diuresis diverticulum cystourethroscope diuresis diverticulum
8. dyspneic ecchymosis extravasation dyspneic ecchymosis extravasation dyspneic
9. flank fossa fulguration flank fossa fulguration flank fossa fulguration flank fossa
10. genitourinary hematuria heme genitourinary hematuria heme genitourinary hematuria
11. hydrocele hydrochlorothiazide hydronephrosis hydrocele hydrochlorothiazide
12. incontinence laminectomy leukocytes incontinence laminectomy leukocytes
13. lithotomy meatus meclizine lithotomy meatus meclizine lithotomy meatus meclizine
14. nephrectomy occlude oophorectomy nephrectomy occlude oophorectomy occlude
15. panendoscope parenchyma periumbilical panendoscope parenchyma periumbilical
16. pessary phallus pyelogram pessary phallus pyelogram pessary phallus pyelogram
17. pyelonephritis pyuria raphe pyelonephritis pyuria raphe pyelonephritis pyuria raphe
18. rectocele resect staghorn rectocele resect staghorn rectocele resect staghorn rectocele
19. suprapubic syncope trabeculation suprapubic syncope trabeculation suprapubic
20. trigone urethrocele urethrotrigonitis trigone urethrocele urethrotrigonitis trigone
21. urogram urosepsis vas deferens urogram urosepsis vas deferens urogram urosepsis
22. vasculature verumontanum vasculature verumontanum vasculature verumontanum
23. Aldactone Bactrim Betadine Aldactone Bactrim Betadine Aldactone Bactrim
24. Calan Cardura Cipro Calan Cardura Cipro Calan Cardura Cipro Calan Cardura Cipro
25. Imodium Lopressor Maxaquin Imodium Lopressor Maxaquin Imodium Lopressor
26. Neptazane Noroxin Propine Neptazane Noroxin Propine Neptazane Noroxin Propine
27. Timoptic Tolinase Toradol Timoptic Tolinase Toradol Timoptic Tolinase Toradol
28. Trimpex Xylocaine Trimpex Xylocaine Trimpex Xylocaine Trimpex Xylocaine

Activity 7-3

Transcribing Medical Sentences

Now you are ready to make the transition from keyboarding medical terms, which is a visual process, to transcribing medical terms, an aural process. You are going to use audiocassette tapes or your CD-ROM rather than printed material. Sentences 74 and 79 contain dangerous abbreviations and need to be transcribed according to the guidelines established in this textbook and the recommendations of *The AAMT Book of Style*, Appendix B.

WORD PROCESSING USERS

Open your word processing package.

Insert the appropriate audiocassette in your transcribing machine and find dictation *7T-1*.

You will be transcribing spelling words in sentence structure.

Listen carefully to each sentence on the audiocassette before transcribing.

Rewind and type (transcribe) the sentences.

Save your work on your student disk.

Refer to the answer key (Appendix E) for immediate feedback.

SOFTWARE USERS

Click on *Chapter 7, Terminology Activity 7-3 (7T-1)*, and follow the directions.

Check Your Progress

Let's pause a minute and see how well you are doing. This section allows you to evaluate your mastery of keyboarding and spelling of selected terms and drugs found in the family practice specialty.

TEXTBOOK USERS

Select the correctly spelled term that matches its definition.
Refer to the answer key (Appendix E) for immediate feedback.

SOFTWARE USERS

Click on *Chapter 7, Terminology Check Your Progress*, and follow the directions.

CHECK YOUR PROGRESS

Directions: Select the correctly spelled term that matches its definition.

1. Generic name for a bactericidal antibiotic:
   (a) bacitracin
   (b) bactracine
   (c) meclizine
   (d) mecizine

2. A colorless blood corpuscle:
   (a) occlude
   (b) oclude
   (c) leukocyte
   (d) leuocyte

3. A cystoscope that gives a wide-angle view of the bladder:
   (a) syncope
   (b) synscope
   (c) pandoscope
   (d) panendoscope

4. A discharge or escape of fluid from a vessel into the tissues:
   (a) extravasation
   (b) extrevasation
   (c) fulguration
   (d) fulgeration

5. Generic name for a diuretic, antihypertensive agent:
   (a) hydrochlorozide
   (b) hydrochlorothiazide
   (c) hydrocele
   (d) hydrosele

6. A diagnostic x-ray study of kidneys, ureters, and bladder:
   (a) nephrogram
   (b) nepherogram
   (c) urogram
   (d) urologram

7. A hernia protrusion of part of the rectum into the vagina:
   (a) cystocele
   (b) cystosele
   (c) rectosele
   (d) rectocele

8. A hollow or depressed area:
   (a) fossa
   (b) fosa
   (c) meatus
   (d) metus

9. A normal alkaline constituent of urine and blood:
   (a) creatinine
   (b) creatine
   (c) incontinence
   (d) incontinance

10. An accumulation of fluid in a sac-like cavity:
    (a) hydrosele
    (b) hydrocele
    (c) urethrosele
    (d) urethrocele

11. A radiograph of an artery:
    (a) arterogram
    (b) arterigram
    (c) arteriogram
    (d) arteiogram

12. A sac or pouch in the walls of a canal or organ:
    (a) verumontanum
    (b) verumonum
    (c) diverticulum
    (d) diverticum

13. A seam or ridge noting the line of junction of halves of a part:
    (a) coapte
    (b) coapt
    (c) rafe
    (d) raphe

14. A skin discoloration caused by a hemorrhage:
    (a) hydronephrosis
    (b) hydronphrosis
    (c) ecchymosis
    (d) echymosis

15. A small beam or supporting structure:
    (a) trabeculation
    (b) traculation
    (c) concomitant
    (d) concommitant

CHECK YOUR PROGRESS *(cont'd)*

16. A triangular area:
    (a) staghorn
    (b) staghorne
    (c) trigon
    (d) trigone

17. Above the pubis:
    (a) periumbilical
    (b) supraumbilical
    (c) suprapubic
    (d) peripubic

18. An abnormal concretion, stone:
    (a) calculus
    (b) calcus
    (c) coudé
    (d) coudus'

19. Generic name for an angiotensin-converting enzyme inhibitor:
    (a) captopril
    (b) amoxicillin
    (c) catopril
    (d) amoxcillin

20. Generic name for an antibiotic:
    (a) captopril
    (b) amoxicillin
    (c) catopril
    (d) amoxcillin

21. Generic name for an antiemetic, antihistamine, motion sickness relief:
    (a) bacitracin
    (b) bactracine
    (c) meclizine
    (d) mecizine

22. An endoscope especially designed for passing through the urethra into the bladder:
    (a) cystoscope
    (b) cystourethroscope
    (c) cystscope
    (d) cystourescope

23. An incision of a duct or organ for the removal of calculi:
    (a) laminectomy
    (b) laminotomy
    (c) lithotomy
    (d) lithectomy

24. An instrument for examining the posterior urethra and bladder:
    (a) cystoscope
    (b) cystourethroscope
    (c) cystscope
    (d) cystourescope

25. An instrument placed in the vagina to support the uterus or rectum:
    (a) pessary
    (b) pesary
    (c) pissary
    (d) pisary

26. An opening:
    (a) fossa
    (b) fosa
    (c) meatus
    (d) metus

27. Around the umbilicus:
    (a) periumbilical
    (b) supraumbilical
    (c) suprapubic
    (d) peripubic

28. Bent or elbowed:
    (a) calculus
    (b) calcus
    (c) coudé
    (d) coudus'

29. Labored or difficult breathing:
    (a) dispnea
    (b) dyspnea
    (c) diuresis
    (d) dyuresis

30. Pertaining to the atrium and ventricle of the heart:
    (a) vas deferens
    (b) atriventricular
    (c) vas defens
    (d) atrioventricular

CHECK YOUR PROGRESS (cont'd)

31. Pertains to the genitalia and urinary organs:
    (a) genitorinary
    (b) genitourinary
    (c) pyruia
    (d) pyuria

32. Pus in the urine:
    (a) genitorinary
    (b) genitorinary
    (c) pyruia
    (d) pyuria

33. Taking place at the same time:
    (a) trabeculation
    (b) traculation
    (c) concomitant
    (d) concommitant

34. A calculus of the renal pelvis usually extending into multiple calices:
    (a) staghorn
    (b) staghorne
    (c) trigon
    (d) trigone

35. Removal of the gallbladder:
    (a) cholecystectomy
    (b) cystometrography
    (c) chocystectomy
    (d) cystorography

36. Destruction of living tissue by electric sparks generated by a high-frequency current:
    (a) extravasation
    (b) extrevasation
    (c) fulguration
    (d) fulgeration

37. Discharge of blood in the urine:
    (a) heme
    (b) hematuria
    (c) heman
    (d) hemeturia

38. Distention of the renal pelvis and calices with urine:
    (a) hydronephrosis
    (b) hydronphrosis
    (c) ecchymosis
    (d) echymosis

39. Elevation on the floor of the prostatic portion of the urethra where the seminal ducts enter:
    (a) verumontanum
    (b) verumonum
    (c) diverticulum
    (d) diverticum

40. The essential elements of an organ:
    (a) perenchyma
    (b) parenchyma
    (c) bardycardia
    (d) bradycardia

41. To cut a portion of a tissue or organ:
    (a) flank
    (b) flanke
    (c) desect
    (d) resect

42. The excision of one or both ovaries:
    (a) oophorectomy
    (b) colporrhaphy
    (c) ophorectomy
    (d) colporhaphy

43. The excretory duct of the testis:
    (a) vas deferens
    (b) atriventricular
    (c) vas defens
    (d) atrioventricular

44. X-ray study of the renal pelvis and ureters:
    (a) pyelogram
    (b) pyleogram
    (c) urogram
    (d) urologram

45. The graphic record of the pressure in the bladder at varying stages of filling:
    (a) cholecystectomy
    (b) cystometrography
    (c) chocystectomy
    (d) cystorography

46. Herniation of the urinary bladder into the vagina:
    (a) cystocele
    (b) cystosele
    (c) rectosele
    (d) rectocele

CHECK YOUR PROGRESS *(cont'd)*

47. The inability to control excretory functions:
    (a) creatinine
    (b) creatine
    (c) incontinence
    (d) incontinance

48. Increased excretion of urine:
    (a) dispneic
    (b) dyspneic
    (c) diuresis
    (d) dyuresis

49. Inflammation of the gallbladder:
    (a) cystitis
    (b) cystisis
    (c) cholcystitis
    (d) cholecystitis

50. Inflammation of the kidney and renal pelvis:
    (a) urethrogonitis
    (b) urethrotrigonitis
    (c) pyelonephritis
    (d) pyelonphritis

51. Inflammation of the urethra and trigone of the bladder:
    (a) urethrogonitis
    (b) urethrotrigonitis
    (c) pyelonephritis
    (d) pyelonphritis

52. Inflammation of the urinary bladder:
    (a) cystitis
    (b) cystisis
    (c) cholcystitis
    (d) cholecystitis

53. The nonprotein, insoluble, iron constituent of hemoglobin:
    (a) heme
    (b) hematuria
    (c) heman
    (d) hemeturia

54. The penis:
    (a) fallus
    (b) fallis
    (c) phalus
    (d) phallus

55. Poisoning from retained and absorbed urinary substances:
    (a) urosepsis
    (b) urethrocele
    (c) urethepsis
    (d) urothcele

56. Prolapse of the female urethra through the urinary meatus:
    (a) urosepsis
    (b) urethrocele
    (c) urethepsis
    (d) urothcele

57. The area between the ribs and ilium:
    (a) flank
    (b) flanke
    (c) desect
    (d) resect

58. Slowness of the heartbeat:
    (a) perenchyma
    (b) parenchyma
    (c) bardycardia
    (d) bradycardia

59. The supply of vessels to a specific region:
    (a) vasculature
    (b) vaculature
    (c) nephrectomy
    (d) neprectomy

60. Surgical excision of the lamina:
    (a) laminectomy
    (b) laminotomy
    (c) lithotomy
    (d) lithectomy

61. Surgical removal of the kidney:
    (a) vasculature
    (b) vaculature
    (c) nephrectomy
    (d) neprectomy

62. Suturing of the vagina:
    (a) oophorectomy
    (b) colporrhaphy
    (c) ophorectomy
    (d) colporhaphy

CHECK YOUR PROGRESS *(cont'd)*

63. Temporary suspension of consciousness; fainting:
    (a) syncope
    (b) synscope
    (c) pandoscope
    (d) panendoscope

64. To bring together, as in suturing a laceration:
    (a) coapte
    (b) coapt
    (c) rafe
    (d) raphe

65. To close tight:
    (a) occlude
    (b) oclude
    (c) leukocyte
    (d) leuocyte

66. Trade name for a diuretic:
    (a) Calen
    (b) Calan
    (c) Aldatone
    (d) Aldactone

67. Trade name for a diuretic, antiglaucoma agent:
    (a) Neptazane
    (b) Netazane
    (c) Noroxin
    (d) Norxin

68. Trade name for an antibacterial, urinary tract anti-infective:
    (a) Neptazane
    (b) Netazane
    (c) Noroxin
    (d) Norxin

69. Trade name for a fluoroquinolone antibiotic, antibacterial:
    (a) Maxquine
    (b) Maxaquin
    (c) Lopressor
    (d) Lopresor

70. Trade name for a fluoroquinolone antibiotic, antibacterial:
    (a) Ciprro
    (b) Cipro
    (c) Cardura
    (d) Carduro

71. Trade name for an anesthetic, antiarrhythmic:
    (a) Xylocine
    (b) Perpine
    (c) Propine
    (d) Xylocaine

72. Trade name for a nonsteroidal anti-inflammatory drug; analgesic for acute, moderately severe pain:
    (a) Toradol
    (b) Torodol
    (c) Tolinase
    (d) Tolenase

73. Trade name for a topical antiglaucoma agent:
    (a) Timoptic
    (b) Timptic
    (c) Trimpix
    (d) Trimpex

74. Trade name for an antianginal, antiarrhythmic, antihypertensive:
    (a) Calen
    (b) Calan
    (c) Aldatone
    (d) Aldactone

75. Trade name for an antianginal, antihypertensive:
    (a) Maxquine
    (b) Maxaquin
    (c) Lopressor
    (d) Lopresor

76. Trade name for an antidiarrheal:
    (a) Imadium
    (b) Imodium
    (c) Emadium
    (d) Emodium

77. Trade name for an antiglaucoma agent; eye drops:
    (a) Xylocine
    (b) Perpine
    (c) Propine
    (d) Xylocaine

78. Trade name for an antihypertensive, antiadrenergic:
    (a) Ciprro
    (b) Cipro
    (c) Cardura
    (d) Carduro

CHECK YOUR PROGRESS *(cont'd)*

79. Trade name for an antibacterial, antibiotic:
    (a) Timoptic
    (b) Timptic
    (c) Trimpix
    (d) Trimpex

80. Trade name for an antibiotic:
    (a) Bactrim
    (b) Betadine
    (c) Backrim
    (d) Betdine

81. Trade name for a topical antibacterial, antiseptic:
    (a) Bactrim
    (b) Betadine
    (c) Backrim
    (d) Betdine

82. Trade name for an antidiabetic agent:
    (a) Toradol
    (b) Torodol
    (c) Tolinase
    (d) Tolenase

Professional transcriptionists proofread their own work. Can you?

WORD PROCESSING USERS

Open your word processing package.

Insert the appropriate audiocassette in your transcribing machine and find
  dictation *7T-2*.

Transcribe and proofread dictation *7T-2*, using formatting guidelines established in
  Chapter 2.

Identify and correct all errors.

Save your work on your student disk.

After completing the transcription, refer to the answer key.

Manually complete the error analysis chart.

Manually complete the Production for Pay summary.

SOFTWARE USERS

Click on *Chapter 7, Proofreading Pretest (7T-2)*, and follow the directions.

Finding your own errors and correcting them is not easy, but it is an essential skill for your success as a medical transcriptionist. The two worksheets in this activity will help you develop your proofreading skills.

TEXTBOOK USERS

Proofread and correct errors in the medical documents shown in *Activities 7-4 and 7-5*.

Refer to the answer key (Appendix E) for immediate feedback.

Manually complete the error analysis chart for each document.

SOFTWARE USERS

Click on *Chapter 7, Activity 7-4*, and follow the directions.

Follow the same process for *Chapter 7, Activity 7-5*.

PROOFREADING

ACTIVITY 7-4
Proofreading Worksheet

Directions: Proofread this medical document, which contains multiple errors. Use open punctuation and all other formatting guidelines established in this textbook.

CONSULTATION REPORT

Patient Name: Barnes, Franklyn
File Number: 003416
Date of Birth: February 13, 19xx
Examination Date: *current date*
Requesting Physician: Izzy Sertoli, MD

HISTORY OF PRESENT ILLNESS

This 22 year old gentleman fell approximately twenty seven ft off a scaffold. He landed on a stack of concete blocks, and sustained a abrasion of his right flank. The patient informs me that he did not have much pain immediately after the fall and therefore did not come to see you for evaluation until later in the day. A urine analyses performed in your office showed 20-50 rbc's. Due to your concern about fight flank trauma I was asked to evaluate the patient.

The patient is alerted and oriented. There is no tenderness over the abdomen. There is a left flank abrasion measuring about 4 c.m. No hemotoma or echymosis are noted. The left flank area is smooth and un-remarkable. There is no tenderness in the lower abdomen. The testicles are normal. The prostrate is 1+, smooth and non-tender. His hemogloben is fourteen.

An IVP was performed that showed a large gass pattern over the entire adbomen. The left kidney functions promply and is smooth. The right kidney shows good function in both the upper and lower poles. There is some decreased filing of the renal penvis but there is good excetion of contast. The renal pelvis does not really fill out will in the entire mid-line area which I think is consistent with a renal contrusion. Thre is no sign of any exvasation.

A renal sonagram also shows the kidney to be totally entact. No deformity to the parencyma or fluid loss is noted. It is essentially a normal appearing kidney.

IMPRESSION
Right renal contusion. No signs of any exvasation.
PLAN
The patient will be admitted to university hospital and placed on bedrest, with observation. I will order a urine culture, and sensitivity test. He will be started on IV antibiotics and I will follow along with you in his care. Thank you for refering this patient to us.

Benjamin Keytone, MD
Bk:xx, d: current date, t: current date

ACTIVITY 7-5
Proofreading Worksheet

Directions: Proofread this medical document, which contains multiple errors. Use open punctuation and all other formatting guidelines established in this textbook.

OPERATIVE REPORT

Patient Name: Cruise, Jason
File Number: 0045612
Date of Birth: March 16, 1967
Examination Date: *current date*

Operation
FLEXIBLE CYSTOSCOPY
PREOPERATIVE DIAGNOSIS
Carcinoma of the prostrate.
POSTOPERATIVE DIAGNOSIS
Carcinoma of the prostrate.
PROCEDURE
Flexible cystioscopy
The patient was identified by me prepped and drapped in the usual fashion. The panindoscopy was performed with a number sixteen french flexible panendoscope. The anterior urethra was unremarkable. The membranous urethra is entact. There is no evidence of any structure.

The prostratic fosa demonstrates grade 2/IV obstruction as viewed from the verue. This probably represents fifteen to twenty grams of resectable adenoma. Thre is no evidence of tumor within the prostratic fosa. The bladder neck anatomy is unremarkable. The bladder mucosa is healthy thruout. There were no stones, tumors, or diverticula identified.

Right and left ureteral orifices were in normal position and normal configuration. Clear refflux is seen bilaterally. The bladder neck anatomy isunremarkable as noted from a retroflex postion. There is no evidence of any tumor envasion into the bladder base.

The scope was withdrawn. The patent tolerated the procedure well.
PLAN
Trimpex 100 mgs. bid Schedule a followup appointment in 2 weeks to discuss treatment options for carcinoma of the prostrate.

Theodore Trigone, MD

xx
D: current date
T: current date

PROOFREADING

Proofreading Transcription Exercises (7T-3 and 7T-4)

Now you are ready to make the transition from simply proofreading printed material to both transcribing and proofreading dictated material. This is the time to concentrate on building your medical vocabulary, which ultimately will improve your speed and accuracy. There are two activities in this section.

WORD PROCESSING USERS

Open your word processing package.

Insert the appropriate audiocassette in your transcribing machine and find dictation *7T-3*.

Step 1: Listen to the entire dictation to gain an understanding of the medical concepts and terms involved in the report. Rewind the tape to the beginning of the dictation and transcribe what you hear. Do not worry about formatting, style, or speed. Simply type what you hear being dictated, using correct punctuation, capitalization, and spelling. Stop as needed to look up words you do not understand or cannot spell. Adjust the speed control of the transcriber to a comfortable level, starting slowly to ensure that no dictated words are missed, and then increase the speed as your accuracy improves.

Step 2: Rewind the tape and transcribe dictation *7T-3* again, including correct spacing and formatting. Proofread the report. Identify and correct all errors. Save your work on your student disk. Refer to the answer key, and manually complete the error analysis chart and Production for Pay summary.

Follow the same process for dictation *7T-4*.

SOFTWARE USERS

Click on *Chapter 7, Activity 7-6 (7T-3), Step 1,* and follow the directions. When you feel comfortable with the dictation, click on *Chapter 7, Activity 7-6 (7T-3), Step 2,* and follow the directions.

Follow the same process for *Chapter 7, Activity 7-7 (7T-4), Step 1* and *Chapter 7, Activity 7-7 (7T-4), Step 2.*

PROOFREADING

Let's pause a minute and see how well you are doing. This section allows you to evaluate your success at transcribing and proofreading urology reports.

WORD PROCESSING USERS

Open your word processing package.

Insert the appropriate audiocassette in your transcribing machine and find dictation 7T-2.

Transcribe and proofread dictation 7T-2, using the formatting guidelines established in Chapter 2.

Identify and correct all errors.

Save your work on your student disk.

After completing the transcription, refer to the answer key.

Manually complete the error analysis chart.

Manually complete the Production for Pay summary.

SOFTWARE USERS

Click on *Chapter 7, Proofreading Check Your Progress (7T-2)*, and follow the directions.

Professional transcriptionists can transcribe and proofread their own work. Can you?

WORD PROCESSING USERS

Open your word processing package.

Insert the appropriate audiocassette in your transcribing machine and find dictation 7T-5.

Transcribe and proofread dictation 7T-5, using the formatting guidelines established in Chapter 2.

Save your work on your student disk.

Identify and correct all errors.

After completing the transcription, refer to the answer key.

Manually complete the error analysis chart.

Manually complete the Production for Pay summary.

Follow the same process for dictation 7T-6.

SOFTWARE USERS

Click on *Chapter 7, Transcription Pretest (7T-5)*, and follow the directions.

Follow the same process for *Chapter 7, Transcription Pretest (7T-6)*.

You have been hired as a transcriptionist at FedDes Wellness Center in the urology division. Your supervisor has asked you to transcribe today's dictation.

TEXT BOOK USERS

Open your word processing package.

Insert the appropriate audiocassette in your transcribing machine and find dictation *7T-7*.

Create or use an existing template as necessary for the six types of reports (chart note, chart note using history and physical format, history and physical examination report, x-ray report, procedure report, consultation letter).

Transcribe and proofread dictation *7T-7*, using the formatting guidelines established in Chapter 2.

Identify and correct all errors.

Save your work on your student disk.

After completing the transcription, refer to the answer key.

Manually complete the error analysis chart.

Manually complete the Production for Pay summary.

Follow the same process for dictations *7T-8* through *7T-15*.

SOFTWARE USERS

Click on *Chapter 7, Transcription at FedDes Wellness Center, Dictation 7T-7*, and follow the directions.

Follow the same process for each of the remaining dictations (*7T-8* through *7T-15*).

Remember to follow the guidelines pertaining to capitalization, numbers, punctuation, abbreviations, measurements, symbols, and use of templates. This material is reviewed in Unit I.

7T-7

Consultation Report
Patient's Name: Jason Stewartson
Requesting Physician: Charles P. Davis, MD
Physician: Benjamin Keytone, MD

Transcription Tips

- A hyphen is used between numbers and *year old*.
    You hear the dictator say: twenty four year old mother.
    You transcribe as: 24-year-old mother.
- Generic drugs are not capitalized: amoxicillin.
- Words beginning with *pre, re, post*, and *non* are generally not hyphenated: nontender.

7T-8

Operative Report
Patient's Name: Soshia Yonie
Ordering Physician: Charles P. Davis, MD
Physician: Helen Loop, MD

Transcription Tips

- A hyphen is used to join two or more words when used as an adjective that precedes a noun. The following word pair is dictated in this report: three-month.
- The following drugs are dictated in this report:
    Betadine: trade name for a topical antibacterial, antiseptic
    Xylocaine: trade name for an anesthetic, antiarrhythmic

7T-9

History and Physical Examination Report
Patient's Name: Roal Diaz
Physician: Benjamin Keytone, MD

Transcription Tips

- The following abbreviations are dictated in this report:
    TURP: transurethral resection of the prostate
    BPH: benign prostatic hypertrophy
- A hyphen is used when two or more words are viewed as a single word: well-developed.
- Figures are used to express the day of the month and the year.
    You hear the dictator say: The patient underwent prostatic resection and hernia repair in nineteen ninety eight.
    You transcribe as: The patient underwent prostatic resection and hernia repair in 1998.
- Words beginning with *pre, re, post*, and *non* are generally not hyphenated: noncontributory.

7T-10

Chart Note using History and Physical Format
Patient's Name: Betty Ann Jackson-Jones
Physician: Helen Loop, MD

Transcription Tips

- A period is used to separate a decimal fraction from its whole number and is used to take the place of the word *point*.
    You hear the dictator say: Her WBC is six point eight.
    You transcribe as: Her WBC is 6.8.
- Figures are used to express vital signs. Commas are used to separate vital signs.
    You hear the dictator say: Temperature ninety seven point eight pulse seventy nine respirations twenty two per minute blood pressure one hundred fifty seven over eighty six.
    You transcribe as: Temperature 97.8, pulse 79, respirations 22/min, BP 157/86.

TRANSCRIPTION

- A hyphen is used to join two or more words when used as an adjective that precedes a noun. The following word pairs are dictated in this report: follow-up, high-powered.
- The following abbreviations are dictated in this report:
    WBC: white blood count
    CVA: costovertebral angle
- The following drug is dictated in this report:
    Noroxin: trade name for an antibacterial, urinary tract anti-infective
- A hyphen is used to take the place of the words *to* or *through* to identify ranges.
    You hear the dictator say: Urinalysis reveals three to five white cells.
    You transcribe as: Urinalysis reveals 3-5 white cells.
- Words beginning with *pre, re, post*, and *non* are generally not hyphenated: nonpalpable, rebound.
- The following procedure is dictated in this report:
    Marshall-Marchetti-Krantz bladder neck suspension: procedure performed to correct a cystocele and urinary incontinence

7T-11

History and Physical Examination Report
Patient's Name: Julia Pierre
Physician: Helen Loop, MD

Transcription Tips
- The following abbreviation is dictated in this report:
    CT: computed tomography
- The following diseases are dictated in this report:
    Crohn's disease: inflammation of the terminal portion of the ileum
    diverticulitis: inflammation of the diverticula of the colon
- The following drugs are dictated in this report:
    Lopressor: trade name for an antianginal, antihypertensive
    Aldactone: trade name for a diuretic
    Imodium: trade name for an antidiarrheal
- Words beginning with *pre, re, post*, and *non* are generally not hyphenated: noncontributory, nontender, pretibial.

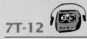

7T-12

History and Physical Examination Report
Patient's Name: Dawson, Thomas
Physician: Theodore Trigone, MD

Transcription Tips
- The following drugs are dictated in this report:
    Bactrim: trade name for an antibiotic
    Trimpex: trade name for an antibacterial, antibiotic
- Figures are used with the + or − symbols.
    You hear the dictator say: Urinalysis shows two plus leukocytes.
    You transcribe as: Urinalysis shows 2 + leukocytes.
    You hear the dictator say: three plus heme.
    You transcribe as: 3 + heme.
- A hyphen is used to join two or more words when used as an adjective that precedes a noun. The following word pair is dictated in this report: follow-up.
- Figures are used for Latin terms. Latin terms are expressed in lower case letters.
    You hear the dictator say: a follow up appointment in three months or P R N basis.
    You transcribe as: a follow-up appointment in 3 months or p.r.n. basis.
- The letter *x* is used to abbreviate the word *by* and the word *times* when it precedes a number or another abbreviation. The dosage of medicine is never separated by line spacing.
    You hear the dictator say: The patient will resume a regimen of Bactrim DS one b eye d times ten days.
    You transcribe as: The patient will resume a regimen of Bactrim DS 1 b.i.d. × 10 days.
- The following disease is dictated in this report:
    Parkinson's disease: slowly progressive disease characterized by degeneration within the nuclear masses of the extrapyramidal system
- The following abbreviations are dictated in this report:
    CVA: costovertebral angle
    UA: urinalysis
    C&S: culture and sensitivity

7T-13

Consultation Letter
Patient's Name: Ross, Mary
Requesting Physician: J. Thomas Geiger, MD
Physician: Helen Loop, MD

Transcription Tips
- A hyphen is used in place of *to* or *through* to identify ranges.
    You hear the dictator say: vague abdominal pain three to four days ago.

You transcribe as: vague abdominal pain 3-4 days ago.

- Capitalize the name of specific departments or sections in a hospital or institution.

    You hear the dictator say: She presented to the university hospital emergency room last night.

    You transcribe as: She presented to the University Hospital Emergency Room last night.

- Quotation marks are used to indicate a direct quote.

    You hear the dictator say: The urinalysis was described as turbid yellow.

    You transcribe as: The urinalysis was described as "turbid yellow."

- The following abbreviations are dictated in this report:

    KUB: kidneys, ureters, bladder

    CVA: costovertebral angle

7T-14

History and Physical Examination Report
Patient's Name: Resch, Gladys
Physician: Helen Loop, MD

Transcription Tips

- The following procedure is dictated in this report:

    Marshall test: performed to determine stress-related urinary incontinence

- The following device is dictated in this report:

    Gellhorn pessary: an inflexible device made of acrylic resin or plastic in the form of a large collar button. It has a canal through the stem that allows drainage of vaginal secretions.

- A hyphen is used when two or more words are viewed as a single word: well-developed, well-nourished.

- The following generic drugs are dictated in this report:

    hydrochlorothiazide: diuretic, antihypertensive agent

    meclizine: antiemetic, antihistamine, motion sickness relief

7T-15

Consultation Report
Patient's Name: Sever, Jed
Requesting Physician: Izzy Sertoli, MD
Physician: Benjamin Keytone, MD

Transcription Tips

- Dangerous abbreviations are dictated within this transcript:

    You will hear the dictator say: The ballon was inflated with 10 cc of saline.

    You should transcribe as: The ballon was inflated with 10 mL of saline.

    You will hear the dictator say: The patient was started on Maxaquin 400 mg p.o.q.d. for a 7-day course.

    You should transcribe as: The patient was started on Maxaquin 400 mg p.o. daily for a 7-day course.

- The following drug is dictated in this report:

    Maxaquin: trade name for a fluoroquinolone antibiotic, antibacterial

- A hyphen is used to join two or more words when used as an adjective that precedes a noun. The following word pairs are dictated in this report: worm-like, moderate-sized, seven-day, blood-tinged.

- The number or pound sign (#) is used to abbreviate the word *number* followed by a medical instrument or apparatus.

    You hear the dictator say: He had a number eighteen french foley catheter.

    You transcribe as: He had a #18 French Foley catheter.

- Words beginning with *pre, re, post,* and *non* are generally not hyphenated: nondraining.

Professional transcriptionists can transcribe and proofread their own work with speed and accuracy. Have you mastered the urology transcription rotation at FedDes Wellness Center?

WORD PROCESSING USERS

Open your word processing package.

Insert the appropriate audiocassette in your transcribing machine and find dictation *7T-5*.

Transcribe and proofread dictation *7T-5*, using the formatting guidelines established in Chapter 2.

Save your work on your student disk.

Identify and correct all errors.

After completing the transcription, refer to the answer key.

Manually complete the error analysis chart.

Manually complete the Production for Pay summary.

Follow the same process for dictation *7T-6*.

SOFTWARE USERS

Click on *Chapter 7, Transcription Check Your Progress (7T-5)*, and follow the directions.

Follow the same process for *Chapter 7, Transcription Check Your Progress (7T-6)*.

Chapter 8

Office Medical Transcription from the Pulmonary Medicine Practice

OBJECTIVES

At the completion of Chapter 8, you should be able to do the following:
1. Match medical terms associated with the pulmonary medicine specialty with their definitions.
2. Spell medical terms associated with the pulmonary medicine specialty.
3. Transcribe medical terms in sentence structure.
4. Proofread, edit, and correct medical documents associated with the pulmonary medicine specialty that contain various errors.
5. Transcribe and proofread authentic medical documents associated with the pulmonary medicine specialty.

What's Ahead

The FedDes Wellness Center has three pulmonologists, or specialists in pulmonary medicine, on staff. Pulmonary medicine is the study of the respiratory system and its organs, including the nose, mouth, pharynx, epiglottis, esophagus, trachea, lungs, bronchi, bronchioles, and alveoli.

The pulmonologist assesses abnormalities that decrease the amount of air entry, cause restrictive breathing, and affect lung parenchyma. The physicians in FedDes Pulmonary medicine division perform laboratory tests and procedures, including pulmonary function tests, bronchoscopy, metabolic cart study, indirect calorimetry, thoracentesis, and pleural biopsy.

In this unit, you assume the role of a medical transcriptionist employed at FedDes Wellness Center. Please remember to follow the guidelines pertaining to capitalization, numbers, punctuation, abbreviations, measurements, symbols, and use of templates to create medical reports at FedDes Wellness Center. This material is reviewed in Unit I. The transcription exercises list the type of report, patient's name, and physician(s) as well as the associated transcription tips.

You will work with the textbook and CD-ROM or accompanying audiocassettes. Your mastery of pulmonary medicine transcription is assessed through worksheets, timed transcription exercises, the error analysis chart, and the Production for Pay summary.

All the answer keys are found in the textbook (Appendix E) and CD-ROM, providing immediate feedback. After transcribing a report, you will proofread your work and correct any errors. Then you will compare your proofread work against a master transcript, categorize all errors, and tabulate the errors on the error analysis chart. The Production for Pay summary correlates your production to the FedDes Wellness Center pay scale. The scale is also linked to your grade. This system allows you to assess your mastery of transcription skills in a real-world scenario.

Let's find out if you can define and spell selected terminology and drugs of the pulmonary medicine specialty that are included in this chapter.

TEXTBOOK USERS

Select the correctly spelled term that matches its definition.
Refer to the answer key (Appendix E) for immediate feedback.

SOFTWARE USERS

Click on *Chapter 8, Terminology Pretest*, and follow the directions.

TERMINOLOGY

PRETEST

Directions: Select the correctly spelled term that matches its definition.

1. Ability to control urination and defecation urges:
   (a) continent
   (b) contenint
   (c) empiric
   (d) impiric

2. Abnormal crackle sound heard on chest auscultation:
   (a) rale
   (b) rub
   (c) ralle
   (d) rube

3. Abnormal heart condition characterized by increased size of the right ventricle:
   (a) cor pulmonale
   (b) cor pulmonary
   (c) pulmonary toilet
   (d) pulmon toilet

4. Abnormal heart rhythm:
   (a) sequela
   (b) gallop
   (c) sequelia
   (d) galop

5. Abnormal slowing or stopping of fluid flowing through a vessel:
   (a) atelectasis
   (b) stasis
   (c) atellectasis
   (d) stacis

6. Abnormal sound heard on chest auscultation that results from an obstructed airway:
   (a) hemotysis
   (b) hemoptysis
   (c) rhonchus
   (d) ronchus

7. Abnormally fast heartbeat:
   (a) tachycardia
   (b) dyrhythmia
   (c) tachcardia
   (d) dysrhythmia

8. Accumulation of excess fluid in the tissues of the body:
   (a) sputum
   (b) edena
   (c) spitum
   (d) edema

9. Accumulation of fluid in the peritoneal cavity:
   (a) caries
   (b) ascites
   (c) caires
   (d) acites

10. Act of closure or state of being closed:
    (a) oclusion
    (b) auscultation
    (c) auscutation
    (d) occlusion

11. Act of fainting:
    (a) somnolence
    (b) somolence
    (c) syncope
    (d) synscope

12. Act of listening for sounds produced within the body with an unaided ear or with a stethoscope:
    (a) oclusion
    (b) auscultation
    (c) auscutation
    (d) occlusion

13. Affecting both sides:
    (a) afebrile
    (b) bilateral
    (c) afevrile
    (d) bilaral

14. Any abnormal condition that follows and is the result of a disease, treatment, or injury:
    (a) erythema
    (b) sequea
    (c) erytema
    (d) sequela

PRETEST *(cont'd)*

15. Any drug that has the capability of increasing the capacity of the pulmonary air passages and improving ventilation to the lungs:
    (a) efflusion
    (b) bronchidilator
    (c) bronchodilator
    (d) effusion

16. Aspiration of fluid from the chest cavity:
    (a) metastasis
    (b) thoracentesis
    (c) metasis
    (d) thorasis

17. Bluish purple discoloration of the skin due to lack of oxygenated blood:
    (a) cyanesis
    (b) cyanosis
    (c) emesis
    (d) enesis

18. Calf pain with dorsiflexion of foot:
    (a) Homan's sign
    (b) theophylline
    (c) Homans' sign
    (d) theophyline

19. Cleansing of the trachea and bronchial tree:
    (a) cor pulmonale
    (b) cor pulmonary
    (c) pulmonary toilet
    (d) pulmon toilet

20. Collapse of a portion of the lung:
    (a) atelectasis
    (b) stasis
    (c) atellectasis
    (d) stacis

21. Compound containing water molecules:
    (a) hydrate
    (b) hidrate
    (c) infiltrate
    (d) enfiltrate

22. Condition of decay and destruction of a tooth:
    (a) caries
    (b) ascites
    (c) caires
    (d) acites

23. Containing pus:
    (a) pedol
    (b) purlent
    (c) purulent
    (d) pedal

24. Coughing or spitting up blood from the respiratory tract:
    (a) hemotysis
    (b) hemoptysis
    (c) rhonchus
    (d) ronchus

25. Cramping pains of the calves caused by poor circulation to the leg muscles:
    (a) dention
    (b) claudication
    (c) caudication
    (d) dentition

26. Decreased supply of oxygenated blood to a body part:
    (a) ischemia
    (b) ischema
    (c) dyspneia
    (d) dyspnea

27. Diagnostic procedure using ultrasound to study heart structure and motion:
    (a) echocardiogram
    (b) echiocardogram
    (c) arteriogram
    (d) arterogram

28. Disordered rhythm:
    (a) rhonchus
    (b) dyrhythmia
    (c) ronchis
    (d) dysrhythmia

29. Drowsiness:
    (a) somnolence
    (b) somolence
    (c) syncope
    (d) synscope

PRETEST *(cont'd)*

30. Enlargement of the glands, especially the lymph nodes:
    (a) thyromegaly
    (b) adenogaly
    (c) adenopathy
    (d) thyropathy

31. Enlargement of the thyroid gland:
    (a) thyromegaly
    (b) adenogaly
    (c) adenopathy
    (d) thyropathy

32. Escape of fluid into a body cavity:
    (a) efflusion
    (b) bronchidilator
    (c) bronchodilator
    (d) effusion

33. Fluid, cells, or other substances passing into tissue spaces:
    (a) hydrate
    (b) hidrate
    (c) infiltrate
    (d) enfiltrate

34. Generic name for an antianxiety drug:
    (a) lorazepam
    (b) lorasepam
    (c) isorbide
    (d) isosorbide

35. Generic name for a calcium channel blocker:
    (a) haperin
    (b) heparin
    (c) nifedipin
    (d) nifedipine

36. Generic name for a corticosteroid:
    (a) prednisone
    (b) prenisone
    (c) cephalosporin
    (d) cephalsporin

37. Generic name for a broad-spectrum antibiotic:
    (a) nitroglyserin
    (b) erythromycin
    (c) nitroglycerin
    (d) erythromysin

38. Generic name for a bronchodilator:
    (a) Homan's sign
    (b) theophylline
    (c) Homans' sign
    (d) theophyline

39. Generic name for a coronary vasodilator, antianginal:
    (a) nitroglyserin
    (b) erythromycin
    (c) nitroglycerin
    (d) erythromysin

40. Generic name for a nitrate-based antianginal agent:
    (a) lorazepam
    (b) lorasepam
    (c) isorbide
    (d) isosorbide

41. Generic name for an aminopenicillin antibiotic:
    (a) amoxicillin
    (b) amoxicilin
    (c) doxepin
    (d) dozepin

42. Generic name for an anticoagulant:
    (a) haperin
    (b) heparin
    (c) nifedipin
    (d) nifedipine

43. Generic name for an antidepressant:
    (a) amoxicillin
    (b) amoxicilin
    (c) doxepin
    (d) dozepin

44. Generic name for any of a large group of broad-spectrum antibiotics:
    (a) prednisone
    (b) prenisone
    (c) cephalosporin
    (d) cephalsporin

45. Increased excretion of urine:
    (a) duiresis
    (b) diuresis
    (c) duiretic
    (d) diuretic

PRETEST (cont'd)

46. Involuntary, rapid, rhythmic movement of the eyeball:
    (a) nystagus
    (b) nystagmus
    (c) adencarcinoma
    (d) adenocarcinoma

47. Labored or difficult breathing:
    (a) ischemia
    (b) ischema
    (c) dyspneia
    (d) dyspnea

48. Localized dilatation of the wall of a blood vessel:
    (a) aneurysm
    (b) embolus
    (c) aneruysm
    (d) emblous

49. Malignant tumor of the glands:
    (a) nystagus
    (b) nystagmus
    (c) adencarcinoma
    (d) adenocarcinoma

50. Mass that is brought by the blood from another vessel and that obstructs blood circulation:
    (a) aneurysm
    (b) embolus
    (c) aneruysm
    (d) emblous

51. Material coughed up from the lungs and ejected through the mouth:
    (a) sputum
    (b) edena
    (c) spitum
    (d) edema

52. Normally occurring microorganisms living within the body that provide natural immunity against certain organisms:
    (a) fora
    (b) saphenous
    (c) flora
    (d) sapenous

53. Occurring at night:
    (a) intrauterine
    (b) nocturnal
    (c) interuterine
    (d) noctural

54. Pertaining to the two main superficial veins of the lower leg:
    (a) fora
    (b) saphenous
    (c) flora
    (d) sapenous

55. Position and condition of the teeth:
    (a) dention
    (b) claudication
    (c) caudication
    (d) dentition

56. Presence of air or gas in the pleural cavity:
    (a) pneumontomy
    (b) pneumonectomy
    (c) pneumotorax
    (d) pneumothorax

57. Radiographic visualization of an artery after injection of a contrast medium:
    (a) echocardiogram
    (b) echiocardogram
    (c) arteriogram
    (d) arterogram

58. Redness of the skin:
    (a) erythema
    (b) sequea
    (c) erytema
    (d) sequela

59. Relating to the foot:
    (a) pedol
    (b) purlent
    (c) purulent
    (d) pedal

60. Situated or occurring above the ventricles:
    (a) superventricular
    (b) supraventricular
    (c) suberventricular
    (d) suparventricular

61. Sound caused by the rubbing together of two surfaces:
    (a) rale
    (b) rub
    (c) ralle
    (d) rube

TERMINOLOGY

PRETEST *(cont'd)*

62. Sound or murmur heard on auscultation:
    (a) bruit
    (b) gallop
    (c) briut
    (d) galop

63. Substance that promotes the excretion of urine:
    (a) duiresis
    (b) diuresis
    (c) duiretic
    (d) diuretic

64. Surgical removal of all or a segment of the lung:
    (a) pneumontomy
    (b) pneumonectomy
    (c) pneumotorax
    (d) pneumothorax

65. An act or instance of vomiting:
    (a) cyanesis
    (b) cyanesis
    (c) emesis
    (d) enesis

66. Transfer of disease from one organ or part to another not directly connected with it:
    (a) metastasis
    (b) thoracentesis
    (c) metasis
    (d) thorasis

67. Treating a disease based on observation and experience rather than reasoning alone:
    (a) continent
    (b) contenint
    (c) empiric
    (d) impiric

68. Treatment by a spray:
    (a) nebulization
    (b) nebullization
    (c) fibrillation
    (d) fibrilation

69. Uncoordinated twitching of muscle fibers:
    (a) nebulization
    (b) nebullization
    (c) fibrillation
    (d) fibrilation

70. Within the uterus:
    (a) intrauterine
    (b) nocturnal
    (c) interuterine
    (d) noctural

71. Without fever:
    (a) afebrile
    (b) bilateral
    (c) afevrile
    (d) bilaral

72. Trade name for a bronchodilator; metered-dose inhaler:
    (a) Proventil
    (b) Provintel
    (c) Vanceril
    (d) Vanseril

73. Trade name for a bronchodilator:
    (a) Ventlin
    (b) Ventolin
    (c) Paxil
    (d) Pasil

74. Trade name for a bronchodilator:
    (a) Theo-Dur
    (b) Xanaz
    (c) Xanax
    (d) Theo-Dure

75. Trade name for a bulk-forming laxative:
    (a) Dilantin
    (b) Dylantin
    (c) FiberCon
    (d) Fiberkon

76. Trade name for a calcium channel blocker for atrial fibrillation:
    (a) Cardizem
    (b) Cardisem
    (c) Colase
    (d) Colace

77. Trade name for a coronary vasodilator:
    (a) Procardia
    (b) Serevent
    (c) Procariodia
    (d) Servent

PRETEST *(cont'd)*

78. Trade name for a corticosteroid used to prevent or treat bronchial asthma:
    (a) Azamcort
    (b) Bumex
    (c) Azmacort
    (d) Bumez

79. Trade name for a corticosteroid:
    (a) Proventil
    (b) Provintel
    (c) Vanceril
    (d) Vanseril

80. Trade name for a loop diuretic:
    (a) Azamcort
    (b) Bumex
    (c) Azmacort
    (d) Bumez

81. Trade name for a narcotic analgesic:
    (a) Compazine
    (b) Darvon
    (c) Compasine
    (d) Darvin

82. Trade name for a bronchodilator; nasal spray:
    (a) Ascriptin
    (b) Asriptin
    (c) Atrovent
    (d) Atovent

83. Trade name for an analgesic and anti-inflammatory:
    (a) Ascriptin
    (b) Asriptin
    (c) Atrovent
    (d) Atovent

84. Trade name for a sedative-hypnotic:
    (a) Pepsid
    (b) Restoril
    (c) Pepcid
    (d) Restoral

85. Trade name for a stool softener:
    (a) Cardizem
    (b) Cardisem
    (c) Colase
    (d) Colace

86. Trade name for a tranquilizer, antiemetic:
    (a) Compazine
    (b) Darvon
    (c) Compasine
    (d) Darvin

87. Trade name for an acid controller for heartburn and acid indigestion:
    (a) Pepsid
    (b) Restoril
    (c) Pepcid
    (d) Restoral

88. Trade name for an acid controller for heartburn and acid indigestion:
    (a) Zantac
    (b) Vasotec
    (c) Zantak
    (d) Vasotek

89. Trade name for an aerosol bronchodilator:
    (a) Procardia
    (b) Serevent
    (c) Procariodia
    (d) Servent

90. Trade name for an antianxiety agent:
    (a) Theo-Dur
    (b) Xanaz
    (c) Xanax
    (d) Theo-Dure

91. Trade name for an anticonvulsant used to treat epilepsy:
    (a) Dilantin
    (b) Dylantin
    (c) FiberCon
    (d) Fiberkon

92. Trade name for an antidepressant:
    (a) Ventlin
    (b) Ventolin
    (c) Paxil
    (d) Pasil

93. Trade name for an antihyperlipidemic:
    (a) Lopressor
    (b) Metacor
    (c) Lopressar
    (d) Mevacor

PRETEST *(cont'd)*

94. Trade name for an antihypertensive:
    (a) Lopressor
    (b) Metacor
    (c) Lopressar
    (d) Mevacor

95. Trade name for an antihypertensive:
    (a) Zantac
    (b) Vasotec
    (c) Zantak
    (d) Vasotek

96. Trade name for a cephalosporin antibiotic:
    (a) Ancef IV
    (b) Ansef IV
    (c) NPH
    (d) PNH

97. Trade name for an extended-release bronchodilator:
    (a) Slow-bid
    (b) Slo-bide
    (c) Slow-bide
    (d) Slo-Bid

98. Trade name for an insulin that decreases blood sugar:
    (a) Ancef IV
    (b) Ansef IV
    (c) NPH
    (d) PNH

Activity 8-1

Keyboarding Medical Terms and Definitions

Let's learn to spell and define selected terminology and drugs of the pulmonary medicine specialty that are included in this chapter. Keyboarding these terms is an effective way to improve your skills.

Word Processing Users

Open your word processing package.
Read and type each word and its definition as shown below.
Save your work on your student disk.

1. Adenocarcinoma (ade-no-kar-si-<u>no</u>-mah) is a malignant tumor of the glands.
2. Adenopathy (ade-<u>nop</u>-ah-the) is the enlargement of the glands, especially the lymph nodes.
3. Afebrile (a-<u>feb</u>-ril) means without fever.
4. Amoxicillin (ah-moks-i-<u>sil</u>-in) is a generic name for an aminopenicillin antibiotic.
5. Aneurysm (<u>an</u>-u-rizm) is a localized dilatation of the wall of a blood vessel.
6. Arteriogram (ar-<u>te</u>-re-o-gram) is the radiographic visualization of an artery after injection of a contrast medium.
7. Ascites (ah-<u>si</u>-tez) is the accumulation of fluid in the peritoneal cavity.
8. Atelectasis (ate-<u>lek</u>-tah-sis) is the collapse of a portion of the lung.
9. Auscultation (aw-skul-<u>ta</u>-shun) is the act of listening for sounds produced within the body with an unaided ear or with a stethoscope.
10. Bilateral (bi-<u>lat</u>-er-al) is affecting both sides.
11. Bronchodilator (brong-ko-di-<u>la</u>-tor) is any drug that has the capability of increasing the capacity of the pulmonary air passages and improving ventilation to the lungs.
12. Bruit (broo <u>e</u>) is a sound or murmur heard on auscultation.
13. Caries (<u>kar</u>-ez) is the condition of decay and destruction of a tooth.
14. Cephalosporin (sef-ah-lo-<u>spor</u>-in) is a generic name for any of the large group of broad-spectrum antibiotics.
15. Claudication (klaw-di-<u>ka</u>-shun) is cramping pains of the calves caused by poor circulation to the leg muscles.
16. Continent (<u>kon</u>-ti-ent) is the ability to control urination and defecation urges.
17. Cor pulmonale (kor pul-mo-<u>na</u>-le) is an abnormal heart condition characterized by increased size of the right ventricle.
18. Cyanosis (si-ah-<u>no</u>-sis) is the bluish purple discoloration of the skin due to lack of oxygenated blood.
19. Dentition (den-<u>tish</u>-un) refers to the position and condition of the teeth.
20. Diuresis (di-u-<u>re</u>-sis) is increased urine excretion.
21. Diuretic (di-u-<u>ret</u>-ik) is a substance that promotes the excretion of urine.
22. Doxepin (<u>dok</u>-se-pin) is a generic name for an antidepressant.
23. Dyspnea (disp-<u>ne</u>-ah) is labored or difficult breathing.
24. Dysrhythmia (dis-<u>rith</u>-me-ah) is a disordered rhythm.
25. Echocardiogram (eko-<u>kar</u>-de-o-gram) is a diagnostic procedure using ultrasound to study heart structure and motion.
26. Edema (e-<u>de</u>-mah) is the accumulation of excess fluid in the tissues of the body.
27. Effusion (e-<u>fu</u>-zhun) is the escape of fluid into a body cavity.
28. Embolus (<u>em</u>-bo-lus) is a mass that is brought by the blood from another vessel and that obstructs blood circulation.
29. Emesis (<u>em</u>-e-sis) is an act or instance of vomiting.
30. Empiric (em-<u>pir</u>-ik) means treating a disease based on observation and experience rather than reasoning alone.
31. Erythema (eri-<u>the</u>-mah) is redness of the skin.
32. Erythromycin (e-<u>rith</u>-ro-<u>mi</u>-sin) is a generic name for a broad-spectrum antibiotic.
33. Fibrillation (fi-bri-<u>la</u>-shun) is the uncoordinated twitching of muscle fibers.
34. Flora (<u>flo</u>-rah) are normally occurring microorganisms living within the body that provide natural immunity against certain organisms.
35. Gallop (<u>gal</u>-op) is an abnormal heart rhythm.
36. Hemoptysis (he-<u>mop</u>-ti-sis) is the coughing or spitting up of blood from the respiratory tract.
37. Heparin (<u>hep</u>-ah-rin) is a generic name for an anticoagulant.
38. Homans' sign (<u>ho</u>-manz sin) is calf pain with dorsiflexion of foot.

TERMINOLOGY

39. Hydrate (hi-drate) is a compound containing water molecules.
40. Infiltrate (in-fil-trate) is fluid, cells, or other substances passing into tissue spaces.
41. Intrauterine (in-trah-u-ter-in) is within the uterus.
42. Ischemia (is-ke-me-ah) is a decreased supply of oxygenated blood to a body part.
43. Isosorbide (i-so-sor-bid) is a generic name for a nitrate-based antianginal agent.
44. Lorazepam (lor-az-eh-pam) is a generic antianxiety drug.
45. Metastasis (me-tas-tah-sis) is the transfer of disease from one organ or part to another not directly connected with it.
46. Nebulization (neb-u-li-za-shun) is a treatment by a spray.
47. Nifedipine (ni-fed-i-pen) is a generic name for a calcium channel blocker.
48. Nitroglycerin (ni-tro-glis-er-in) is a generic name for a coronary vasodilator and antianginal.
49. Nocturnal (nok-tur-nal) means occurring at night.
50. Nystagmus (nis-tag-mus) is the involuntary, rapid, rhythmic movement of the eyeball.
51. Occlusion (o-kloo-zhun) is the act of closure or state of being closed.
52. Pedal (ped-al) means relating to the foot.
53. Pneumonectomy (nu-mo-nek-to-me) is the surgical removal of all or a segment of the lung.
54. Pneumothorax (nu-mo-tho-raks) is the presence of air or gas in the pleural cavity.
55. Prednisone (pred-ni-son) is a generic corticosteroid.
56. Pulmonary toilet (pul-mo-ner-e toi-let) is the cleansing of the trachea and bronchial tree.
57. Purulent (pu-roo-lent) means containing pus.
58. Rale (rahl) is an abnormal crackle sound heard on chest auscultation.
59. Rhonchus (rong-kus) is an abnormal sound heard on chest auscultation that results from an obstructed airway.
60. Rub (rub) is a sound caused by the rubbing together of two surfaces.
61. Saphenous (sah-fe-nus) pertains to the two main superficial veins of the lower leg.
62. Sequela (se-kwel-lah) is any abnormal condition that follows and is the result of a disease, treatment, or injury.
63. Somnolence (som-no-lens) means drowsiness.
64. Sputum (spu-tum) is the material coughed up from the lungs and ejected through the mouth.
65. Stasis (sta-sis) is an abnormal slowing or stopping of fluid flowing through a vessel.
66. Supraventricular (soo-prah-ven-trik-u-lar) means situated or occurring above the ventricles.
67. Syncope (sing-ko-pe) is the act of fainting.
68. Tachycardia (take-kar-de-ah) is an abnormally fast heartbeat.
69. Theophylline (the-o-fil-in) is a generic name for a bronchodilator.
70. Thoracentesis (tho-rah-sen-te-sis) is the aspiration of fluid from the chest cavity.
71. Thyromegaly (thi-ro-meg-ah-le) is the enlargement of the thyroid gland.
72. Ancef IV (an-sef) is the trade name for a cephalosporin antibiotic.
73. Ascriptin (ah-skrip-tin) is the trade name for an analgesic and anti-inflammatory.
74. Atrovent (at-ro-vent) is the trade name for a bronchodilator nasal spray.
75. Azmacort (az-ma-kort) is the trade name for a corticosteroid used to prevent or treat bronchial asthma.
76. Bumex (bu-meks) is the trade name for a loop diuretic.
77. Cardizem (kar-di-zem) is the trade name for a calcium channel blocker used for atrial fibrillation.
78. Colace (ko-las) is the trade name for a stool softener.
79. Compazine (kom-pah-zen) is the trade name for a tranquilizer and antiemetic.
80. Darvon (dar-von) is the trade name for a narcotic analgesic.
81. Dilantin (di-lan-tin) is the trade name for an anticonvulsant used to treat epilepsy.
82. FiberCon (fi-ber-kon) is the trade name for a bulk-forming laxative.
83. Lopressor (lo-pres-or) is the trade name for an antihypertensive.
84. Mevacor (me-va-kor) is the trade name for an antihyperlipidemic.
85. NPH (neutral protamine Hagedorn) insulin is the trade name for an insulin that decreases blood sugar.
86. Paxil (pak-sil) is the trade name for an antidepressant.
87. Pepcid (pep-sid) is the trade name for an acid controller for heartburn and acid indigestion.
88. Procardia (pro-kar-de-ah) is the trade name for a coronary vasodilator.
89. Proventil (pro-ven-til) is a trade name for a bronchodilator and metered-dose inhaler.
90. Restoril (res-to-ril) is the trade name for a sedative-hypnotic.
91. Serevent (ser-e-vent) is the trade name for an aerosol bronchodilator.

92. Slo-Bid (<u>slo</u>-bid) is the trade name for an extended-release bronchodilator.
93. Theo-Dur (<u>the</u>-o-dur) is the trade name for a bronchodilator.
94. Vanceril (<u>van</u>-ser-il) is the trade name for a corticosteroid.
95. Vasotec (<u>vah</u>-so-tek) is the trade name for an antihypertensive.
96. Ventolin (<u>ven</u>-to-lin) is the trade name for a bronchodilator.
97. Xanax (<u>zan</u>-aks) is the trade name for an antianxiety agent.
98. Zantac (<u>zan</u>-tak) is the trade name for an acid controller for heartburn and acid indigestion.

Do you remember back in school when you had to write each spelling word ten times? Because you had to physically write each word, your mind and body were focused on the assignment, and the method worked. Let's follow this successful method by reinforcing the spelling of selected terms and drugs found in the pulmonary medicine specialty through keyboarding drills.

Word Processing Users

Open your word processing package.
Read, mentally spell, and type each word in its sequence.
Save your work on your student disk.

1. adenocarcinoma adenopathy afebrile adenocarcinoma adenopathy afebrile adenocarcinoma
2. amoxicillin aneurysm arteriogram amoxicillin aneurysm arteriogram amoxicillin aneurysm
3. ascites atelectasis auscultation ascites atelectasis auscultation ascites atelectasis auscultation
4. bilateral bronchodilator bruit bilateral bronchodilator bruit bilateral bronchodilator bruit
5. caries cephalosporin claudication caries cephalosporin claudication caries cephalosporin
6. continent cor pulmonale cyanosis continent cor pulmonale cyanosis continent cor pulmonale
7. dentition diuresis diuretic dentition diuresis diuretic dentition diuresis diuretic dentition
8. doxepin dyspnea dysrhythmia doxepin dyspnea dysrhythmia doxepin dyspnea dysrhythmia
9. echocardiogram edema effusion echocardiogram edema effusion echocardiogram edema
10. embolus emesis empiric embolus emesis empiric embolus emesis empiric embolus emesis
11. erythema erythromycin fibrillation erythema erythromycin fibrillation erythema fibrillation
12. flora gallop hemoptysis flora gallop hemoptysis flora gallop hemoptysis flora gallop flora
13. heparin Homans' sign hydrate heparin Homans' sign hydrate heparin Homans' sign hydrate

14. infiltrate intrauterine ischemia infiltrate intrauterine ischemia infiltrate intrauterine ischemia
15. isosorbide lorazepam metastasis isosorbide lorazepam metastasis isosorbide lorazepam
16. nebulization nifedipine nitroglycerin nebulization nifedipine nitroglycerin nebulization
17. nocturnal nystagmus occlusion nocturnal nystagmus occlusion nocturnal nystagmus
18. pedal pneumonectomy pneumothorax pedal pneumonectomy pneumothorax pneumonectomy
19. prednisone pulmonary toilet purulent prednisone pulmonary toilet purulent prednisone
20. rale rhonchus rub rale rhonchus rub rale rhonchus rub rale rhonchus rub rale rhonchus rub
21. saphenous sequela somnolence saphenous sequela somnolence saphenous sequela
22. sputum stasis supraventricular sputum stasis supraventricular sputum stasis supraventricular
23. syncope tachycardia theophylline syncope tachycardia theophylline syncope tachycardia
24. thoracentesis thyromegaly thoracentesis thyromegaly thoracentesis thyromegaly
25. Ancef IV Ascriptin Atrovent Ancef IV Ascriptin Atrovent Ancef IV Ascriptin Atrovent
26. Azmacort Bumex Cardizem Azmacort Bumex Cardizem Azmacort Bumex Cardizem
27. Colace Compazine Darvon Colace Compazine Darvon Colace Compazine Darvon Colace
28. Dilantin FiberCon Lopressor Dilantin FiberCon Lopressor Dilantin FiberCon Lopressor
29. Mevacor Paxil Pepcid Mevacor Paxil Pepcid Mevacor Paxil Pepcid Mevacor Paxil Pepcid
30. Procardia Proventil Restoril Procardia Proventil Restoril Procardia Proventil
31. Serevent Slo-Bid Theo-Dur Serevent Slo-Bid Theo-Dur Serevent Slo-Bid Theo-Dur Serevent
32. Vanceril Vasotec Ventolin Vanceril Vasotec Ventolin Vanceril Vasotec Ventolin Vanceril
33. Xanax Zantac Xanax Zantac Xanax Zantac Xanax Zantac Xanax Zantac Xanax Zantac

Now you are ready to make the transition from keyboarding medical terms, which is a visual process, to transcribing medical terms, an aural process. You are going to use audiocassette tapes or your CD-ROM rather than printed material. Sentences 84, 95, and 98 contain dangerous abbreviations and need to be transcribed according to the guidelines established in this textbook and the recommendations of *The AAMT Book of Style*, Appendix B.

WORD PROCESSING USERS

Open your word processing package.

Insert the appropriate audiocassette in your transcribing machine and find dictation 8*T-1*.

You will be transcribing spelling words in sentence structure.

Listen carefully to each sentence on the audiocassette before transcribing.

Rewind and type (transcribe) the sentences.

Save your work on your student disk.

Refer to the answer key (Appendix E) for immediate feedback.

SOFTWARE USERS

Click on *Chapter 8, Terminology Activity 8-3 (8T-1)*, and follow the directions.

Let's pause a minute and see how well you are doing. This section allows you to evaluate your mastery of keyboarding and spelling selected terms and drugs found in the pulmonary medicine specialty.

TEXTBOOK USERS

Select the correctly spelled term that matches its definition.
Refer to the answer key (Appendix E) for immediate feedback.

SOFTWARE USERS

Click on *Chapter 8, Terminology Check Your Progress*, and follow the directions.

CHECK YOUR PROGRESS

Directions: Select the correctly spelled term that matches its definition.

1. Increased excretion of urine:
    (a) duiresis
    (b) diuresis
    (c) duiretic
    (d) diuretic

2. Involuntary, rapid, rhythmic movement of the eyeball:
    (a) nystagus
    (b) nystagmus
    (c) adencarcinoma
    (d) adenocarcinoma

3. Labored or difficult breathing:
    (a) ischemia
    (b) ischema
    (c) dyspneia
    (d) dyspnea

4. Localized dilatation of the wall of a blood vessel:
    (a) aneurysm
    (b) embolus
    (c) aneruysm
    (d) emblous

5. Malignant tumor of the glands:
    (a) nystagus
    (b) nystagmus
    (c) adencarcinoma
    (d) adenocarcinoma

6. Containing pus:
    (a) pedol
    (b) purlent
    (c) purulent
    (d) pedal

7. Coughing or spitting up blood from the respiratory tract:
    (a) hemotysis
    (b) hemoptysis
    (c) rhonchus
    (d) ronchus

8. Cramping pains of the calves caused by poor circulation to the leg muscles:
    (a) dention
    (b) claudication
    (c) caudication
    (d) dentition

9. Any drug that has the capability of increasing the capacity of the pulmonary air passages and improving ventilation to the lungs:
    (a) efflusion
    (b) bronchidilator
    (c) bronchodilator
    (d) effusion

10. Aspiration of fluid from the chest cavity:
    (a) metastasis
    (b) thoracentesis
    (c) metasis
    (d) thorasis

11. Bluish purple discoloration of the skin due to lack of oxygenated blood:
    (a) cyanesis
    (b) cyanosis
    (c) emesis
    (d) enesis

12. Calf pain with dorsiflexion of foot:
    (a) Homan's sign
    (b) theophylline
    (c) Homans' sign
    (d) theophyline

13. Accumulation of fluid in the peritoneal cavity:
    (a) caries
    (b) ascites
    (c) caires
    (d) acites

14. Act of closure or state of being closed:
    (a) oclusion
    (b) auscultation
    (c) auscutation
    (d) occlusion

CHECK YOUR PROGRESS *(cont'd)*

15. Act of fainting:
    (a) somnolence
    (b) somolence
    (c) syncope
    (d) synscope

16. Abnormal heart condition characterized by increased size of the right ventricle:
    (a) cor pulmonale
    (b) cor pulmonary
    (c) pulmonary toilet
    (d) pulmon toilet

17. Abnormal heart rhythm:
    (a) sequela
    (b) gallop
    (c) sequelia
    (d) galop

18. Abnormal slowing or stopping of fluid flowing through a vessel:
    (a) atelectasis
    (b) stasis
    (c) atellectasis
    (d) stacis

19. Ability to control urination and defecation urges:
    (a) continent
    (b) contenint
    (c) empiric
    (d) impiric

20. Abnormal crackle sound heard on chest auscultation:
    (a) rale
    (b) rub
    (c) ralle
    (d) rube

21. Abnormal sound heard on chest auscultation that results from an obstructed airway:
    (a) hemotysis
    (b) hemoptysis
    (c) rhonchus
    (d) ronchus

22. Abnormally fast heartbeat:
    (a) tachycardia
    (b) dyrhythmia
    (c) tachcardia
    (d) dysrhythmia

23. Accumulation of excess fluid in the tissues of the body:
    (a) sputum
    (b) edena
    (c) spitum
    (d) edema

24. Act of listening for sounds produced within the body with an unaided ear or with a stethoscope:
    (a) oclusion
    (b) auscultation
    (c) auscutation
    (d) occlusion

25. Drowsiness:
    (a) somnolence
    (b) somolence
    (c) syncope
    (d) synscope

26. Enlargement of the glands, especially the lymph nodes:
    (a) thyromegaly
    (b) adenogaly
    (c) adenopathy
    (d) thyropathy

27. Enlargement of the thyroid gland:
    (a) thyromegaly
    (b) adenogaly
    (c) adenopathy
    (d) thyropathy

28. Escape of fluid into a body cavity:
    (a) efflusion
    (b) bronchidilator
    (c) bronchodilator
    (d) effusion

CHECK YOUR PROGRESS *(cont'd)*

29. Affecting both sides:
    (a) afebrile
    (b) bilateral
    (c) afevrile
    (d) bilaral

30. Any abnormal condition that follows and is the result of a disease, treatment, or injury:
    (a) erythema
    (b) sequea
    (c) erytema
    (d) sequela

31. Cleansing of the trachea and bronchial tree:
    (a) cor pulmonale
    (b) cor pulmonary
    (c) pulmonary toilet
    (d) pulmon toilet

32. Collapse of a portion of the lung:
    (a) atelectasis
    (b) stasis
    (c) atellectasis
    (d) stacis

33. Decreased supply of oxygenated blood to a body part:
    (a) ischemia
    (b) ischema
    (c) dyspneia
    (d) dyspnea

34. Mass that is brought by the blood from another vessel and that obstructs blood circulation:
    (a) aneurysm
    (b) embolus
    (c) aneruysm
    (d) emblous

35. Material coughed up from the lungs and ejected through the mouth:
    (a) sputum
    (b) edena
    (c) spitum
    (d) edema

36. Normally occurring microorganisms living within the body that provide natural immunity against certain organisms:
    (a) fora
    (b) saphenous
    (c) flora
    (d) sapenous

37. Occurring at night:
    (a) intrauterine
    (b) nocturnal
    (c) interuterine
    (d) noctural

38. Pertaining to the two main superficial veins of the lower leg:
    (a) fora
    (b) saphenous
    (c) flora
    (d) sapenous

39. Diagnostic procedure using ultrasound to study heart structure and motion:
    (a) echocardiogram
    (b) echiocardogram
    (c) arteriogram
    (d) arterogram

40. Disordered rhythm:
    (a) rhonchus
    (b) dyrhythmia
    (c) ronchis
    (d) dysrhythmia

41. Treatment by a spray:
    (a) nebulization
    (b) nebullization
    (c) fibrillation
    (d) fibrilation

42. Uncoordinated twitching of muscle fibers:
    (a) nebulization
    (b) nebullization
    (c) fibrillation
    (d) fibrilation

CHECK YOUR PROGRESS *(cont'd)*

43. Within the uterus:
    (a) intrauterine
    (b) nocturnal
    (c) interuterine
    (d) noctural

44. Without fever:
    (a) afebrile
    (b) bilateral
    (c) afevrile
    (d) bilaral

45. Compound containing water molecules:
    (a) hydrate
    (b) hidrate
    (c) infiltrate
    (d) enfiltrate

46. Condition of decay and destruction of a tooth:
    (a) caries
    (b) ascites
    (c) caires
    (d) acites

47. Generic name for an antianxiety drug:
    (a) lorazepam
    (b) lorasepam
    (c) isorbide
    (d) isosorbide

48. Generic name for a nitrate-based antianginal agent:
    (a) lorazepam
    (b) lorasepam
    (c) isorbide
    (d) isosorbide

49. Generic name for an aminopenicillin antibiotic:
    (a) amoxicillin
    (b) amaxicillin
    (c) doxepin
    (d) dozepin

50. Generic name for an anticoagulant:
    (a) haperin
    (b) heparin
    (c) nifedipin
    (d) nifedipine

51. Generic name for an antidepressant:
    (a) amoxicillin
    (b) amoxicilin
    (c) doxepin
    (d) dozepin

52. Position and condition of the teeth:
    (a) dention
    (b) claudication
    (c) caudication
    (d) dentition

53. Situated or occurring above the ventricles:
    (a) superventricular
    (b) supraventricular
    (c) suberventricular
    (d) suparventricular

54. Sound caused by the rubbing together of two surfaces:
    (a) rale
    (b) rub
    (c) ralle
    (d) rube

55. Sound or murmur heard on auscultation:
    (a) bruit
    (b) gallop
    (c) briut
    (d) galop

56. Substance that promotes the excretion of urine:
    (a) duiresis
    (b) diuresis
    (c) duiretic
    (d) diuretic

57. Surgical removal of all or part of the lung:
    (a) pneumontomy
    (b) pneumonectomy
    (c) pneumotorax
    (d) pneumothorax

58. An act or instance of vomiting:
    (a) cyanesis
    (b) cyanosis
    (c) emesis
    (d) enesis

CHECK YOUR PROGRESS *(cont'd)*

59. Transfer of disease from one organ or part to another not directly connected with it:
    (a) metastasis
    (b) thoracentesis
    (c) metasis
    (d) thorasis

60. Treating a disease based on observation and experience rather than reasoning alone:
    (a) continent
    (b) contenint
    (c) empiric
    (d) impiric

61. Presence of air or gas in the pleural cavity:
    (a) pneumontomy
    (b) pneumonectomy
    (c) pneumotorax
    (d) pneumothorax

62. Radiographic visualization of an artery after injection of a contrast medium:
    (a) echocardiogram
    (b) echiocardogram
    (c) arteriogram
    (d) arterogram

63. Redness of the skin:
    (a) erythema
    (b) sequea
    (c) erytema
    (d) sequela

64. Relating to the foot:
    (a) pedol
    (b) purlent
    (c) purulent
    (d) pedal

65. Generic name for any of a large group of broad-spectrum antibiotics:
    (a) prednisone
    (b) prenisone
    (c) cephalosporin
    (d) cephalsporin

66. Generic name for a calcium channel blocker:
    (a) haperin
    (b) heparin
    (c) nifedipin
    (d) nifedipine

67. Generic name for a corticosteroid:
    (a) prednisone
    (b) prenisone
    (c) cephalosporin
    (d) cephalsporin

68. Generic name for a broad-spectrum antibiotic:
    (a) nitroglyserin
    (b) erythromycin
    (c) nitroglycerin
    (d) erythromysin

69. Generic name for a bronchodilator:
    (a) Homan's sign
    (b) theophylline
    (c) Homans' sign
    (d) theophyline

70. Generic name for a coronary vasodilator, antianginal:
    (a) nitroglyserin
    (b) erythromycin
    (c) nitroglycerin
    (d) erythromysin

71. Trade name for a bronchodilator, metered-dose inhaler:
    (a) Proventil
    (b) Provintel
    (c) Vanceril
    (d) Vanseril

72. Trade name for a bronchodilator:
    (a) Ventlin
    (b) Ventolin
    (c) Paxil
    (d) Pasil

73. Trade name for a bronchodilator:
    (a) Theo-Dur
    (b) Xanaz
    (c) Xanax
    (d) Theo-Dure

CHECK YOUR PROGRESS (cont'd)

74. Trade name for a bulk-forming laxative:
    (a) Dilantin
    (b) Dylantin
    (c) FiberCon
    (d) Fiberkon

75. Trade name for a calcium channel blocker used for atrial fibrillation:
    (a) Cardizem
    (b) Cardisem
    (c) Colase
    (d) Colace

76. Trade name for a coronary vasodilator:
    (a) Procardia
    (b) Serevent
    (c) Procariodia
    (d) Servent

77. Trade name for a corticosteroid used to prevent or treat bronchial asthma:
    (a) Azamcort
    (b) Bumex
    (c) Azmacort
    (d) Bumez

78. Trade name for a corticosteroid:
    (a) Proventil
    (b) Provintel
    (c) Vanceril
    (d) Vanseril

79. Trade name for a loop diuretic:
    (a) Azamcort
    (b) Bumex
    (c) Azmacort
    (d) Bumez

80. Trade name for a narcotic analgesic:
    (a) Compazine
    (b) Darvon
    (c) Compasine
    (d) Darvin

81. Trade name for a bronchodilator, nasal spray:
    (a) Ascriptin
    (b) Asriptin
    (c) Atrovent
    (d) Atovent

82. Trade name for an analgesic and anti-inflammatory:
    (a) Ascriptin
    (b) Asriptin
    (c) Atrovent
    (d) Atovent

83. Trade name for a sedative-hypnotic:
    (a) Pepsid
    (b) Restoril
    (c) Pepcid
    (d) Restoral

84. Trade name for a stool softener:
    (a) Cardizem
    (b) Cardisem
    (c) Colase
    (d) Colace

85. Trade name for a tranquilizer and antiemetic:
    (a) Compazine
    (b) Darvon
    (c) Compasine
    (d) Darvin

86. Trade name for an acid controller for heartburn and acid indigestion:
    (a) Pepsid
    (b) Restoril
    (c) Pepcid
    (d) Restoral

87. Trade name for an acid controller for heartburn and acid indigestion:
    (a) Zantac
    (b) Vasotec
    (c) Zantak
    (d) Vasotek

88. Trade name for an aerosol bronchodilator:
    (a) Procardia
    (b) Serevent
    (c) Procariodia
    (d) Servent

89. Trade name for an antianxiety agent:
    (a) Theo-Dur
    (b) Xanaz
    (c) Xanax
    (d) Theo-Dure

CHECK YOUR PROGRESS *(cont'd)*

90. Trade name for an anticonvulsant used in the treatment of epilepsy:
    (a) Dilantin
    (b) Dylantin
    (c) FiberCon
    (d) Fiberkon

91. Trade name for an antidepressant:
    (a) Ventlin
    (b) Ventolin
    (c) Paxil
    (d) Pasil

92. Trade name for an antihyperlipidemic:
    (a) Lopressor
    (b) Metacor
    (c) Lopressar
    (d) Mevacor

93. Trade name for an antihypertensive:
    (a) Lopressor
    (b) Metacor
    (c) Lopresor
    (d) Mevacor

94. Trade name for an antihypertensive:
    (a) Zantac
    (b) Vasotec
    (c) Zantak
    (d) Vasotek

95. Trade name for a cephalosporin antibiotic:
    (a) Ancef IV
    (b) Ansef IV
    (c) NPH
    (d) PNH

96. Trade name for an extended-release bronchodilator:
    (a) Slow-bid
    (b) Slo-bide
    (c) Slow-bide
    (d) Slo-Bid

97. Trade name for an insulin that decreases blood sugar:
    (a) Ancef IV
    (b) Ansef IV
    (c) NPH
    (d) PNH

98. An abnormal heart rhythm:
    (a) galop
    (b) rale
    (c) gallop
    (d) ralle

WORD PROCESSING USERS

Open your word processing package.

Insert the appropriate audiocassette in your transcribing machine and find dictation *8T-2*.

Transcribe and proofread dictation *8T-2*, using the formatting guidelines established in Chapter 2.

Identify and correct all errors.

Save your work on your student disk.

After completing the transcription, refer to the answer key.

Manually complete the error analysis chart.

Manually complete the Production for Pay summary.

SOFTWARE USERS

Click on *Chapter 8, Proofreading Pretest (8T-2)*, and follow the directions.

TEXTBOOK USERS

Proofread and correct errors in the medical documents shown in *Activities 8-4 and 8-5*.

Refer to the answer key (Appendix E) for immediate feedback.

Manually complete the error analysis chart for each document.

SOFTWARE USERS

Click on *Chapter 8, Activity 8-4*, and follow the directions.

Follow the same process for *Chapter 8, Activity 8-5*.

ACTIVITY 8-4
Proofreading Worksheet

Directions: Proofread this medical document using all formatting guidelines established in this textbook.

CONSULTATION REPORT

Patient Name: Calabretta, Gregory
File Number: 09451
Date of Birth: January 15, 19xx
Examination Date: *current date*
Requesting Physician: Izzy Sertoli, MD

HISTORY OF PRESENT ILLNESS
The patient is a 42 year old white male who presented to the Hospital with some vague chest pain as well as a history of shortness of breathe. The patient states to me that he has had shortness of breathe for approximately a year and 1/2. The dispnea is worse on excursion especially when climbing stairs and doing his job as a janitor. He has had a dry cough which on occasion was productive of clear sputume but has not been productive of blood or puss. Her complains of vague substernal left sided chest pain. The pain is worse with movement or papation of the area.

PAST HISTORY
Her past history is significant for asthma. He had a bilateral hernia repair 3 yrs ago.

REVIEW OF SYSTEMS
Neg.

PHYSICAL EXAMINATION
GENERAL: His blood pressure is 120 over 70 pulse seventy respirations 12 per minute.
HEENT: Negative. Neck veins are not extended. Trachea is mid line. There are noknodes in the superclavicular or cervical chain.
CHEST: Breath sounds reveal some krackles at the basis but are otherwise negative.
HEART: Heart sounds are normal but distant.
EXTREMITIES: No clubing cyanosis or edema noted.

LABORATORY DATA
Room air abg shows a po2 of fifty nine without co2 retention. Chest x-ray reveals a diffuse inter-stitial process with no hilar knodes

continued

ACTIVITY 8-4 *(cont'd)*

CONSULTATION REPORT
Patient Name: Calabretta, Gregory
File Number: 09451
Page 2

IMPRESSION
I suspect that we are dealing with an inflammatory precess in his lungs. A illness such as sarciod is a extinct possibility as we discussed on the phone last night. Additionally this could be chf although clinically it does not look like it. We will have an answer if the next chest x ray results show improvement with dyuresis. If it does not than a more intensive work up shall take place. Clinically I doubt an infection. I suspect we end up doing a bronchscopy with a biopsy.

PLAN
If there is no improvement on tomorrows x-ray we will proceed with a more agressive workup. The patient states she has no previous chest x-rays for comparison.

Allan Bolus MD

ACTIVITY 8-5
Proofreading Worksheet

Directions: Proofread this medical document using all formatting guidelines established in this textbook.

current date

Charles P. Davis, MD
FedDes Wellness Center
Family Practice Division, Suite 300
101 Wellness Way Drive
New York, NY 10036

Re: Lawrence a. Rabia

Date of Birth: Janaury 20, 19xx

Dear Dr. Davis

Mr. Rabai is a 62 year old white male with a past history of smoking. He is 6 weeks status post aortic aneurysm repair. Postoperatively she did well and was discharged. At home, she has been fairly home bound but not bedridden. He was in his usual state of health without an upper respiratory illness cough congestion or aches when he developed the a cute on set of left sided pleuritic chest pain. The pleurtic component of the pain has entensified and is actually positional at this time. He denied any hemotysis. He has some mild shortness of breathe and mild dispnea or exertion. He has no history of ankle edema or deep vein thrombsis all though he has had coronary artery by pass grafting and a safenous vein harvest on the left side.

On physical examination the patients temperature was ninety nine. His other vital signs were stable. HENT was benign. Neck showed no mass or adenpathy. Lungs showed diminished breathe sounds bilaterally with scratchie rublike sounds on the left side. Cardiovascular exam shows SI SII within normal limits and grade 1 over 6 systolic injection murmur at the lower left sternal border. There was no cardiac rub. Adbomen was soft. Extremities showed no edema. Calfs were benign and non-tender.

Chest x ray showed no evidence of neumothorax with some hyper inflation and chronic obstructive pulmonary disease changes. Her ventilation prefusion scan showed an abnormal perfusion study with 3 matched defects.

PROOFREADING

ACTIVITY 8-5 *(cont'd)*

Lawrence a. Rabia
current date
Page 3

IMPRESSION: Pleuritic left sided chest pain 6 weeks post operative and an abnormal perfusion scan. Given the indeterminate scan I suspect there is a substantial chance this may yet be a pulmonary imbolus. I would empirically haperinize at this time and procede with pulmonary angoigraphy. I have discussed this with the patient and he understands and agrees.

Thank-you for this referral.

Sincerely

Allan Bolus MD

xx

PROOFREADING

Activities 8-6 and 8-7

Proofreading Transcription Exercises (8T-3 and 8T-4)

Now you are ready to make the transition from simply proofreading printed material to both transcribing and proofreading dictated material. There are two activities in this section.

WORD PROCESSING USERS

Open your word processing package.

Insert the appropriate audiocassette in your transcribing machine and find dictation *8T-3*.

Step 1: Listen to the entire dictation to gain an understanding of the medical concepts and terms involved in the report. Rewind the tape to the beginning of the dictation, and transcribe what you hear. Do not worry about formatting, style, or speed. Simply type what you hear being dictated, using correct punctuation, capitalization, and spelling. Stop as needed to look up words you do not understand or cannot spell. Adjust the speed control of the transcriber to a comfortable level, starting slowly to ensure no dictated words are missed, and then increase the speed as your accuracy improves.

Step 2: Rewind the tape and transcribe dictation *8T-3* again, including correct spacing and formatting. Proofread the report. Identify and correct all errors. Save your work on your student disk. Refer to the answer key, and manually complete the error analysis chart and Production for Pay summary.

Follow the same process for dictation *8T-4*.

SOFTWARE USERS

Click on *Chapter 8, Activity 8-6 (8T-3), Step 1*, and follow the directions. When you feel comfortable with the dictation, click on *Chapter 8, Activity 8-6 (8T-3), Step 2*, and follow the directions.

Follow the same process for *Chapter 8, Activity 8-7 (8T-4), Step 1* and *Chapter 8, Activity 8-7 (8T-4), Step 2*.

Let's pause a minute and see how well you are doing. This section allows you to evaluate your success at transcribing and proofreading pulmonary medicine reports.

WORD PROCESSING USERS

Open your word processing package.

Insert the appropriate audiocassette in your transcribing machine and find dictation *8T-2*.

Transcribe and proofread dictation *8T-2*, using the formatting guidelines established in Chapter 2.

Identify and correct all errors.

Save your work on your student disk.

After completing the transcription, refer to the answer key.

Manually complete the error analysis chart.

Manually complete the Production for Pay summary.

SOFTWARE USERS

Click on *Chapter 8, Proofreading Check Your Progress (8T-2)*, and follow the directions.

PROOFREADING

Professional transcriptionists can transcribe and proofread their own work. Can you?

WORD PROCESSING USERS

Open your word processing package.

Insert the appropriate audiocassette in your transcribing machine and find dictation *8T-5*.

Transcribe and proofread dictation *8T-5*, using the formatting guidelines established in Chapter 2.

Save your work on your student disk.

Identify and correct all errors.

After completing the transcription, refer to the answer key.

Manually complete the error analysis chart.

Manually complete the Production for Pay summary.

Follow the same process for dictation *8T-6*.

SOFTWARE USERS

Click on *Chapter 8, Transcription Pretest (8T-5)*, and follow the directions.

Follow the same process for *Chapter 8, Transcription Pretest (8T-6)*.

TRANSCRIPTION

You have been hired as a transcriptionist at FedDes Wellness Center in the Pulmonary Medicine Division. Your supervisor has asked you to transcribe today's dictation.

WORD PROCESSING USERS

Open your word processing package.

Insert the appropriate audiocassette in your transcribing machine and find dictation *8T-7*.

Create or use an existing template as necessary for the six types of reports (chart note, chart note using history and physical format, history and physical examination report, x-ray report, procedure report, consultation letter).

Transcribe and proofread dictation *8T-7*, using the formatting guidelines established in Chapter 2.

Identify and correct all errors.

Save your work on your student disk.

After completing the transcription, refer to the answer key.

Manually complete the error analysis chart.

Manually complete the Production for Pay summary.

Follow the same process for dictations *8T-8* through *8T-12*.

SOFTWARE USERS

Click on *Chapter 8, Transcription at FedDes Wellness Center, Dictation 8T-7*, and follow the directions.

Follow the same process for each of the remaining transcriptions (*8T-8* through *8T-12*).

INDEX OF DICTATIONS AND ASSOCIATED TRANSCRIPTION TIPS

Remember to follow the guidelines pertaining to capitalization, numbers, punctuation, abbreviations, measurements, symbols, and use of templates to create medical reports at FedDes Wellness Center. This material is reviewed in Unit I.

 8T-7

History and Physical Examination Report
Patient's Name: Francine Banks
Physician: Allan Bolus, MD

Transcription Tips

- A hyphen is used between numbers and *year old*.
    You hear the dictator say: This is a twenty eight year old white female.
    You transcribe as: This is a 28-year-old white female.
- A hyphen is used to take the place of the words *to* or *through* to identify ranges.
    You hear the dictator say: respiratory infection of seven to ten days duration.
    You transcribe as: respiratory infection of 7-10 days' duration.
- A hyphen is used to join two or more words when used as an adjective that precedes a noun.
    The following word pairs are dictated in this report: blood-tinged, follow-up.
- The following drugs are dictated in this report:
    erythromycin: generic name for a broad-spectrum antibiotic
    Proventil inhaler: trade name for a bronchodilator, metered-dose inhaler
- Words beginning with *pre, re, post*, and *non* are generally not hyphenated: noncontributory.
- A period is used to take the place of the word *point*.
    You hear the dictator say: Temperature was one hundred point four.
    You transcribe as: Temperature was 100.4.
- Figures are used for age, weight, height, blood pressure, pulse, and respiration. The diagonal (/) is used to indicate the word *per* in laboratory values and respirations or the word *over* in blood pressure.
    You hear the dictator say: b p one hundred ten over sixty. Respiratory rate twenty to twenty four per minute.

You transcribe as: BP 110/60. Respiratory rate 20-24/min.
- The following abbreviations are dictated in this report. The plurals of all-capital abbreviations are formed by adding the letter *s*.
    TMs: tympanic membranes
    WBC: white blood count
- Figures and capital letters are used to refer to the vertebral column and spinal nerves.
    You hear the dictator say: sinus tachycardia without murmur or s three.
    You transcribe as: Sinus tachycardia without murmur or S3.

 8T-8

Consultation Report
Patient's Name: Heather Williams
Requesting Physician: Charles P. Davis, MD
Physician: Douglas Sputum, MD

Transcription Tips

- A hyphen is used to join two or more words when used as an adjective that precedes a noun.
    The following word pair is dictated in this report: innocent-sounding.
- Figures are used to refer to grade, phase, and pregnancy and delivery.
    You hear the dictator say: There is a short grade two over six innocent-sounding aortic ejection murmur.
    You transcribe as: There is a short grade 2/6 innocent-sounding aortic ejection murmur.
- Figures are used with the + or − symbols.
    You hear the dictator say: There is one plus dependent edema.
    You transcribe as: There is 1 + dependent edema.
- The following procedure is dictated in this report:
    dobutamine MUGA scan: multiple-gated acquisition scan, nuclear medicine imaging

 8T-9

History and Physical Examination Report
Patient's Name: Quinetta Nelson
Physician: Neal Alveoli, MD

TRANSCRIPTION

Transcription Tips

- The following abbreviations are dictated in this report. The plurals of all-capital abbreviations are formed by adding the letter *s*.
    - DJD: degenerative joint disease
    - TIAs: transient ischemic attacks
    - AV: atrioventricular
    - TMs: tympanic membranes
    - JVD: jugular venous distention
    - COPD: chronic obstructive pulmonary disease
- Words beginning with *pre, re, post*, and *non* are generally not hyphenated: postabdominal, non-tender.
- The following drugs are dictated in this report:
    - Proventil: trade name for a bronchodilator, metered-dose inhaler
    - Vanceril: trade name for a corticosteroid
    - Atrovent: trade name for a nasal spray, bronchodilator
    - nitroglycerin spray: generic name for a coronary vasodilator, antianginal
    - Darvon: trade name for a narcotic analgesic
    - Slo-Bid: trade name for an extended-release bronchodilator
    - lorazepam: generic antianxiety drug
- A hyphen is used when two or more words are viewed as a single word. The following word pair is dictated in this report: three-quarters.
- Capital letters are used for electrocardiographic leads, waves, and segments. Waves include P, Q, R, S, T, and U and their combinations.
    - You hear the dictator say: increased p two with a midsystolic murmur.
    - You transcribe as: Increased P2 with a midsystolic murmur.
- The following disease is dictated in this report:
    - cor pulmonale: a serious cardiac condition with right ventricular heart failure

8T-10

Consultation Report
Patient's Name: Marty Waye
Requesting Physician: Izzy Sertoli, MD
Physician: Allan Bolus, MD

Transcription Tips

- A hyphen joins two or more words as an adjective that precedes a noun.
    - The following word pair is dictated in this report: left-sided.
- The following abbreviations are dictated in this report:
    - CT: computed tomography

- ENT: ear, nose, throat
- MI: myocardial infarction
- JVD: jugular venous distention
- HEENT: head, eyes, ears, nose, throat
- PT: prothrombin time
- The following procedure is dictated in this report:
    - thoracentesis: surgical puncture and drainage of the thoracic cavity
- The following drug is dictated in this report:
    - cephalosporin: generic name for any of a large group of broad-spectrum antibiotics

8T-11

Consultation Report
Patient's Name: John Washington
Requesting Physician: Adam Valence, MD
Physician: Douglas Sputum, MD

Transcription Tips

- Words beginning with *pre, re, post*, and *non* are generally not hyphenated: preoperatively, noncontributory, nontender.
- The percent sign (%) is used with words and figures.
    - You hear the dictator say: found to have a seventy percent distal left main occlusion.
    - You transcribe as: found to have a 70% distal left main occlusion.
- The following drugs are dictated in this report:
    - nitroglycerin: generic name for a coronary vasodilator, antianginal
    - heparin: generic name for an anticoagulant
- The following abbreviations are dictated in this report:
    - TB: tuberculosis
    - AP: anteroposterior
    - FEV1: forced expiratory volume; pulmonary function test that measures the volume of air expired at 1 second. The patient is instructed to inhale as slowly and deeply as possible and then to exhale as quickly and completely as possible into the mouthpiece of a spirometer. The procedure is repeated three times, and the largest volume is recorded.
- BUN: blood urea nitrogen
- Figures and capital letters are used to refer to the vertebral column and spinal nerves.
    - You hear the dictator say: Cardiac exam reveals soft *s* four gallop.
    - You transcribe as: Cardiac exam reveals soft S4 gallop.
- A period is used to take the place of the word *point*.

You hear the dictator say: hemoglobin of eleven point two.

You transcribe as: hemoglobin of 11.2.

- A comma is used to punctuate large numbers with five or more digits in units of three.

  You hear the dictator say: white count ten thousand eight hundred.

  You transcribe as: white count 10,800.

- An apostrophe is used to form the possessive of singular and plural nouns.

  You hear the dictator say: The patients pulmonary function tests.

  You transcribe as: The patient's pulmonary function tests.

Transcription Tips

- The following abbreviations are dictated in this report:

  TB: tuberculosis

  URI: upper respiratory infection

  MUGA scan: multiple-gated acquisition scan

- Ordinal numbers are used to indicate order or position in a series rather than quantity. As with all numbers in medical reports, AAMT recommends using numerals (figures).

  You hear the dictator say: normal first and second sounds.

  You transcribe as: normal 1st and 2nd sounds.

- Figures are used with the + or − symbols.

  You hear the dictator say: There is three plus edema.

  You transcribe as: There is 3 + edema.

8T-12

Consultation Report
Patient's Name: Brenda McMurray
Requesting Physician: Charles P. Davis, MD
Physician: Neal Alveoli, MD

Professional transcriptionists can transcribe and proofread their own work with speed and accuracy. Have you mastered the pulmonary medicine transcription rotation at FedDes Wellness Center?

WORD PROCESSING USERS

Open your word processing package.

Insert the appropriate audiocassette in your transcribing machine and find dictation *8T-5*.

Transcribe and proofread dictation *8T-5*, using the formatting guidelines established in Chapter 2.

Save your work on your student disk.

Identify and correct all errors.

After completing the transcription, refer to the answer key.

Manually complete the error analysis chart.

Manually complete the Production for Pay summary.

Follow the same process for dictation *8T-6*.

SOFTWARE USERS

Click on *Chapter 8, Transcription Check Your Progress (8T-5)*, and follow the directions.

Follow the same process for *Chapter 8, Transcription Check Your Progress (8T-6)*.

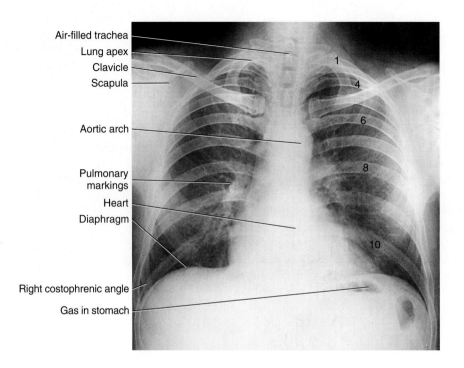

Air-filled trachea
Lung apex
Clavicle
Scapula

Aortic arch

Pulmonary markings

Heart
Diaphragm

Right costophrenic angle

Gas in stomach

1
4
6
8
10

Figure 8-1 Posteroanterior (PA) chest projection. *(From Ballinger PW, Frank ED: Merrill's atlas of radiographic positions and radiologic procedures, ed 9, St Louis, 1999, Mosby.)*

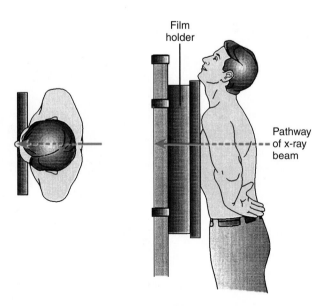

Film holder

Pathway of x-ray beam

Figure 8-2 Posteroanterior (PA) projection.

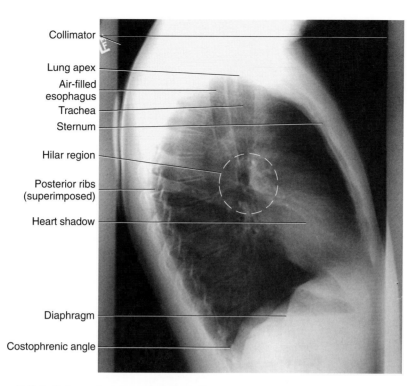

Collimator

Lung apex

Air-filled esophagus

Trachea

Sternum

Hilar region

Posterior ribs (superimposed)

Heart shadow

Diaphragm

Costophrenic angle

Figure 8-3 Left lateral chest. *(From Ballinger PW, Frank ED:* Merrill's atlas of radiographic positions and radiologic procedures, *ed 10, St Louis, 2003, Mosby.)*

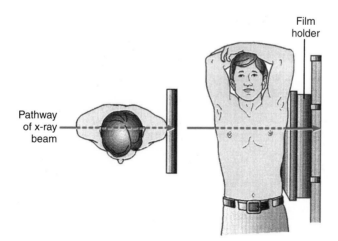

Film holder

Pathway of x-ray beam

Figure 8-4 Patient in an erect, left lateral position resulting in a lateral x-ray projection.

Chapter 9

Office Medical Transcription from the Gastroenterology Practice

OBJECTIVES

At the completion of Chapter 9, you should be able to do the following:

1. Match medical terms associated with the gastroenterology specialty with their definitions.
2. Spell medical terms associated with the gastroenterology specialty.
3. Transcribe medical terms in sentence structure.
4. Proofread, edit, and correct medical documents associated with the gastroenterology specialty that contain various errors.
5. Transcribe and proofread authentic medical documents associated with the gastroenterology specialty.

INTRODUCTION TO THE GASTROENTEROLOGY ROTATION

What's Ahead

INTRODUCTION TO THE GASTROENTEROLOGY ROTATION

The FedDes Wellness Center has three gastroenterologists, or specialists in gastroenterology, on staff. Gastroenterology is the study of the digestive tract, liver, and pancreas. The gastroenterologist assesses the function of these organs by performing invasive and noninvasive testing.

Assessment of gastrointestinal problems begin with the patient's complete history, from the mouth and teeth to bowel habits. The gastrointestinal tract examination encompasses many organs, including the mouth and pharynx, esophagus, stomach, duodenum, liver, gallbladder, pancreas, small intestine, colon, and rectum.

The physicians in FedDes Gastroenterology Division perform laboratory tests and procedures using an endoscope, including gastroscopy, exploratory laparoscopy, colonoscopy, and flexible sigmoidoscopy. Other diagnostic tests include an upper GI (gastrointestinal) series and a lower GI series (barium enema). Both these common x-ray studies use barium sulfate to image the alimentary tract.

In this unit, you assume the role of a medical transcriptionist employed at FedDes Wellness Center.

Please follow the guidelines pertaining to capitalization, numbers, punctuation, abbreviations, measurements, symbols, and use of templates to create medical reports at FedDes Wellness Center. This material is reviewed in Unit I. The transcription exercises list the type of report, patient's name, and physician(s) as well as the associated transcription tips.

You will work with the textbook and CD-ROM or accompanying audiocassettes. Your mastery of gastroenterology transcription is assessed through worksheets, timed transcription exercises, the error analysis chart, and the Production for Pay summary.

All the answer keys are found on the CD-ROM, providing immediate feedback. After transcribing a report, you will proofread your work and correct any errors. Then you will compare your proofread work against a master transcript, categorize all errors, and tabulate the errors on the error analysis chart. The Production for Pay summary correlates your production to the FedDes Wellness Center pay scale. The scale is also linked to your grade. This system allows you to assess your mastery of transcription skills in a real-world scenario.

Let's find out if you can define and spell selected terminology and drugs of the gastroenterology specialty that are included in this chapter.

TEXTBOOK USERS

Select the correctly spelled term that matches its definition.
Refer to the answer key (Appendix E) for immediate feedback.

SOFTWARE USERS

Click on *Chapter 9, Terminology Pretest*, and follow the directions.

PRETEST

Directions: Select the correctly spelled term that matches its definition.

1. A 37% aqueous solution of formaldehyde:
   (a) forlate
   (b) formalen
   (c) formalin
   (d) forlaten

2. A backward or return flow:
   (a) stent
   (b) reflux
   (c) stant
   (d) refluxe

3. A normal component of urine:
   (a) keytone
   (b) ketone
   (c) creatine
   (d) creatinine

4. Generic name for a corticosteroid:
   (a) meclizane
   (b) meclazane
   (c) hydrocortsone
   (d) hydrocortisone

5. A gland in the male that surrounds the neck of the bladder and urethra:
   (a) prostate
   (b) tirate
   (c) postate
   (d) titrate

6. Enlargement of the thyroid gland:
   (a) hepatasplenmegaly
   (b) thyromegaly
   (c) hepatosplenomegaly
   (d) thyomegaly

7. A mold for keeping a skin graft in place:
   (a) stent
   (b) reflux
   (c) stant
   (d) refluxe

8. A radiographic record of an artery after injection of a contrast medium:
   (a) pinna
   (b) arterogram
   (c) pina
   (d) arteriogram

9. Ability to move spontaneously:
   (a) bilary
   (b) biliary
   (c) motility
   (d) molity

10. After a meal:
    (a) postprandial
    (b) prophylatic
    (c) posprandial
    (d) prophyacic

11. An agent that tends to ward off disease:
    (a) postprandial
    (b) prophylactic
    (c) posprandial
    (d) prophyacic

12. Generic name for an anticoagulant:
    (a) heparin
    (b) lidocaine
    (c) heparen
    (d) lidacaine

13. Generic name for an anti-inflammatory, antiallergic agent:
    (a) prenisone
    (b) prednisone
    (c) lidocaine
    (d) lidocain

14. Generic name for an antinauseant:
    (a) meclizine
    (b) mecizine
    (c) nitroglycerin
    (d) nitoglycerin

15. An elongated endoscope, usually fiberoptic:
    (a) fiberscope
    (b) fiveroscope
    (c) colonoscope
    (d) colonscope

16. An endoscope for use in sigmoidoscopy:
    (a) sigmoidoscope
    (b) sigmiodoscope
    (c) colonoscope
    (d) colonscope

PRETEST (cont'd)

17. An increase in the severity of a disease or symptoms:
    (a) retroflexion
    (b) retroflesion
    (c) exacerbation
    (d) exacerbasion

18. An opening created by surgery, disease, or trauma between two or more organs or structures:
    (a) anastomosis
    (b) anastamosis
    (c) stenosis
    (d) stenasis

19. Any compound containing carbon oxide:
    (a) keytone
    (b) ketone
    (c) creatine
    (d) creatinine

20. Any growth or mass protruding from a mucous membrane:
    (a) polyp
    (b) polpa
    (c) scera
    (d) sclera

21. Any solution compound that conducts electricity:
    (a) lumen
    (b) lumin
    (c) electrilyte
    (d) electrolyte

22. Cavity or channel within a tube:
    (a) lumen
    (b) lumin
    (c) electrilyte
    (d) electrolyte

23. Darkening of the feces by blood pigments:
    (a) malena
    (b) erythema
    (c) melena
    (d) erthema

24. Difficulty in swallowing:
    (a) hematochezia
    (b) dysphagia
    (c) hemotachesia
    (d) dysphogia

25. Disease of the lymph nodes:
    (a) laminectomy
    (b) lymphadenopathy
    (c) lamenectomy
    (d) lympanopathy

26. Enlargement of the liver and spleen:
    (a) hepatasplenmegaly
    (b) thyromegaly
    (c) hepatosplenomegaly
    (d) thyomegaly

27. Establishment of a new opening into the stomach:
    (a) gastriparesis
    (b) gastroparesis
    (c) gastristomy
    (d) gastrostomy

28. Feeling of uneasiness:
    (a) targor
    (b) turgor
    (c) malaise
    (d) malise

29. Folic acid:
    (a) folate
    (b) formalen
    (c) formalin
    (d) forlaten

30. Hernia of the bladder, usually into the vagina and introitus:
    (a) rectocele
    (b) recocele
    (c) cystocele
    (d) cestocele

31. Hernial protrusion of part of the rectum into the vagina:
    (a) rectocele
    (b) recocele
    (c) cystocele
    (d) cestocele

32. Inflammation of the colon:
    (a) colitis
    (b) colotis
    (c) proctitis
    (d) protitis

TERMINOLOGY

PRETEST *(cont'd)*

33. Inflammation of the inner ear:
    (a) labrinithitis
    (b) gasritis
    (c) gastritis
    (d) labyrinthitis

34. Inflammation of the rectum:
    (a) colitis
    (b) colotis
    (c) proctitis
    (d) protitis

35. Inflammation of the stomach, especially the mucosa:
    (a) labrinithitis
    (b) gasritis
    (c) gastritis
    (d) labyrinthitis

36. Involuntary, rapid, rhythmic movement of the eyeball:
    (a) adenomatous
    (b) adenamatous
    (c) nistagmus
    (d) nystagmus

37. Jaundice:
    (a) decubitus
    (b) decubetus
    (c) icterus
    (d) ictreus

38. Generic name for a local anesthetic, antiarrhythmic:
    (a) heparin
    (b) lidocaine
    (c) heparen
    (d) lidacaine

39. Muscular pain:
    (a) myalgia
    (b) odynophagia
    (c) myelgia
    (d) oynophagia

40. One of the forms of vitamin B-6:
    (a) occult
    (b) ocult
    (c) pyridxine
    (d) pyridoxine

41. Burning, squeezing pain while swallowing:
    (a) myalgia
    (b) odynophagia
    (c) myelgia
    (d) oynophagia

42. Projecting part of the ear lying outside the head:
    (a) pinna
    (b) arterogram
    (c) pina
    (d) arteriogram

43. Redness of the skin due to capillary dilatation:
    (a) malena
    (b) erythema
    (c) melena
    (d) erthema

44. Pertaining to bile or the biliary tract:
    (a) bilary
    (b) biliary
    (c) motility
    (d) molity

45. Pertaining to the stomach and esophagus:
    (a) gastroesophageal
    (b) gasointestinal
    (c) gasoesophageal
    (d) gastrointestinal

46. Pertaining to some types of glandular hyperplasia:
    (a) adenomatous
    (b) adenamatous
    (c) nistagmus
    (d) nystagmus

47. Pertaining to the stomach and the intestines:
    (a) gastroesophageal
    (b) gasointestinal
    (c) gasoesophageal
    (d) gastrointestinal

48. Removal of the right or left side of the colon:
    (a) hemicolectomy
    (b) hemacolectomy
    (c) cholecystectomy
    (d) colecystectomy

PRETEST *(cont'd)*

49. Slight degree of gastroparalysis:
    (a) gastriparesis
    (b) gastroparesis
    (c) gastristomy
    (d) gastrostomy

50. Specimen hidden from view:
    (a) occult
    (b) ocult
    (c) pyridxine
    (d) pyridoxine

51. Surgical excision of the lamina:
    (a) laminectomy
    (b) lymphadenopathy
    (c) lamenectomy
    (d) lympanopathy

52. The bending of an organ so that its top is thrust backward:
    (a) retroflexion
    (b) retroflesion
    (c) exacerbation
    (d) exacerbasion

53. The condition of fullness; the expected resiliency of the skin:
    (a) targor
    (b) turgor
    (c) malaise
    (d) malise

54. The cul-de-sac, about 6 cm in depth, lying below the terminal ileum, forming the first part of the large intestine:
    (a) heme
    (b) cecum
    (c) hema
    (d) cecam

55. Direct examination of the interior of the sigmoid colon:
    (a) endoscopy
    (b) sigmiodoscopy
    (c) endioscopy
    (d) sigmoidoscopy

56. Establishment of an artificial opening into the colon:
    (a) colonscopy
    (b) colonoscopy
    (c) colostomy
    (d) colonstomy

57. Examination of the interior of a canal or hollow viscus by means of an endoscope:
    (a) endoscopy
    (b) viscosopy
    (c) endioscopy
    (d) viscuscopy

58. The narrowing of a body passage or opening:
    (a) anastomosis
    (b) anastamosis
    (c) stenosis
    (d) stenasis

59. The oxygen-carrying, color-furnishing group of hemoglobin:
    (a) heme
    (b) cecum
    (c) hema
    (d) cecam

60. The passage of bloody stools:
    (a) hematochezia
    (b) dysphagia
    (c) hemotachesia
    (d) dysphogia

61. Position when recumbent:
    (a) decubitus
    (b) decubetus
    (c) icterus
    (d) ictreus

62. Surgical removal of the gallbladder:
    (a) hemicolectomy
    (b) hemacolectomy
    (c) cholecystectomy
    (d) colecystectomy

63. The tough, white outer coat of the eyeball:
    (a) polyp
    (b) polpa
    (c) scera
    (d) sclera

PRETEST *(cont'd)*

64. Visual examination of the inner surface of the colon by means of a colonoscope:
    (a) colonscopy
    (b) colonoscopy
    (c) colostomy
    (d) colonstomy

65. To analyze a given solution component by adding a liquid reagent:
    (a) prostate
    (b) tirate
    (c) postate
    (d) titrate

66. Generic name for a vasodilator used to relieve certain types of pain:
    (a) meclizine
    (b) mecizine
    (c) nitroglycerin
    (d) nitoglycerin

67. Vomiting of blood indicating upper gastrointestinal bleeding:
    (a) hematemesis
    (b) hemetemesis
    (c) emasis
    (d) emesis

68. An act or instance of vomiting:
    (a) hematemesis
    (b) hemetemesis
    (c) emasis
    (d) emesis

69. Trade name for an antianxiety agent:
    (a) Ativan
    (b) Atevan
    (c) Bumex
    (d) Bumix

70. Trade name for an antagonist used to treat gastric and duodenal ulcers:
    (a) Axid
    (b) Cheme-7
    (c) Chem-7
    (d) Axide

71. Trade name for a loop diuretic:
    (a) Ativan
    (b) Atevan
    (c) Bumex
    (d) Bumix

72. Trade name for a profile of seven different chemical laboratory tests:
    (a) Axid
    (b) Cheme-7
    (c) Chem-7
    (d) Axide

73. Trade name for an anticoagulant:
    (a) Demerol
    (b) Coumadin
    (c) Demirol
    (d) Doumaden

74. Trade name for a synthetic narcotic analgesic:
    (a) Demerol
    (b) Coumadin
    (c) Demirol
    (d) Doumaden

75. Trade name for an anticonvulsant used to treat epilepsy:
    (a) Delantin
    (b) Dilantin
    (c) Elavil
    (d) Elevil

76. Trade name for an antidepressant:
    (a) Delantin
    (b) Dilantin
    (c) Elavil
    (d) Elevil

77. Trade name for a guaiac test for occult blood:
    (a) Humilin
    (b) Hemoccult
    (c) Humulin
    (d) Hemocult

78. Trade name for an antidiabetic:
    (a) Humilin
    (b) Hemoccult
    (c) Humulin
    (d) Hemocult

PRETEST *(cont'd)*

79. Trade name for an antihypertensive used to treat benign prostatic hyperplasia:
    (a) Indocin
    (b) Indicin
    (c) Hitrin
    (d) Hytrin

80. Trade name for a nonsteroidal anti-inflammatory drug (NSAID):
    (a) Indocin
    (b) Indicin
    (c) Hitrin
    (d) Hytrin

81. Trade name for a potassium supplement:
    (a) K-Dur
    (b) Lopressor
    (c) K-Dura
    (d) Lopressar

82. Trade name for an antihypertensive:
    (a) K-Dur
    (b) Lopressor
    (c) K-Dura
    (d) Lopressar

83. Trade name for a urinary bacteriostatic:
    (a) Mazide
    (b) Maxzide
    (c) Macroid
    (d) Macrobid

84. Trade name for a diuretic, antihypertensive:
    (a) Mazide
    (b) Maxzide
    (c) Macroid
    (d) Macrobid

85. Trade name for a bulk laxative:
    (a) Metamacil
    (b) Naporsyn
    (c) Metamucil
    (d) Naprosyn

86. Trade name for an NSAID:
    (a) Metamacil
    (b) Naporsyn
    (c) Metamucil
    (d) Naprosyn

87. Trade name for an antianginal, antihypertensive:
    (a) Paxil
    (b) Pasil
    (c) Norvasc
    (d) Norasc

88. Trade name for an antidepressant:
    (a) Paxil
    (b) Pasil
    (c) Norvasc
    (d) Norasc

89. Trade name for an acid controller for heartburn and acid indigestion:
    (a) Maxzide
    (b) Pepcid
    (c) Maxside
    (d) Pepid

90. Trade name for a gastric acid secretion inhibitor:
    (a) Priosec
    (b) K-Dure
    (c) Prilosec
    (d) K-Dur

91. Trade name for a coronary vasodilator:
    (a) Regan
    (b) Procardia
    (c) Porcardia
    (d) Reglan

92. Trade name for a gastrointestinal stimulant, antiemetic:
    (a) Regan
    (b) Procardia
    (c) Porcardia
    (d) Reglan

93. Trade name for a mild central nervous system stimulant, antidepressant:
    (a) Ritalin
    (b) Ritilin
    (c) Synthroid
    (d) Synroid

94. Trade name for a thyroid hormone:
    (a) Ritalin
    (b) Ritilin
    (c) Synthroid
    (d) Synroid

PRETEST *(cont'd)*

95. Trade name for an antihypertensive:
    (a) Tenormin
    (b) Tenorrmin
    (c) Terramycin
    (d) Teramycin

96. Trade name for an antibiotic:
    (a) Tenormin
    (b) Tenorrmin
    (c) Terramycin
    (d) Teramycin

97. Trade name for an antiemetic:
    (a) Timoptic
    (b) Tiggan
    (c) Timptic
    (d) Tigan

98. Trade name for a beta blocker, antiglaucoma agent:
    (a) Timoptic
    (b) Tiggan
    (c) Timptic
    (d) Tigan

99. Trade name for an antihypertensive:
    (a) Vastec
    (b) Versed
    (c) Vasotec
    (d) Verse

100. Trade name for a short-acting benzodiazepine, general anesthetic adjunct for preoperative sedation:
    (a) Vastec
    (b) Versed
    (c) Vasotec
    (d) Verse

101. Trade name for a reductase inhibitor for hypercholesterolemia and coronary heart disease:
    (a) Zoccor
    (b) Zokur
    (c) Zochor
    (d) Zocor

Let's learn to spell and define selected terminology and drugs of the gastroenterology specialty that are included in this chapter. Keyboarding these terms is an effective way to improve your skills.

Word Processing Users

Open your word processing package.
Read and type each word and its definition as shown below.
Save your work on your student disk.

1. Adenomatous (ad-e-<u>no</u>-ma-tus) pertains to some types of glandular hyperplasia.
2. Anastomosis (a-nas-to-<u>mo</u>-sis) is an opening created by surgery, disease, or trauma between two or more organs or structures.
3. Arteriogram (ar-<u>ter</u>-e-o-gram) is a radiographic record of an artery after injection of a contrast medium.
4. Biliary (<u>bil</u>-e-ar-e) pertains to bile or the biliary tract.
5. Cecum (<u>se</u>-kum) is the cul-de-sac, about 6 cm in depth, lying below the terminal ileum, forming the first part of the large intestine.
6. Cholecystectomy (<u>ko</u>-le-sis-<u>tek</u>-to-me) is the surgical removal of the gallbladder.
7. Colitis (ko-<u>li</u>-tis) is inflammation of the colon.
8. Colonoscope (ko-<u>lon</u>-o-skop) is an elongated endoscope, usually fiberoptic.
9. Colonoscopy (ko-lon-<u>os</u>-ko-pe) is the visual examination of the inner surface of the colon by means of a colonoscope.
10. Colostomy (ko-<u>los</u>-to-me) is the establishment of an artificial opening into the colon.
11. Creatinine (kre-<u>at</u>-i-nen) is a normal component of urine.
12. Cystocele (<u>sis</u>-to-sel) is a hernia of the bladder, usually into the vagina and introitus.
13. Decubitus (de-<u>kyu</u>-bi-tus) is a recumbent or horizontal position.
14. Dysphagia (dis-<u>fa</u>-je-a) is difficulty in swallowing.
15. Electrolytes (e-<u>lek</u>-tro-lights) is any solution compound that conducts electricity.
16. Emesis (<u>em</u>-e-sis) is an act or instance of vomiting.
17. Endoscopy (en-<u>dos</u>-ko-pe) is the examination of the interior of a canal or hollow viscus by means of an endoscope.
18. Erythema (er-i-<u>the</u>-ma) is redness of the skin due to capillary dilatation.
19. Exacerbation (eg-zas-er-<u>ba</u>-shun) is an increase in the severity of a disease or symptoms.
20. Folate (<u>fo</u>-lat) is folic acid.
21. Formalin (<u>for</u>-ma-lin) is a 37% aqueous solution of formaldehyde.
22. Gastritis (gas-<u>tri</u>-tis) is inflammation of the stomach, especially the mucosa.
23. Gastroesophageal (<u>gas</u>-tro-e-sof-a-je-al) pertains to both the stomach and the esophagus.
24. Gastrointestinal (<u>gas</u>-tro-in-tes-tin-al) pertains to the stomach and the intestines.
25. Gastroparesis (gas-tro-pa-<u>re</u>-sis) is a slight degree of gastroparalysis.
26. Gastrostomy (gas-<u>tros</u>-to-me) is the establishment of a new opening into the stomach.
27. Hematemesis (he-ma-<u>tem</u>-e-sis) is the vomiting of blood indicating upper gastrointestinal bleeding.
28. Hematochezia (<u>he</u>-ma-to-<u>ke</u>-ze-a) is the passage of bloody stools.
29. Heme (hem) is the oxygen-carrying, color-furnishing group of hemoglobin.
30. Hemicolectomy (<u>hem</u>-e-ko-<u>lek</u>-to-me) is the removal of the right or left side of the colon.
31. Heparin (<u>hep</u>-ah-rin) is a generic name for an anticoagulant.
32. Hepatosplenomegaly (hep-ah-to-sple-no-<u>meg</u>-ah-le) is the enlargement of the liver and spleen.
33. Hydrocortisone (hi-dro-<u>kor</u>-ti-son) is a generic name for a corticosteroid.
34. Icterus (<u>ik</u>-ter-us) is jaundice.
35. Ketone (<u>ke</u>-tone) is any compound containing carbon oxide.
36. Labyrinthitis (lab-i-rin-<u>thi</u>-tis) is inflammation of the inner ear.
37. Laminectomy (lam-i-<u>nek</u>-to-me) is the surgical excision of the lamina.
38. Lidocaine (<u>li</u>-do-cane) is a generic name for a local anesthetic and antiarrhythmic.
39. Lumen (<u>lu</u>-men) is a cavity or channel within a tube.
40. Lymphadenopathy (lim-fad-e-<u>nop</u>-ah-the) is disease of the lymph nodes.
41. Malaise (mal-<u>az</u>) is a feeling of uneasiness.
42. Meclizine (<u>mek</u>-li-zen) is a generic name for an antinauseant.
43. Melena (me-<u>le</u>-nah) is darkening of the feces by blood pigments.
44. Motility (mo-<u>til</u>-i-te) is the ability to move spontaneously.
45. Myalgia (mi-<u>al</u>-je-ah) is muscular pain.
46. Nitroglycerin (ni-tro-<u>glis</u>-er-in) is a generic name for a vasodilator used to relieve certain types of pain.

47. Nystagmus (nis-tag-mus) is the involuntary, rapid, rhythmic movement of the eyeball.
48. Occult (o-kult) is hidden from view.
49. Odynophagia (o-din-o-fa-je-ah) is burning, squeezing pain while swallowing
50. Pinna (pin-ah) is the projecting part of the ear lying outside the head.
51. Polyp (pol-ip) is any growth or mass protruding from a mucous membrane.
52. Postprandial (post-pran-de-al) means after a meal.
53. Prednisone (pred-ni-son) is a generic name for an anti-inflammatory and antiallergic agent.
54. Proctitis (prok-ti-tis) is inflammation of the rectum.
55. Prophylactic (pro-fi-lak-tik) is an agent that tends to ward off disease.
56. Prostate (pros-tat) is a gland in the male that surrounds the neck of the bladder and urethra.
57. Pyridoxine (pir-o-dok-sen) is one of the forms of vitamin B-6.
58. Rectocele (rek-to-sel) is the hernial protrusion of part of the rectum into the vagina.
59. Reflux (re-fluks) is a backward or return flow.
60. Retroflexion (ret-ro-flek-shun) is the bending of an organ so that its top is thrust backward.
61. Sclera (skle-rah) is the tough, white outer coat of the eyeball.
62. Sigmoidoscope (sig-moi-do-skop) is an endoscope for use in sigmoidoscopy.
63. Sigmoidoscopy (sig-moi-dos-ko-pe) is the direct examination of the interior of the sigmoid colon.
64. Stenosis (ste-no-sis) is the narrowing of a body passage or opening.
65. Stent is a device placed within the lumen of a vessel to provide support and patency of the vessel.
66. Thyromegaly (thi-ro-meg-ah-le) is enlargement of the thyroid gland.
67. Titrate (ti-trat) is to analyze a given solution component by adding a liquid reagent.
68. Turgor (tur-gor) is the condition of fullness; the expected resiliency of the skin.
69. Ativan (at-i-van) is the trade name for an antianxiety agent.
70. Axid (ak-sid) is the trade name for an antagonist for the treatment of gastric and duodenal ulcers.
71. Bumex (bum-eks) is the trade name for a loop diuretic.
72. Chem-7 is the trade name for a profile of seven different chemical laboratory tests.
73. Coumadin (koo-mah-din) is the trade name for an anticoagulant.
74. Demerol (dem-er-ol) is the trade name for a synthetic narcotic analgesic.
75. Dilantin (di-lan-tin) is the trade name for an anticonvulsant used to treat epilepsy.
76. Elavil (el-ah-vil) is the trade name for an antidepressant.
77. Hemoccult (he-mo-kult) is the trade name for a guaiac test for occult blood.
78. Humulin (hu-mu-lin) is the trade name for an antidiabetic.
79. Hytrin (hi-trin) is the trade name for an antihypertensive used to treat benign prostatic hyperplasia.
80. Indocin (in-do-sin) is the trade name for a nonsteroidal anti-inflammatory drug, NSAID.
81. K-Dur (ka-dur) is the trade name for a potassium supplement.
82. Lopressor (lo-pres-or) is the trade name for an antihypertensive.
83. Macrobid (mak-ro-bid) is the trade name for a urinary bacteriostatic.
84. Maxzide (mak-sid) is the trade name for a diuretic and antihypertensive.
85. Metamucil (met-ah-mu-sil) is the trade name for a bulk laxative.
86. Naprosyn (nah-pro-sin) is the trade name for an NSAID.
87. Norvasc (nor-vask) is the trade name for an antianginal and antihypertensive.
88. Paxil (pa-sil) is the trade name for an antidepressant.
89. Pepcid (pep-sid) is the trade name for an acid controller for heartburn and acid indigestion.
90. Prilosec (pril-o-sek) is the trade name for a gastric acid secretion inhibitor.
91. Procardia (pro-kar-de-ah) is the trade name for a coronary vasodilator.
92. Reglan (reg-lan) is the trade name for a gastrointestinal stimulant and antiemetic.
93. Ritalin (rit-ah-lin) is the trade name for a mild central nervous system stimulant and antidepressant.
94. Synthroid (sin-throid) is the trade name for a thyroid hormone.
95. Tenormin (ten-or-min) is the trade name for an antihypertensive.
96. Terramycin (ter-ah-mi-sin) is the trade name for an antibiotic.
97. Tigan (ti-gan) is the trade name for an antiemetic.
98. Timoptic (tim-op-tik) is the trade name for a beta blocker, antiglaucoma agent.
99. Vasotec (vah-so-tek) is the trade name for an antihypertensive.
100. Versed (ver-sed) is the trade name for a short-acting benzodiazepine and general anesthetic adjunct for preoperative sedation.
101. Zocor (zo-kor) is the trade name for a reductase inhibitor for hypercholesterolemia and coronary heart disease.

Do you remember back in school when you had to write each spelling word ten times? Because you had to physically write each word, your mind and body were focused on the assignment, and the method worked. Let's follow this successful method by reinforcing the spelling of selected terms and drugs found in the gastroenterology specialty through keyboarding drills.

Word Processing Users

Open your word processing package.
Read, mentally spell, and type each word in its sequence.
Save your work on your student disk.

1. adenomatous anastomosis arteriogram adenomatous anastomosis arteriogram
2. biliary cecum cholecystectomy biliary cecum cholecystectomy biliary cecum
3. colitis colonoscope colonoscopy colitis colonoscope colonoscopy colitis
4. colostomy creatinine cystocele colostomy creatinine cystocele colostomy
5. decubitus dysphagia electrolytes decubitus dysphagia electrolytes decubitus
6. emesis endoscopy erythema emesis endoscopy erythema emesis endoscopy
7. exacerbation folate formalin exacerbation folate formalin exacerbation folate
8. gastritis gastroesophageal gastrointestinal gastritis gastroesophageal gastrointestinal
9. gastroparesis gastrostomy hematemesis gastroparesis gastrostomy hematemesis
10. hematochezia heme hemicolectomy hematochezia heme hemicolectomy
11. heparin hepatosplenomegaly hydrocortisone heparin hepatosplenomegaly hydrocortisone
12. icterus ketone labyrinthitis icterus ketone labyrinthitis icterus ketone labyrinthitis
13. laminectomy lidocaine lumen laminectomy lidocaine lumen laminectomy lidocaine
14. lymphadenopathy malaise meclizine lymphadenopathy malaise meclizine

15. melena motility myalgia melena motility myalgia melena motility myalgia melena
16. nitroglycerin nystagmus occult nitroglycerin nystagmus occult nitroglycerin
17. odynophagia pinna polyp odynophagia pinna polyp odynophagia pinna polyp
18. postprandial prednisone proctitis postprandial prednisone proctitis postprandial
19. prophylactic prostate pyridoxine prophylactic prostate pyridoxine prophylactic prostate
20. rectocele reflux retroflexion rectocele reflux retroflexion rectocele reflux retroflexion
21. sclera sigmoidoscope sigmoidoscopy sclera sigmoidoscope sigmoidoscopy sclera
22. stenosis stent thyromegaly stenosis stent thyromegaly stenosis stent thyromegaly
23. titrate turgor titrate turgor titrate turgor titrate turgor titrate turgor titrate turgor titrate
24. Ativan Axid Bumex Ativan Axid Bumex Ativan Axid Bumex Ativan Axid Bumex
25. Chem-7 Coumadin Demerol Chem-7 Coumadin Demerol Chem-7 Coumadin
26. Dilantin Elavil Hemoccult Dilantin Elavil Hemoccult Dilantin Elavil Hemoccult
27. Humulin Hytrin Indocin Humulin Hytrin Indocin Humulin Hytrin Indocin Humulin
28. K-Dur Lopressor Macrobid K-Dur Lopressor Macrobid K-Dur Lopressor Macrobid
29. Maxzide Metamucil Naprosyn Maxzide Metamucil Naprosyn Maxzide Metamucil
30. Norvasc Paxil Pepcid Norvasc Paxil Pepcid Norvasc Paxil Pepcid Norvasc Paxil
31. Prilosec Procardia Reglan Prilosec Procardia Reglan Prilosec Procardia Reglan
32. Ritalin Synthroid Tenormin Ritalin Synthroid Tenormin Ritalin Synthroid Tenormin
33. Terramycin Tigan Timoptic Terramycin Tigan Timoptic Terramycin Tigan Timoptic
34. Vasotec Versed Zocor Vasotec Versed Zocor Vasotec Versed Zocor Vasotec Versed

Now you are ready to make the transition from keyboarding medical terms, which is a visual process, to transcribing medical terms, an aural process. You are going to use audiocassette tapes or your CD-ROM rather than printed material.

WORD PROCESSING USERS

Open your word processing package.

Insert the appropriate audiocassette in your transcribing machine and find dictation *9T-1*.

You will be transcribing spelling words in sentence structure.

Listen carefully to each sentence on the audiocassette before transcribing.

Rewind and type (transcribe) the sentences.

Save your work on your student disk.

Refer to the answer key (Appendix E) for immediate feedback.

SOFTWARE USERS

Click on *Chapter 9, Terminology Activity 9-3 (9T-1)*, and follow the directions.

Let's pause a minute and see how well you are doing. This section allows you to evaluate your mastery of keyboarding and spelling selected terms and drugs found in the gastroenterology specialty.

TEXTBOOK USERS

Select the correctly spelled term that matches its definition.
Refer to the answer key (Appendix E) for immediate feedback.

SOFTWARE USERS

Click on *Chapter 9, Terminology Check Your Progress*, and follow the directions.

NAME _____   DATE _____

CHECK YOUR PROGRESS

Directions: Select the correctly spelled term that matches its definition.

1. Visual examination of the inner surface of the colon by means of a colonoscope:
   (a) colonscopy
   (b) colonoscopy
   (c) colostomy
   (d) colonstomy

2. To analyze a given solution component by adding a liquid reagent:
   (a) prostate
   (b) tirate
   (c) postate
   (d) titrate

3. Generic name for a vasodilator used to relieve certain types of pain:
   (a) meclizine
   (b) mecizine
   (c) nitroglycerin
   (d) nitoglycerin

4. Vomiting of blood indicating upper gastrointestinal bleeding:
   (a) hematemesis
   (b) hemetemesis
   (c) emasis
   (d) emesis

5. The tough, white outer coat of the eyeball:
   (a) polyp
   (b) polpa
   (c) scera
   (d) sclera

6. The passage of bloody stools:
   (a) hematochezia
   (b) dysphagia
   (c) hemotachesia
   (d) dysphogia

7. Position when recumbent:
   (a) decubitus
   (b) decubetus
   (c) icterus
   (d) ictreus

8. Surgical removal of the gallbladder:
   (a) hemicolectomy
   (b) hemacolectomy
   (c) cholecystectomy
   (d) colecystectomy

9. Examination of the interior of a canal or hollow viscus by means of endoscope:
   (a) endoscopy
   (b) sigmiodoscopy
   (c) endioscopy
   (d) sigmoidoscopy

10. The narrowing of a body passage or opening:
    (a) anastomosis
    (b) anastomosis
    (c) stenosis
    (d) stenasis

11. The oxygen-carrying, color-furnishing group of hemoglobin:
    (a) heme
    (b) cecum
    (c) hema
    (d) cecam

12. The bending of an organ so that its top is thrust backward:
    (a) retroflexion
    (b) retroflesion
    (c) exacerbation
    (d) exacerbasion

13. The condition of fullness; the expected resiliency of the skin:
    (a) targor
    (b) turgor
    (c) malaise
    (d) malise

14. The cul-de-sac, about 6 cm in depth, lying below the terminal ileum, forming the first part of the large intestine:
    (a) heme
    (b) cecum
    (c) hema
    (d) cecam

15. Direct examination of the interior of the sigmoid colon:
    (a) endoscopy
    (b) sigmiodoscopy
    (c) endioscopy
    (d) sigmoidoscopy

CHECK YOUR PROGRESS *(cont'd)*

16. Establishment of an artificial opening into the colon:
    (a) colonscopy
    (b) colonoscopy
    (c) colostomy
    (d) colonstomy

17. Generic name for a local anesthetic, antiarrhythmic:
    (a) heparin
    (b) lidocaine
    (c) heparen
    (d) lidacaine

18. Muscular pain:
    (a) myalgia
    (b) odynophagia
    (c) myelgia
    (d) oynophagia

19. One of the forms of vitamin B-6:
    (a) occult
    (b) ocult
    (c) pyridxine
    (d) pyridoxine

20. Burning, squeezing pain while swallowing:
    (a) myalgia
    (b) odynophagia
    (c) myelgia
    (d) oynophagia

21. Projecting part of the ear lying outside the head:
    (a) pinna
    (b) arterogram
    (c) pina
    (d) arteriogram

22. Redness of the skin due to capillary dilatation:
    (a) malena
    (b) erythema
    (c) melena
    (d) erthema

23. Pertaining to bile or the biliary tract:
    (a) bilary
    (b) biliary
    (c) motility
    (d) molity

24. Pertaining to both the stomach and the esophagus:
    (a) gastroesophageal
    (b) gasointestinal
    (c) gasoesophageal
    (d) gastrointestinal

25. Pertaining to some types of glandular hyperplasia:
    (a) adenomatous
    (b) adenamatous
    (c) nistagmus
    (d) nystagmus

26. Pertaining to the stomach and the intestines:
    (a) gastroesophageal
    (b) gasointestinal
    (c) gasoesophageal
    (d) gastrointestinal

27. A 37% aqueous solution of formaldehyde:
    (a) forlate
    (b) formalen
    (c) formalin
    (d) forlaten

28. A backward or return flow:
    (a) stent
    (b) reflux
    (c) stant
    (d) refluxe

29. A normal component of urine:
    (a) keytone
    (b) ketone
    (c) creatine
    (d) creatinine

30. Generic name for a corticosteroid:
    (a) meclizane
    (b) meclazane
    (c) hydrocortsone
    (d) hydrocortisone

31. A gland in the male that surrounds the neck of the bladder and urethra:
    (a) prostate
    (b) tirate
    (c) postate
    (d) titrate

CHECK YOUR PROGRESS *(cont'd)*

32. Enlargement of the thyroid gland:
    (a) hepatasplenmegaly
    (b) thyromegaly
    (c) hepatosplenomegaly
    (d) thyomegaly

33. A device that provides support and patency to a vessel:
    (a) stent
    (b) reflux
    (c) stant
    (d) refluxe

34. A radiographic record of an artery after injection of a contrast medium:
    (a) pinna
    (b) arterogram
    (c) pina
    (d) arteriogram

35. Ability to move spontaneously:
    (a) bilary
    (b) biliary
    (c) motility
    (d) molity

36. After a meal:
    (a) postprandial
    (b) prophylatic
    (c) posprandial
    (d) prophyacic

37. An agent that tends to ward off disease:
    (a) postprandial
    (b) prophylactic
    (c) posprandial
    (d) prophyacic

38. Generic name for an anticoagulant:
    (a) heparin
    (b) lidocaine
    (c) formalin
    (d) lidacaine

39. Generic name for an anti-inflammatory, antiallergic agent:
    (a) prenisone
    (b) prednisone
    (c) lidocaine
    (d) lidocain

40. Generic name for an antinauseant:
    (a) meclizine
    (b) mecizine
    (c) nitroglycerin
    (d) nitoglycerin

41. An elongated endoscope, usually fiberoptic:
    (a) fiberscope
    (b) fiberoscope
    (c) colonoscope
    (d) colonscope

42. An endoscope for use in sigmoidoscopy:
    (a) sigmoidoscope
    (b) sigmiodoscope
    (c) colonoscope
    (d) colonscope

43. An increase in the severity of a disease or symptoms:
    (a) retroflexion
    (b) retroflesion
    (c) exacerbation
    (d) exacerbasion

44. An opening created by surgery, disease, or trauma between two or more organs or structures:
    (a) anastomosis
    (b) anastamosis
    (c) stenosis
    (d) stenasis

45. Any compound containing carbon oxide:
    (a) keytone
    (b) ketone
    (c) creatine
    (d) creatinine

46. Any growth or mass protruding from a mucous membrane:
    (a) polyp
    (b) polpa
    (c) scera
    (d) sclera

47. Any solution compound that conducts electricity:
    (a) lumen
    (b) lumin
    (c) electrilyte
    (d) electrolyte

CHECK YOUR PROGRESS (cont'd)

48. Cavity or channel within a tube:
    (a) lumen
    (b) lumin
    (c) electrilyte
    (d) electrolyte

49. Darkening of the feces by blood pigments:
    (a) malena
    (b) erythema
    (c) melena
    (d) erthema

50. Difficulty in swallowing:
    (a) hematochezia
    (b) dysphagia
    (c) hemotachesia
    (d) dysphogia

51. Disease of the lymph nodes:
    (a) laminectomy
    (b) lymphadenopathy
    (c) lamenectomy
    (d) lympanopathy

52. Enlargement of the liver and spleen:
    (a) hepatasplenmegaly
    (b) thyromegaly
    (c) hepatosplenomegaly
    (d) thyomegaly

53. Establishment of a new opening into the stomach:
    (a) gastriparesis
    (b) gastroparesis
    (c) gastristomy
    (d) gastrostomy

54. Feeling of uneasiness:
    (a) targor
    (b) turgor
    (c) malaise
    (d) malise

55. Folic acid:
    (a) folate
    (b) formalen
    (c) formalin
    (d) forlaten

56. Hernia of the bladder, usually into the vagina and introitus:
    (a) rectocele
    (b) recocele
    (c) cystocele
    (d) cestocele

57. Hernial protrusion of part of the rectum into the vagina:
    (a) rectocele
    (b) recocele
    (c) cystocele
    (d) cestocele

58. Inflammation of the colon:
    (a) colitis
    (b) colotis
    (c) proctitis
    (d) protitis

59. Inflammation of the inner ear:
    (a) labrinithitis
    (b) gasritis
    (c) gastritis
    (d) labyrinthitis

60. Inflammation of the rectum:
    (a) colitis
    (b) colotis
    (c) proctitis
    (d) protitis

61. Inflammation of the stomach, especially the mucosa:
    (a) labrinithitis
    (b) gasritis
    (c) gastritis
    (d) labyrinthitis

62. Involuntary, rapid, rhythmic movement of the eyeball:
    (a) adenomatous
    (b) adenamatous
    (c) nistagmus
    (d) nystagmus

63. Jaundice:
    (a) decubitus
    (b) decubetus
    (c) icterus
    (d) ictreus

CHECK YOUR PROGRESS *(cont'd)*

64. Removal of the right or left side of the colon:
    (a) hemicolectomy
    (b) hemacolectomy
    (c) cholecystectomy
    (d) colecystectomy

65. Slight degree of gastroparalysis:
    (a) gastriparesis
    (b) gastroparesis
    (c) gastristomy
    (d) gastrostomy

66. Specimen hidden from view:
    (a) occult
    (b) ocult
    (c) pyridoxine
    (d) pyridoxine

67. Surgical excision of the lamina:
    (a) laminectomy
    (b) lymphadenopathy
    (c) lamenectomy
    (d) lympanopathy

68. Trade name for an antihypertensive:
    (a) Tenormin
    (b) Tenorrmin
    (c) Terramycin
    (d) Teramycin

69. Trade name for an antibiotic:
    (a) Tenormin
    (b) Tenorrmin
    (c) Terramycin
    (d) Teramycin

70. Trade name for an antiemetic:
    (a) Timoptic
    (b) Tiggan
    (c) Timptic
    (d) Tigan

71. Trade name for a beta blocker, antiglaucoma agent:
    (a) Timoptic
    (b) Tiggan
    (c) Timptic
    (d) Tigan

72. Trade name for an antihypertensive:
    (a) Vastec
    (b) Versed
    (c) Vasotec
    (d) Verse

73. Trade name for a short-acting benzodiazepine, general anesthetic adjunct for preoperative sedation:
    (a) Vastec
    (b) Versed
    (c) Vasotec
    (d) Verse

74. Trade name for a reductase inhibitor for hypercholesterolemia and coronary heart disease:
    (a) Zoccor
    (b) Zokur
    (c) Zochor
    (d) Zocor

75. Trade name for an antihypertensive used to treat benign prostatic hyperplasia:
    (a) Indocin
    (b) Indicin
    (c) Hitrin
    (d) Hytrin

76. Trade name for a nonsteroidal anti-inflammatory drug (NSAID):
    (a) Indocin
    (b) Indicin
    (c) Hitrin
    (d) Hytrin

77. Trade name for a potassium supplement:
    (a) K-Dur
    (b) Lopressor
    (c) K-Dura
    (d) Lopressar

78. Trade name for an antihypertensive:
    (a) K-Dur
    (b) Lopressor
    (c) K-Dura
    (d) Lopressar

CHECK YOUR PROGRESS *(cont'd)*

79. Trade name for a urinary bacteriostatic:
    (a) Mazide
    (b) Maxzide
    (c) Macroid
    (d) Macrobid

80. Trade name for a diuretic, antihypertensive:
    (a) Mazide
    (b) Maxzide
    (c) Macroid
    (d) Macrobid

81. Trade name for a bulk laxative:
    (a) Metamacil
    (b) Naporsyn
    (c) Metamucil
    (d) Naprosyn

82. Trade name for an NSAID:
    (a) Metamacil
    (b) Naporsyn
    (c) Metamucil
    (d) Naprosyn

83. Trade name for an antianginal, antihypertensive:
    (a) Paxil
    (b) Pasil
    (c) Norvasc
    (d) Norasc

84. Trade name for an antidepressant:
    (a) Paxil
    (b) Pasil
    (c) Norvasc
    (d) Norasc

85. Trade name for an acid controller for heartburn and acid indigestion:
    (a) Maxide
    (b) Pepcid
    (c) Maxzide
    (d) Pepid

86. Trade name for a gastric acid secretion inhibitor:
    (a) Priosec
    (b) Pepcid
    (c) Prilosec
    (d) Pepid

87. Trade name for a coronary vasodilator:
    (a) Regan
    (b) Procardia
    (c) Porcardia
    (d) Reglan

88. Trade name for a gastrointestinal stimulant, antiemetic:
    (a) Regan
    (b) Procardia
    (c) Porcardia
    (d) Reglan

89. Trade name for a mild central nervous system stimulant, antidepressant:
    (a) Ritalin
    (b) Ritilin
    (c) Synthroid
    (d) Synroid

90. Trade name for a thyroid hormone:
    (a) Ritalin
    (b) Ritilin
    (c) Synthroid
    (d) Synroid

91. Trade name for an antianxiety agent:
    (a) Ativan
    (b) Atevan
    (c) Bumex
    (d) Bumix

92. Trade name for an antagonist used to treat gastric and duodenal ulcers:
    (a) Axid
    (b) Cheme-7
    (c) Chem-7
    (d) Axide

93. Trade name for a loop diuretic:
    (a) Ativan
    (b) Atevan
    (c) Bumex
    (d) Bumix

94. Trade name for a profile of seven different chemical laboratory tests:
    (a) Axid
    (b) Cheme-7
    (c) Chem-7
    (d) Axide

CHECK YOUR PROGRESS *(cont'd)*

95. Trade name for an anticoagulant:
    (a) Demerol
    (b) Coumadin
    (c) Demirol
    (d) Doumaden

96. Trade name for a synthetic narcotic analgesic:
    (a) Demerol
    (b) Coumadin
    (c) Demirol
    (d) Doumaden

97. Trade name for an anticonvulsant used to treat epilepsy:
    (a) Delantin
    (b) Dilantin
    (c) Elavil
    (d) Elevil

98. Trade name for an antidepressant:
    (a) Delantin
    (b) Dilantin
    (c) Elavil
    (d) Elevil

99. Trade name for a guaiac test for occult blood:
    (a) Humilin
    (b) Hemoccult
    (c) Humulin
    (d) Hemocult

100. Trade name for an antidiabetic:
    (a) Humilin
    (b) Hemoccult
    (c) Humulin
    (d) Hemocult

Professional transcriptionists proofread their own work. Can you?

WORD PROCESSING USERS

Open your word processing package.

Insert the appropriate audiocassette in your transcribing machine and find dictation *9T-2*.

Transcribe and proofread dictation *9T-2*, using the formatting guidelines established in Chapter 2.

Identify and correct all errors.

Save your work on your student disk.

After completing the transcription, refer to the answer key.

Manually complete the error analysis chart.

Manually complete the Production for Pay summary.

SOFTWARE USERS

Click on *Chapter 9, Proofreading, Pretest (9T-2)*, and follow the directions.

PROOFREADING

Finding and correcting your own errors is an essential skill. The worksheets in these activities will help develop your proofreading skills.

TEXTBOOK USERS

Proofread and correct errors in the medical documents shown in *Activities 9-4 and 9-5*.
Refer to the answer key (Appendix E) for immediate feedback.
Manually complete the error analysis chart for each document.

SOFTWARE USERS

Click on *Chapter 9, Activity 9-4*, and follow the directions.
Follow the same process for *Chapter 9, Activity 9-5*.

ACTIVITY 9-4
Proofreading Worksheet

Directions: Proofread this medical document, which contains multiple errors. Use open punctuation and all other formatting guidelines established in this textbook.

HISTORY AND PHYSICAL EXAMINATION
Patient Name: Schupp, Lacey
File Number: 00841
Date of Birth: November 2, 19xx
Examination Date: *current date*
Physician: Anna Bolism, MD
HISTORY
CHEIF COMPLAINT
Melenic stools

HISTORY OF PRESSENT ILLNESS
The patient is a very pleasant 48 year old white male who I have previously saw for constipation that was due to a molity related disturbance as a complication of her polio. He has been taking Naporsyn on a chronic bases and over the last four-five days she has been having melenic stools. During the same time frame she has note progressive fatigue and weakness. A hemmoglobin study performed in Dr. Geiger's office showed that her hemmoglobin was in the six point five range and she was admitted to University Hospital. She denies any adbominal pain. There is know prior history of ulcer disease or hemotemesis. She has lost about three-5 pds. over this same time frame.
PAST MEDICAL HISTORY
She has numerous postpolio complications including a neurogenic bladder and constipation. She has had several back surgerys as well as a wrist operation. He does not smoke or drink..
MEDICATIONS
Naporsyn.
Pasil.
Elevil.
Ativan.
FAMILY HISTORY
Noncontributory.
PHYSICAL EXAMINATION:
GENERAL: A pale white male who is in no a cute distress.
HEART: Negative.
LUNGS: Negative.
ABDOMEN: Negative.
RECTAL: A rectal exam showed know stool available for hemocult evaluation.

continued

HISTORY AND PHYSICAL EXAMINATION
Patient Name: Schupp, Lacey
File Number: 00841
Page 2

LABORATORY DATA
Lab studies show a BUN elevated at thirty three with a creatine of zero point four.
His electrolites were normal as were her platelet count and co-agulation time.
Hemmoglobin was six point nine.

IMPRESION
GI bleed. Its almost certainly upper GI bleeding due to nonsteroid use.

PLAN
1. Transfuse 2 units of packed sells.
2. Perform an upper endoescopy later this morning. We will make farther recomendations after the endoescopy.

Anna Bolism

ACTIVITY 9-5
Proofreading Worksheet

Directions:Proofread this medical document, which contains multiple errors. Use open punctuation and all other formatting guidelines established in this textbook.

OPERATIVE REPORT

Patient Name: Artemis, Jacob
File Number: 00864
Date of Birth: December 12, 1958

PREOPERATIVE DIAGNOSIS
Hepatitis C and mildly elevated liver enzymes.

POSTOPERATIVE DIAGNOSIS
Hepatitis C and mildly elevated liver enzymes.

OPERATION
Percutaneous liver biopsy under ultrasound guidance.

PROCEDURE
The patient was counciled. Potential complications were explained. Concent was obtained. The patient was place supine on the exam table. Ultra-sound was used to scan in the midaxillary line. The liver margins were identified and the best location for the liver boipsy was selected along the mid axilary line at aproximately the tenth inter-coastal space. The skin was then preped and draped in the usual sterile manner. Lidocane one percent was used for tropical anesthesia of the skin sudcutaneous tissue and down to the inter-costal space. A number twenty two gauge spinal needel was used to sound the depth of the liver.

Because of the patients obesity the liver was found to be approximately five centimeters from the skin surface. The Klatskin needle was then attached to a glass syringe filled with sterile saline. The Clatskin needle was inserted into the intercostal space and then subsequently into the liver for a quick suction biopsy. The first past yielded only a five milimeters fragment of tissue. A second pass was therefore performed which yielded a much larger four centimeters peace of tan appearing liver. The liver biopsy was scent in a Formalen jar for pathological analyses. The skin was then dressed and tapped. The patient was then observed four four hours. No immediate complications were observed. Postbiopsy vital signs were normal. The patient tolerated the procedure well with out any complications.

IMPRESSION
Hepatitis C and mildly elevated liver enzymes.
Kate Cobalamin Md.

Now you are ready to make the transition from simply proofreading printed material to both transcribing and proofreading dictated material. This is the time to concentrate on building your medical vocabulary, which ultimately will improve your speed and accuracy.

WORD PROCESSING USERS

Open your word processing package.

Insert the appropriate audiocassette in your transcribing machine and find dictation *9T-3.*

Step 1: Listen to the entire dictation to gain an understanding of the medical concepts and terms involved in the report. Rewind the tape to the beginning of the dictation and transcribe what you hear. Do not worry about formatting, style, or speed. Simply type what you hear being dictated, using correct punctuation, capitalization, and spelling. Stop as needed to look up words you do not understand or cannot spell. Adjust the speed control of the transcriber to a comfortable level, starting slowly to ensure no dictated words are missed, and increase the speed as your accuracy improves.

Step 2: Rewind the tape and transcribe dictation *9T-3* again, including correct spacing and formatting. Proofread the report. Identify and correct all errors. Save your work on your student disk. Refer to the answer key and manually complete the error analysis chart and Production for Pay summary.

Follow the same process for dictation *9T-4.*

SOFTWARE USERS

Click on *Chapter 9, Activity 9-6 (9T-3), Step 1,* and follow the directions. When you feel comfortable with the dictation, click on *Chapter 9, Activity 9-6 (9T-3), Step 2,* and follow the directions.

Follow the same process for *Chapter 9, Activity 9-7 (9T-4), Step 1* and *Chapter 9, Activity 9-7 (9T-4), Step 2.*

Let's pause a minute and see how well you are doing. This section allows you to evaluate your success at transcribing and proofreading gastroenterology reports.

WORD PROCESSING USERS

Open your word processing package.

Insert the appropriate audiocassette in your transcribing machine and find dictation *9T-2*.

Transcribe and proofread dictation *9T-2*, using the formatting guidelines established in Chapter 2.

Identify and correct all errors.

Save your work on your student disk.

After completing the transcription, refer to the answer key.

Manually complete the error analysis chart.

Manually complete the Production for Pay summary.

SOFTWARE USERS

Click on *Chapter 9, Proofreading Check Your Progress (9T-2)*, and follow the directions.

Professional transcriptionists can transcribe and proofread their own work. Can you?

WORD PROCESSING USERS

Open your word processing package.

Insert the appropriate audiocassette in your transcribing machine and find dictation *9T-5*.

Transcribe and proofread dictation *9T-5*, using the formatting guidelines established in Chapter 2.

Identify and correct all errors.

Save your work on your student disk.

After completing the transcription, refer to the answer key.

Manually complete the error analysis chart.

Manually complete the Production for Pay summary.

Follow the same process for dictation *9T-6*.

SOFTWARE USERS

Click on *Chapter 9, Transcription Pretest (9T-5)*, and follow the directions.

Follow the same process for *Chapter 9, Transcription Pretest (9T-6)*.

You have been hired as a transcriptionist at FedDes Wellness Center in the Gastroenterology Division. Your supervisor has asked you to transcribe today's dictation.

WORD PROCESSING USERS

Open your word processing package.

Insert the appropriate audiocassette in your transcribing machine and find dictation 9T-7.

Create or use your existing templates as necessary for the six types of reports (chart note, chart note using history and physical format, history and physical examination report, x-ray report, procedure report, consultation letter).

Transcribe and proofread dictation 9T-7, using the formatting guidelines established in Chapter 2.

Identify and correct all errors.

Save your work on your student disk.

After completing the transcription, refer to the answer key.

Manually complete the error analysis chart.

Manually complete the Production for Pay summary.

Follow the same process for dictations 9T-8 through 9T-15.

SOFTWARE USERS

Click on *Chapter 9, Transcription at FedDes Wellness Center (9T-7),* and follow the directions.

Follow the same process for each of the remaining dictations (*9T-8* through *9T-15*).

INDEX OF DICTATIONS AND ASSOCIATED TRANSCRIPTION TIPS

Remember to follow the guidelines pertaining to capitalization, numbers, punctuation, abbreviations, measurements, symbols, and use of templates to create medical reports at FedDes Wellness Center. This material is reviewed in Unit I.

9T-7

Consultation Letter
Patient's Name: Alice Kier
Requesting Physician: Charles P. Davis, MD
Physician: Kate Cobalamin, MD

Transcription Tips

• A hyphen is used between numbers and *year old*.
  You hear the dictator say: Ms. Kier is a fifty nine year old woman.
  You transcribe as: Ms. Kier is a 59-year-old woman.
• Quotation marks are used to indicate a direct quote.
  You hear the dictator say: Her description of the discomfort is really quite vague stating that the pain jumps around her abdomen.
  You transcribe as: Her description of the discomfort is really quite vague, stating that the pain "jumps around" her abdomen.
• The following medications are dictated in this letter:
  Synthroid: trade name for a thyroid hormone
  hydrocortisone: generic name for a corticosteroid
  K-Dur: trade name for a potassium supplement
  Bumex: trade name for a loop diuretic
  Lopressor: trade name for an antihypertensive
  Vasotec: trade name for an antihypertensive
  Dilantin: trade name for an anticonvulsant used in the treatment of epilepsy
  Prilosec: trade name for a gastric secretion inhibitor
  Zocor: trade name for a reductase inhibitor for hypercholesterolemia and coronary heart disease
  nitroglycerin paste: generic name for a vasodilator used to relieve certain types of pain
• A hyphen is used to join two or more words when used as an adjective that precedes a noun. The following word pairs are dictated in this report: well-appearing, heme-negative.

• Continuation pages for consultation letters must include a 3-line heading beginning at the 1-inch top margin, as shown below:
  Charles P. Davis, MD
  current date
  Page 2
• An apostrophe is used to form the possessive of singular and plural nouns.
  You hear the dictator say: Thank you for the opportunity of sharing in Ms. Kiers care.
  You transcribe as: Thank you for the opportunity of sharing in Ms. Kier's care.

9T-8

Operative Report
Patient's Name: Raymond Dubin
Physician: Gwenn Maltase, MD

Transcription Tips

• Figures are used for measurements and Latin terms. No period follows metric abbreviations unless the abbreviation ends a sentence.
  You hear the dictator say: Sigmoidoscopy was completed to sixty centimeters into the descending colon.
  You transcribe as: Sigmoidoscopy was completed to 60 cm into the descending colon.
• Figures are used almost exclusively as opposed to spelled-out numbers to improve clarity and avoid potential mistakes.
  You hear the dictator say: a repeat colonoscopy is recommended in three years.
  You transcribe as: a repeat colonoscopy is recommended in 3 years.

9T-9

History and Physical Examination
Patient's Name: Chi Chen
Physician: Anna Bolism, MD

Transcription Tips

• The following abbreviations are dictated in this report:
  GI: gastrointestinal
  t.i.d.: three times a day
  RBC: red blood count
  WBC: white blood count

TRANSCRIPTION

- The following medication is dictated in this report:
  Procardia: trade name for a coronary vasodilator
- The following laboratory tests are dictated in this report:
  - Chem-7: trade name for a profile of seven different chemical laboratory tests
  - Partial thromboplastin time: period of time required for clot formation in recalcified blood plasma after contact as well as the activation and addition of platelet substitutes; used to assess the pathways of coagulation

- A hyphen is used to join two or more words when used as an adjective that precedes a noun. The following word pairs are dictated in this report: middle-aged, low-grade.
- Words beginning with *pre*, *re*, *post*, and *non* are generally not hyphenated: nontender.
- The following abbreviations are dictated in this report:
  - CBC: complete blood count
  - BUN: blood urea nitrogen
  - SGOT: serum glutamic-oxaloacetic transaminase
  - GI: gastrointestinal

9T-10

Operative Report
Patient's Name: Ronald Dubinsky
Physician: Gwenn Maltase, MD

Transcription Tip
- The following procedure is dictated in this report: Olympus video sigmoidoscope.

9T-11

Consultation Report
Patient's Name: Micah Landis
Requesting Physician: Matthew Sponch, MD
Physician: Anna Bolism, MD

Transcription Tip
- The following term is dictated in this report: impaction: the condition of being wedged in firmly.

9T-12

History and Physical Examination Report
Patient's Name: Manuelo Rodriquez
Physician: Gwenn Maltase, MD

Transcription Tips
- A hyphen is used to take the place of the words *to* or *through* to identify ranges.
  - You hear the dictator say: On questioning, the patient reports a three to four year history of solid food dysphagia.
  - You transcribe as: On questioning, the patient reports a 3-4 year history of solid food dysphagia.
- The following medications are dictated in this report: Reglan, insulin.

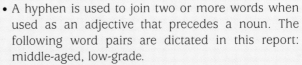

9T-13

Consultation Report
Patient's Name: Alice Chan
Requesting Physician: Izzy Sertoli, MD
Physician: Kate Cobalamin, MD

Transcription Tips
- The following abbreviation is dictated in this report:
  - PEG: percutaneous endoscopic gastrostomy
- Words beginning with *pre*, *re*, *post*, and *non* are generally not hyphenated: postinfarct.
- Capitalize eponyms. Eponyms are surnames teamed with a disease, instrument, or surgical procedure.
  - You hear the dictator say: foley catheter
  - You transcribe as: Foley catheter
- The number or pound sign (#) is used to abbreviate the word *number* followed by medical instrument or apparatus.
  - You hear the dictator say: The nurse placed a number twenty two French Foley catheter to keep the PEG tube tract open.
  - You transcribe as: The nurse placed a #22 French Foley catheter to keep the PEG tube tract open.
- A hyphen is used to join two or more words when used as an adjective that precedes a noun. The following word pair is dictated in this report: fungal-appearing.

9T-14

History and Physical Examination Report
Patient's Name: Ahed Admad
Physician: Gwenn Maltase, MD

Transcription Tips
- The following medications are dictated in this report:
  - Indocin: trade name for a nonsteroidal anti-inflammatory drug

TRANSCRIPTION

nitroglycerin: generic name for a vasodilator used to relieve certain types of pain

Metamucil: trade name for a bulk laxative.

- Words beginning with *pre*, *re*, *post*, and *non* are generally not hyphenated: nonsmoker, nontender.
- Figures and capital letters are used to refer to the vertebral column and spinal nerves.

    You hear the dictator say: Cardiac exam reveals a regular rate and rhythm with a normal s one and s two.

    You transcribe as: Cardiac exam reveals a regular rate and rhythm with a normal S1 and S2.

- Figures are used to refer to grade, phase, and pregnancy and delivery.

    You hear the dictator say: There is a grade two over six systolic murmur at the apex.

    You transcribe as: There is a grade 2/6 systolic murmur at the apex.

- The diagonal (/) is used to indicate the word *per* in laboratory values and respirations or the word *over* in blood pressure.

    You hear the dictator say: There is a grade two over six systolic murmur at the apex.

    You transcribe as: There is a grade 2/6 systolic murmur at the apex.

- The following abbreviations are dictated in this report:

    ECG: electrocardiogram

    CBC: complete blood count

    WBC: white blood count

- The following diagnostic tests/procedures are dictated in this report:

    prothrombin time: test to measure the activity of factors I, II, V, VII, and X, which participate in the extrinsic pathway of coagulation

    Chem-7: trade name for a profile of seven different chemical laboratory tests

Consultation Report
Patient's Name: Ralph Norr
Physician: Anna Bolism, MD

Transcription Tips

- The following medications are dictated in this report:

    Pepcid: trade name for an acid controller for heartburn and acid indigestion

    Tenormin: trade name for an antihypertensive

    Prilosec: trade name for a gastric acid secretion inhibitor

- Words beginning with *pre*, *re*, *post*, and *non* are generally not hyphenated: nonsteroidal.
- A hyphen is used between two "like" vowels: anti-inflammatory.
- The following laboratory tests are dictated in this report:

    prothrombin time: test to measure the activity of factors I, II, V, VII, and X, which participate in the extrinsic pathway of coagulation

    partial thromboplastin time: period required for clot formation in recalcified blood plasma after contact activation and the addition of platelet substitutes; used to assess the pathways of coagulation

    creatine kinase: Presence of this enzyme in the blood is strongly indicative of a recent myocardial infarction.

    lactic dehydrogenase: Presence of this enzyme occurs in elevated concentrations when the tissues are injured.

- Capitalize eponyms. Eponyms are surnames teamed with a disease, instrument, or surgical procedure.

    You hear the dictator say: barretts esophagus

    You transcribe as: Barrett's esophagus

- The following abbreviations are dictated in this report:

    GI: gastrointestinal

    CBC: complete blood count

    EGD: esophagogastroduodenoscopy; endoscopic examination of the interior of the esophagus, stomach, and initial portion of the duodenum

Professional transcriptionists can transcribe and proofread their own work with speed and accuracy. Have you mastered the gastroenterology transcription rotation at FedDes Wellness Center?

WORD PROCESSING USERS

Open your word processing package.

Insert the appropriate audiocassette in your transcribing machine and find dictation *9T-5*.

Transcribe and proofread dictation *9T-5*, using the formatting guidelines established in Chapter 2.

Identify and correct all errors.

Save your work on your student disk.

After completing the transcription, refer to the answer key.

Manually complete the error analysis chart.

Manually complete the Production for Pay summary.

Follow the same process for dictation *9T-6*.

SOFTWARE USERS

Click on *Chapter 9, Transcription Check Your Progress, (9T-5)*, and follow the directions.

Follow the same process for *Chapter 9, Transcription Check Your Progress (9T-6)*.

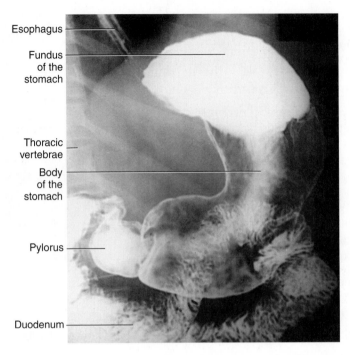

Esophagus

Fundus of the stomach

Thoracic vertebrae

Body of the stomach

Pylorus

Duodenum

Figure 9-1 Double-contrast x-ray view of the stomach. Film obtained with patient in the left posterior oblique (LPO) position. *(From Ballinger PW, Frank ED:* Merrill's atlas of radiographic positions and radiologic procedures, *ed 10, St Louis, 2003, Mosby.)*

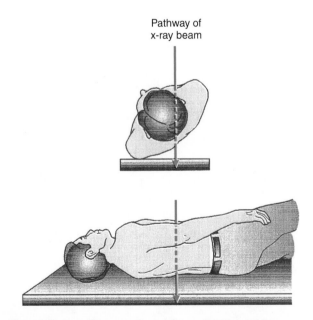

Pathway of x-ray beam

Figure 9-2 Left posterior oblique (LPO) position resulting in an anteroposterior (AP) oblique projection.

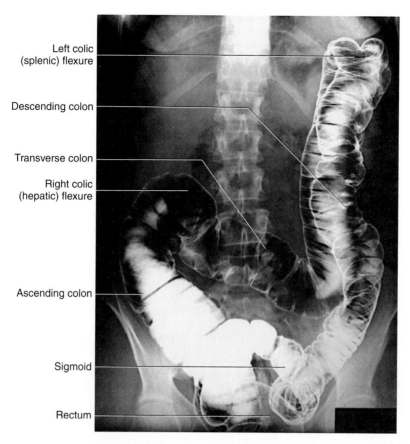

Left colic
(splenic) flexure

Descending colon

Transverse colon

Right colic
(hepatic) flexure

Ascending colon

Sigmoid

Rectum

Figure 9-3 Double-contrast posteroanterior (PA) radiographic view of the large intestine. Film obtained with patient in a prone position. *(From Ballinger PW, Frank ED:* Merrill's atlas of radiographic positions and radiologic procedures, *ed 10, St Louis, 2003, Mosby.)*

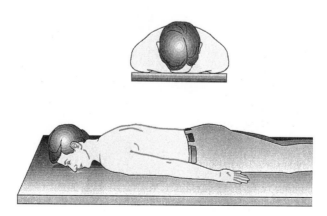

Figure 9-4 Prone body position.

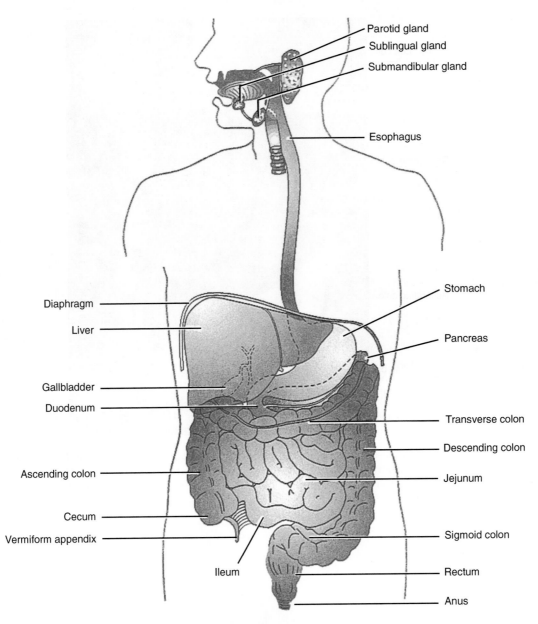

Parotid gland
Sublingual gland
Submandibular gland
Esophagus
Stomach
Pancreas
Diaphragm
Liver
Gallbladder
Duodenum
Transverse colon
Descending colon
Ascending colon
Jejunum
Cecum
Vermiform appendix
Sigmoid colon
Ileum
Rectum
Anus

Figure 9-5 The human digestive system (anterior view).

Chapter 10

Office Medical Transcription from the Cardiology Practice

OBJECTIVES

At the completion of Chapter 10, you should be able to do the following:
1. Match medical terms associated with the cardiology specialty with their definitions.
2. Spell medical terms associated with the cardiology specialty.
3. Transcribe medical terms in sentence structure.
4. Proofread, edit, and correct medical documents associated with the cardiology specialty that contain various errors.
5. Transcribe and proofread authentic medical documents associated with the cardiology specialty.

INTRODUCTION TO THE CARDIOLOGY ROTATION

Terminology
Pretest
Activities
    10-1: Keyboarding Medical Terms and Definitions
    10-2: Spelling Medical Terms
    10-3: Transcribing Medical Sentences, *10T-1*
Check Your Progress

Proofreading
Pretest, *10T-2*
Activities
    10-4: Proofreading Worksheet
    10-5: Proofreading Worksheet
    10-6: Proofreading Transcription Exercise, *10T-3*
    10-7: Proofreading Transcription Exercise, *10T-4*
Check Your Progress, *10T-2*

Transcription
Pretest, *10T-5* and *10T-6*
Cardiology Transcription at FedDes Wellness Center
Index of Dictations and Associated Transcription Tips, *10T-7* through *10T-12*
Check Your Progress, *10T-5* and *10T-6*

Anatomical Illustrations and Medical Images

What's Ahead

The FedDes Wellness Center has three cardiologists, or specialists in cardiology, on staff. Cardiology is the study of the heart and vessels that carry blood throughout the body. The cardiologist assesses the function of the heart by performing invasive and noninvasive testing.

Assessment of cardiovascular problems begins with the patient's abnormal vital signs. The cardiologist will note any bluish coloring around the lips and/or nail beds, which is an indication of decreased oxygen, and clubbing of the fingers, which is an indication of chronic oxygen deficiency. The cardiologist uses palpation to feel for the pulses and auscultation to listen for bruits or other abnormal sounds.

The physicians in FedDes Cardiology Division perform laboratory tests and procedures that include chest x-rays, electrocardiogram (ECG), echocardiogram, and cardiac catheterization.

In this unit, you assume the role of a medical transcriptionist employed at FedDes Wellness Center. Please remember to follow the guidelines pertaining to capitalization, numbers, punctuation, abbreviations, measurements, symbols, and use of templates to create medical reports at FedDes Wellness Center. This material is reviewed in Unit I. The transcription exercises list the type of report, patient's name, and physician(s) as well as the associated transcription tips.

You will work with the textbook and CD-ROM or the accompanying audiocassettes. Your mastery of cardiology transcription is assessed through worksheets, timed transcription exercises, the error analysis chart, and the Production for Pay summary.

All answer keys are found on the CD-ROM, providing immediate feedback. After transcribing a report, you will proofread your work and correct any errors. Then you will compare your proofread work against a master transcript, categorize all errors, and tabulate the errors on the error analysis chart. The Production for Pay summary correlates your production to the FedDes Wellness Center pay scale. The scale is also linked to your grade. This system allows you to assess your mastery of transcription skills in a real-world scenario.

Let's find out if you can define and spell selected terminology and drugs of the cardiology specialty that are included in this chapter.

TEXTBOOK USERS

Select the correctly spelled term that matches its definition.
Refer to the answer key (Appendix E) for immediate feedback.

SOFTWARE USERS

Click on *Chapter 10, Terminology Pretest*, and follow the directions.

PRETEST

Directions: Select the correctly spelled term that matches its definition.

1. Generic name for a cardiotonic agent:
   (a) dobutamine
   (b) dobitamine
   (c) cardiolite
   (d) cardialite

2. Generic name for a cardiotonic:
   (a) digixin
   (b) paroxysm
   (c) digoxin
   (d) paroxism

3. A condition of elevated lipid levels in the blood:
   (a) hyolipidemia
   (b) hyperlipidemia
   (c) hypokalemia
   (d) hyperkalemia

4. Generic name for a coronary vasodilator:
   (a) atrial
   (b) atrilae
   (c) diltiazem
   (d) diltazem

5. Generic name for a coronary vasodilator:
   (a) fibrilla
   (b) verapamil
   (c) fabrille
   (d) verpamil

6. Localized abnormal dilatation of the wall of a blood vessel:
   (a) verapemil
   (b) verpamil
   (c) aneurism
   (d) aneurysm

7. A sound or murmur heard on auscultation:
   (a) digoxin
   (b) digixin
   (c) bruit
   (d) briut

8. A triple cadence to the heart sounds:
   (a) gallop
   (b) galop
   (c) bruit
   (d) briut

9. An abnormally rapid heart rate:
   (a) tachycardia
   (b) tachicardia
   (c) bradicardia
   (d) bradycardia

10. Generic name for an antiarrhythmic agent used to treat atrial flutter, atrial fibrillation, premature ventricular contractions, and tachycardia:
    (a) quindine
    (b) quinidine
    (c) nortrityline
    (d) nortriptyline

11. Generic name for an anticoagulant:
    (a) heparin
    (b) heperin
    (c) paroxysm
    (d) parxysim

12. Generic name for an antidepressant:
    (a) quindine
    (b) quinidine
    (c) nortrityline
    (d) nortriptyline

13. An increase in total red cell mass of blood:
    (a) polycythemia
    (b) pleura
    (c) polycyemia
    (d) pleuria

14. Cavity or channel:
    (a) guot
    (b) sinus
    (c) gout
    (d) sinnus

15. Characterized by low blood pressure or causing a reduction in blood pressure:
    (a) hypercholesterolemia
    (b) hypertensive
    (c) hypocholesterolemia
    (d) hypotensive

16. Continuous dry rattling in the throat due to a partial obstruction, heard on auscultation:
    (a) pectoralis
    (b) rhonchus
    (c) pectalis
    (d) rhionchus

PRETEST (cont'd)

17. Cramp-like pains in the calf; limping:
    (a) caudication
    (b) claudication
    (c) fibrilation
    (d) fibrillation

18. Dark bluish or purplish coloration of the skin due to deficient oxygenation of the blood:
    (a) cyanosis
    (b) diaphoresis
    (c) cyainosis
    (d) diaphorsis

19. Defective rhythm:
    (a) rhonchus
    (b) dysrhythmia
    (c) ronchus
    (d) dysrrhythmia

20. Device used to administer electrical shocks to the heart:
    (a) cardiomyopathy
    (b) cardioverter
    (c) cardomyopathy
    (d) cardoverter

21. Disease of unknown cause:
    (a) idiopathic
    (b) inotropic
    (c) idipathic
    (d) intropic

22. Disorder associated with an inborn error of uric acid metabolism that increases production or interferes with the excretion of uric acid:
    (a) guot
    (b) sinus
    (c) gout
    (d) sinnus

23. Exceedingly rapid contractions of muscle fibrils:
    (a) caudication
    (b) claudication
    (c) fibrilation
    (d) fibrillation

24. Failure to conduct an impulse down one division of the left bundle branch:
    (a) expiratory
    (b) expiratery
    (c) hemblock
    (d) hemiblock

25. Formation of a small depression:
    (a) pitting
    (b) iliac
    (c) piting
    (d) ilac

26. Greater than normal concentration of potassium ions in the blood:
    (a) hyolipidemia
    (b) hyperlipidemia
    (c) hypokalemia
    (d) hyperkalemia

27. Pertaining to the force of muscular contractions:
    (a) idiopathic
    (b) inotropic
    (c) idipathic
    (d) intropic

28. Decreased supply of oxygenated blood to a body part:
    (a) erythemia
    (b) erythema
    (c) ischema
    (d) ischemia

29. Mass of tissues and organs separating the sternum in front and the vertebral column behind:
    (a) mediastinum
    (b) venous
    (c) medastinum
    (d) veinous

30. Having a normal-sized head; mesocephalic:
    (a) atherosclerotic
    (b) atheriosclerotic
    (c) normocephalic
    (d) normiocephalic

31. Perspiration:
    (a) cyanosis
    (b) diaphoresis
    (c) cyainosis
    (d) diaphorsis

PRETEST *(cont'd)*

32. Pertaining to a location situated below and to the side:
    (a) colleratal
    (b) inferolateral
    (c) coleratal
    (d) inferlateral

33. Pertaining to the atrium:
    (a) afebrile
    (b) afebril
    (c) atrail
    (d) atrial

34. Pertaining to the chest or breast:
    (a) pectoralis
    (b) rhonchus
    (c) pectalis
    (d) rhionchus

35. Pertaining to the foot or feet:
    (a) pedal
    (b) padel
    (c) carotid
    (d) cariotid

36. Pertaining to the muscular tissue of the heart:
    (a) myocardial
    (b) myocardal
    (c) thromosis
    (d) thrombosis

37. Pertaining to the veins:
    (a) mediastinum
    (b) venous
    (c) medastinum
    (d) veinous

38. Radiograph of an artery after injection of a contrast medium:
    (a) arthrography
    (b) artherography
    (c) arteriography
    (d) arteriography

39. Radiographic visualization of blood vessels after injection of a contrast agent:
    (a) angiography
    (b) angography
    (c) athrography
    (d) atherography

40. Redness of the skin due to capillary dilatation:
    (a) erythemia
    (b) erythema
    (c) ischema
    (d) ischemia

41. Pertaining to exhalation:
    (a) expiratory
    (b) expiratery
    (c) hemblock
    (d) hemiblock

42. Pertaining to the duodenum, the first division of the small intestine:
    (a) intimal
    (b) intomal
    (c) doudenal
    (d) duodenal

43. Pertaining to the ilium:
    (a) pitting
    (b) iliac
    (c) piting
    (d) ilac

44. Pertaining to the inner coat of a vessel:
    (a) intimal
    (b) intomal
    (c) doudenal
    (d) duodenal

45. Pertaining to the principal artery of the neck:
    (a) pedal
    (b) padel
    (c) carotid
    (d) cariotid

46. Serous membrane investing the lungs and lining the walls of the thoracic cavity:
    (a) polycythemia
    (b) pleura
    (c) polycyemia
    (d) pleuria

47. A secondary or accessory blood pathway:
    (a) collateral
    (b) inferolateral
    (c) coleratal
    (d) inferlateral

PRETEST *(cont'd)*

48. Coughing or spitting of blood from the respiratory tract:
    (a) hemptysis
    (b) hemoptysis
    (c) epiphysis
    (d) epiphtysis

49. Sudden insufficiency of arterial or venous blood supply:
    (a) heparin
    (b) heperin
    (c) infarction
    (d) infartion

50. Sudden recurrence or increase in intensity of symptoms; spasm or seizure:
    (a) paroxysm
    (b) paroxism
    (c) aneurism
    (d) aneurysm

51. Surgical removal of the gallbladder:
    (a) cholecystectomy
    (b) endartertomy
    (c) cholcystectomy
    (d) endarterectomy

52. Temporary suspension of consciousness; fainting:
    (a) syncope
    (b) echocardiogram
    (c) synscope
    (d) echocardogram

53. Disease process of the heart muscle:
    (a) cardiomyopathy
    (b) cardioverter
    (c) cardomyopathy
    (d) cardoverter

54. The center for ossification of the proximal and distal ends of a long bone:
    (a) hemptysis
    (b) hemoptysis
    (c) epiphysis
    (d) epiphtysis

55. Formation of a blood clot within the vascular system:
    (a) myocardial
    (b) myocardal
    (c) thromosis
    (d) thrombosis

56. Loss of sight without an apparent lesion of the eye:
    (a) stensis
    (b) stenosis
    (c) amarosis
    (d) amaurosis

57. Hardening of an artery due to deposits of plaque within the vessel:
    (a) atherosclerotic
    (b) atheriosclerotic
    (c) normocephalic
    (d) normiocephalic

58. The narrowing or contraction of a body passage:
    (a) stensis
    (b) stenosis
    (c) amarosis
    (d) amaurosis

59. The presence of an abnormally large amount of cholesterol in the cells and plasma of the blood:
    (a) hypercholesterolemia
    (b) hypertensive
    (c) hypocholesterolemia
    (d) hypotensive

60. Slowness of the heartbeat:
    (a) tachycardia
    (b) tachicardia
    (c) bradicardia
    (d) bradycardia

61. Surgical procedure done to clear a blocked artery:
    (a) cholecystectomy
    (b) endartertomy
    (c) cholcystectomy
    (d) endarterectomy

62. Diagnostic procedure using ultrasound to study heart structure and motion:
    (a) syncope
    (b) echocardiogram
    (c) synscope
    (d) echocardogram

63. Variation from the normal rhythm of the heartbeat:
    (a) arhythmia
    (b) bruit
    (c) arrhythmia
    (d) bruite

64. Without fever:
    (a) afebrile
    (b) afebril
    (c) atrail
    (d) atrial

65. Trade name for an antihypertensive:
    (a) Capoten
    (b) Capatin
    (c) Zyloprim
    (d) Zylaprim

66. Trade name for myocardial perfusion agent for cardiac SPECT imaging:
    (a) Cardolite
    (b) Xanax
    (c) Cardiolite
    (d) Xanix

67. Trade name for a calcium channel blocker for atrial fibrillation:
    (a) Vasotec
    (b) Vasotic
    (c) Cardisem
    (d) Cardizem

68. Trade name for an anticoagulant:
    (a) Coumadim
    (b) Coumadin
    (c) Trentil
    (d) Trental

69. Trade name for a nonsteroidal anti-inflammatory drug (NSAID), used to prevent gastric ulcers:
    (a) Cycotec
    (b) Terramycin
    (c) Cytotec
    (d) Teramycin

70. Trade name for an analgesic, anti-inflammatory:
    (a) Ecotrin
    (b) Icotrin
    (c) Lasix
    (d) Laxis

71. Trade name for an NSAID:
    (a) Indocin
    (b) Endocin
    (c) Lotensin
    (d) Lotinsen

72. Trade name for an antianginal:
    (a) Lescol
    (b) Lescil
    (c) Isordol
    (d) Isordil

73. Trade name for a potassium supplement:
    (a) Theo-Dur
    (b) K-Dur
    (c) T-Dur
    (d) Kheo-Dur

74. Trade name for an antiarrhythmic, cardiotonic that increases cardiac output:
    (a) Lanoxin
    (b) Lanozin
    (c) Tenormin
    (d) Tenorrmin

75. Trade name for a diuretic:
    (a) Ecotrin
    (b) Icotrin
    (c) Lasix
    (d) Laxis

76. Trade name for a reductase inhibitor for hypercholesterolemia:
    (a) Lescol
    (b) Lescil
    (c) Isordol
    (d) Isordil

PRETEST (cont'd)

77. Trade name for an antihypertensive:
    (a) Indocin
    (b) Endocin
    (c) Lotensin
    (d) Lotinsen

78. Trade name for a reductase inhibitor for hypercholesterolemia:
    (a) Metavor
    (b) Mevacor
    (c) Synthroid
    (d) Syntoid

79. Trade name for a coronary vasodilator:
    (a) Persantine
    (b) Reglan
    (c) Presantine
    (d) Relan

80. Trade name for estrogen replacement therapy:
    (a) Provera
    (b) Prevera
    (c) Permarin
    (d) Premarin

81. Trade name for progestin for secondary amenorrhea and abnormal uterine bleeding:
    (a) Provera
    (b) Prevera
    (c) Permarin
    (d) Premarin

82. Trade name for an antiarrhythmic:
    (a) Quinidex
    (b) Senekot
    (c) Quindez
    (d) Senokot

83. Trade name for a gastrointestinal stimulant, antiemetic:
    (a) Persantine
    (b) Reglan
    (c) Presantine
    (d) Relan

84. Trade name for a laxative:
    (a) Quinidex
    (b) Senekot
    (c) Quindez
    (d) Senokot

85. Trade name for a thyroid hormone:
    (a) Metavor
    (b) Mevacor
    (c) Synthroid
    (d) Syntoid

86. Trade name for a beta blocker, antihypertensive agent:
    (a) Lanoxin
    (b) Lanozin
    (c) Tenormin
    (d) Tenorrmin

87. Trade name for an antibiotic:
    (a) Cycotec
    (b) Terramycin
    (c) Cytotec
    (d) Teramycin

88. Trade name for a bronchodilator:
    (a) Theo-Dur
    (b) K-Dur
    (c) T-Dur
    (d) Kheo-Dur

89. Trade name for an oral hemorheologic drug:
    (a) Xanex
    (b) Zanax
    (c) Trentil
    (d) Trental

90. Trade name for an antihypertensive agent:
    (a) Vasotec
    (b) Vasotic
    (c) Zyloprim
    (d) Zyloprime

91. Trade name for an antianxiety agent:
    (a) Cardolite
    (b) Xanax
    (c) Cardiolite
    (d) Xanix

92. Trade name for an antigout agent:
    (a) Capoten
    (b) Capatin
    (c) Zyloprim
    (d) Zylaprim

Let's learn to spell and define selected terminology and drugs of the cardiology specialty that are included in this chapter. Keyboarding these terms is an effective way to improve your skills. Read and key each word and its definition.

Word Processing Users

Open your word processing package. Read and type each word and its definition as shown below. Save your work on your student disk.

1. Afebrile (a-<u>feb</u>-ril) is without fever.
2. Amaurosis (am-aw-<u>ro</u>-sis) is the loss of sight without an apparent lesion of the eye.
3. Aneurysm (<u>an</u>-u-rizm) is the localized abnormal dilatation of the wall of a blood vessel.
4. Angiography (an-je-<u>og</u>-rah-fe) is the radiographic visualization of a blood vessel after injecting a contrast agent.
5. Arrhythmia (ah-<u>rith</u>-me-ah) is the variation from the normal rhythm of the heartbeat.
6. Arteriography (ar-te-re-<u>og</u>-rah-fe) is the radiographic visualization of an artery after injection of a contrast agent.
7. Atherosclerosis (ath-er-o-skle-<u>ro</u>-sis) is the hardening of an artery due to deposits of plaque within the vessel.
8. Atrial (<u>a</u>-tre-al) pertains to the atrium.
9. Bradycardia (brad-e-<u>kar</u>-de-ah) is slowness of the heartbeat.
10. Bruit (broo e *or* broot) is a sound or murmur heard on auscultation.
11. Cardiomyopathy (kar-de-o-mi-<u>op</u>-ah-the) is a disease process of the heart muscle.
12. Cardioverter (<u>kar</u>-de-o-ver-ter) is a device used to administer electrical shocks to the heart.
13. Carotid (kah-<u>rot</u>-id) pertains to the principal artery of the neck.
14. Cholecystectomy (ko-le-sis-<u>tek</u>-to-me) is the surgical removal of the gallbladder.
15. Claudication (klaw-di-<u>ka</u>-shun) is the cramp-like pains in the calf; limping.
16. Collateral (ko-<u>lat</u>-er-al) is a secondary or accessory blood pathway.
17. Cyanosis (si-a-<u>no</u>-sis) is a dark bluish or purplish coloration of the skin due to deficient oxygenation of the blood.
18. Diaphoresis (di-a-fo-<u>re</u>-sis) is perspiration.
19. Digoxin (di-<u>jok</u>-sin) is a generic name for a cardiotonic.
20. Diltiazem (<u>dil</u>-ti-a-zem) is a generic name for a coronary vasodilator.
21. Dobutamine (do-<u>byu</u>-ta-men) is a generic name for a cardiotonic agent.
22. Duodenal (du-o-<u>de</u>-nal) pertains to the duodenum, the first division of the small intestine.
23. Dysrhythmia (dis-<u>rith</u>-me-a) is a defective heart rhythm.
24. Echocardiogram (ek-o-<u>kar</u>-de-o-gram) is a diagnostic procedure using ultrasound to study heart structure and motion.
25. Endarterectomy (end-ar-ter-<u>ek</u>-to-me) is a surgical procedure to clear a blocked artery.
26. Epiphysis (e-<u>pif</u>-i-sis) is the center for ossification of the proximal and distal ends of a long bone.
27. Erythema (er-i-<u>the</u>-ma) is the redness of the skin due to capillary dilatation.
28. Expiratory (ek-<u>spi</u>-ra-to-re) pertains to exhalation.
29. Fibrillation (fi-bri-<u>la</u>-shun) is the rapid, irregular, uncoordinated contractions of muscle fibers.
30. Gallop (<u>gal</u>-op) is a triple cadence to the heart sounds.
31. Gout (gowt) is a disorder associated with an inborn error of uric acid metabolism that increases production or interferes with the excretion of uric acid.
32. Hemiblock (<u>hem</u>-e-blok) is the failure to conduct an impulse down one division of the left bundle branch.
33. Hemoptysis (he-<u>mop</u>-ti-sis) is the coughing or spitting of blood from the respiratory tract.
34. Heparin (<u>hep</u>-a-rin) is a generic name for an anticoagulant.
35. Hypercholesterolemia (<u>hi</u>-per-ko-<u>les</u>-ter-ol-e-me-a) is the presence of an abnormally large amount of cholesterol in the cells and plasma of the blood.
36. Hyperkalemia (<u>hi</u>-per-kal-<u>e</u>-ma-a) is the greater than normal concentration of potassium ions in the blood.
37. Hyperlipidemia (<u>hi</u>-per-lip-i-<u>de</u>-me-a) is a condition of elevated lipid levels in the blood.
38. Hypotensive (<u>hi</u>-po-<u>ten</u>-siv) is characterized by low blood pressure or causing a reduction in blood pressure.
39. Idiopathic (<u>id</u>-e-o-<u>path</u>-ik) is a disease of unknown cause.
40. Iliac (<u>il</u>-e-ak) pertains to the ilium.

41. Infarction (in-fark-shun) is the sudden insufficiency of arterial or venous blood supply.
42. Inferolateral (in-fer-o-lat-e-ral) pertains to a location situated below and to the side.
43. Inotropic (in-o-trop-ik) pertains to the force of muscular contractions.
44. Intimal (in-ti-mal) relates to the inner coat of a vessel.
45. Ischemia (is-ke-me-a) is the decreased supply of oxygenated blood to a body part.
46. Mediastinum (me-de-ah-sti-num) is the mass of tissues and organs separating the sternum in front and the vertebral column behind.
47. Myocardial (mi-o-kar-de-al) pertains to the muscular tissue of the heart.
48. Normocephalic (nor-mo-se-fal-ik) means having a normal-sized head; mesocephalic.
49. Nortriptyline (nor-trip-ti-lin) is a generic name for an antidepressant.
50. Paroxysm (par-ok-sism) is the sudden recurrence or increase in the intensity of symptoms; spasm or seizure.
51. Pectoralis (pek-to-ra-lis) pertains to the chest or breast.
52. Pedal (ped-al) pertains to the foot or feet.
53. Pitting (pit-ing) is the formation of a small depression.
54. Pleura (ploo-rah) is the serous membrane investing the lungs and lining the walls of the thoracic cavity.
55. Polycythemia (pol-e-si-the-me-ah) is an increase in the total red cell mass of the blood.
56. Quinidine (kwin-i-den) is a generic name for an antiarrhythmic agent used to treat atrial flutter, atrial fibrillation, premature ventricular contractions, and tachycardia.
57. Rhonchus (rong-kus) is a continuous dry rattling in the throat or bronchial tube due to a partial obstruction, heard on auscultation.
58. Sinus (si-nus) is a cavity or channel.
59. Stenosis (ste-no-sis) is the narrowing or contraction of a body passage.
60. Syncope (sing-ko-pe) is a temporary suspension of consciousness; fainting.
61. Tachycardia (tak-e-kar-de-ah) is an abnormally rapid heart rate.
62. Thrombosis (throm-bo-sis) is the formation of a blood clot within the vascular system.
63. Venous (ve-nus) pertains to the veins.
64. Verapamil (ver-ah-pam-il) is a generic name for a coronary vasodilator.
65. Capoten (kap-o-ten) is the trade name for an antihypertensive.
66. Cardiolite (kar-de-o-lit) is the trade name for a myocardial perfusion agent for cardiac SPECT imaging.
67. Cardizem (kar-di-zem) is the trade name for a calcium channel blocker for atrial fibrillation.
68. Coumadin (koo-mah-din) is the trade name for an anticoagulant.
69. Cytotec (si-to-tek) is the trade name for a nonsteroidal anti-inflammatory drug (NSAID) used to prevent gastric ulcers.
70. Ecotrin (ek-o-trin) is the trade name for an analgesic and anti-inflammatory.
71. Indocin (in-do-sin) is the trade name for a nonsteroidal anti-inflammatory drug (NSAID).
72. Isordil (i-sor-dil) is the trade name for an antianginal.
73. K-Dur (Kay-dur) is the trade name for a potassium supplement.
74. Lanoxin (lah-nok-sin) is the trade name for an antiarrhythmic and cardiotonic used to increase cardiac output.
75. Lasix (la-ziks) is the trade name for a diuretic.
76. Lescol (le-zkol) is the trade name for a reductase inhibitor for hypercholesterolemia.
77. Lotensin (lo-ten-sin) is the trade name for an antihypertensive.
78. Mevacor (mev-a kor) is the trade name for a reductase inhibitor for hypercholesterolemia.
79. Persantine (per-san-ten) is the trade name for a coronary vasodilator.
80. Premarin (prem-ah-rin) is the trade name for estrogen replacement therapy.
81. Provera (pro-ver-ah) is the trade name for progestin for secondary amenorrhea and abnormal uterine bleeding.
82. Quinidex (kwin-i-deks) is the trade name for an antiarrhythmic.
83. Reglan (reg-lan) is the trade name for a gastrointestinal stimulant and antiemetic.
84. Senokot (se-no-kot) is the trade name for a laxative.
85. Synthroid (sin-throid) is the trade name for a thyroid hormone.
86. Tenormin (ten-or-min) is the trade name for a beta blocker and antihypertensive agent.
87. Terramycin (ter-ah-mi-sin) is the trade name for an antibiotic.
88. Theo-Dur (the-o-dur) is the trade name for a bronchodilator.
89. Trental (tren-tal) is the trade name for an oral hemorheologic drug.
90. Vasotec (vah-o-tek) is the trade name for an antihypertensive agent.
91. Xanax (zan-aks) is the trade name for an anti-anxiety agent.
92. Zyloprim (zi-lo-prim) is the trade name for an antigout agent.

Do you remember back in school when you had to write each spelling word ten times? Because you had to physically write each word, your mind and body were focused on the assignment, and the method worked. Let's follow this successful method by reinforcing the spelling of selected terms and drugs found in the cardiology specialty through keyboarding drills.

Word Processing Users

Open your word processing package.
Read, mentally spell, and type each word in its sequence.
Save your work on your student disk.

1. afebrile amaurosis aneurysm afebrile amaurosis aneurysm afebrile amaurosis aneurysm
2. angiography arrhythmia arteriography angiography arrhythmia arteriography angiography
3. atherosclerotic atrial bradycardia atherosclerotic atrial bradycardia atherosclerotic atrial
4. bruit cardiomyopathy cardioverter bruit cardiomyopathy cardioverter bruit cardiomyopathy
5. carotid cholecystectomy claudication carotid cholecystectomy claudication carotid
6. collateral cyanosis diaphoresis collateral cyanosis diaphoresis collateral cyanosis diaphoresis
7. digoxin diltiazem dobutamine digoxin diltiazem dobutamine digoxin diltiazem dobutamine
8. duodenal dysrhythmia echocardiogram duodenal dysrhythmia echocardiogram duodenal
9. endarterectomy epiphysis erythema endarterectomy epiphysis erythema endarterectomy
10. expiratory fibrillation gallop expiratory fibrillation gallop expiratory fibrillation gallop
11. gout hemiblock hemoptysis gout hemiblock hemoptysis gout hemiblock hemoptysis gout
12. heparin hypercholesterolemia hyperkalemia heparin hypercholesterolemia hyperkalemia

13. hyperlipidemia hypotensive idiopathic hyperlipidemia hypotensive idiopathic hyperlipidemia
14. iliac infarction inferolateral iliac infarction inferolateral iliac infarction inferolateral iliac
15. inotropic ischemia intimal inotropic ischemia intimal inotropic ischemia intimal inotropic
16. mediastinum myocardial normocephalic mediastinum myocardial normocephalic
17. nortriptyline paroxysm pectoralis nortriptyline paroxysm pectoralis nortriptyline paroxysm
18. pedal pitting pleura pedal pitting pleura pedal pitting pleura pedal pitting pleura pedal pitting
19. polycythemia quinidine rhonchus polycythemia quinidine rhonchus polycythemia quinidine
20. sinus stenosis syncope sinus stenosis syncope sinus stenosis syncope sinus stenosis syncope
21. tachycardia thrombosis venous verapamil tachycardia thrombosis venous verapamil
22. Capoten Cardiolite Cardizem Capoten Cardiolite Cardizem Capoten Cardiolite Cardizem
23. Coumadin Cytotec Ecotrin Coumadin Cytotec Ecotrin Coumadin Cytotec Ecotrin Coumadin
24. Indocin Isordil K-Dur Indocin Isordil K-Dur Indocin Isordil K-Dur Indocin Isordil K-Dur
25. Lanoxin Lasix Lescol Lanoxin Lasix Lescol Lanoxin Lasix Lescol Lanoxin Lasix Lescol
26. Lotensin Mevacor Persantine Lotensin Mevacor Persantine Lotensin Mevacor Persantine
27. Premarin Provera Quinidex Premarin Provera Quinidex Premarin Provera Quinidex Premarin
28. Reglan Senokot Synthroid Reglan Senokot Synthroid Reglan Senokot Synthroid Reglan
29. Tenormin Terramycin Theo-Dur Tenormin Terramycin Theo-Dur Tenormin Terramycin
30. Trental Vasotec Xanax Zyloprim Trental Vasotec Xanax Zyloprim Trental Vasotec Xanax

Now you are ready to make the transition from keyboarding medical terms, which is a visual process, to transcribing medical terms, an aural process. You are going to use audiocassette tapes or your CD-ROM rather than printed material. Sentences 49, 70, 74, 76, 85, and 88 contain dangerous abbreviations and need to be transcribed according to the guidelines established in this textbook and the recommendations of *The AAMT Book of Style*, Appendix B.

WORD PROCESSING USERS

Open your word processing package.

Insert the appropriate audiocassette in your transcribing machine and find dictation *10T-1*.

You will be transcribing spelling words in sentence structure.

Listen carefully to each sentence on the audiocassette before transcribing.

Rewind and type (transcribe) the sentences.

Save your work on your student disk.

Refer to the answer key (Appendix E) for immediate feedback.

SOFTWARE USERS

Click on *Chapter 10, Activity 10-3 (10T-1)*, and follow the directions.

Let's pause a minute and see how well you are doing. This section allows you to evaluate your mastery of keyboarding and spelling selected terms and drugs found in the cardiology specialty.

TEXTBOOK USERS

Select the correctly spelled term that matches its definition.
Refer to the answer key (Appendix E) for immediate feedback.

SOFTWARE USERS

Click on *Chapter 10, Terminology Check Your Progress*, and follow the directions.

CHECK YOUR PROGRESS

Directions: Select the correctly spelled term that matches its definition.

1. Without fever:
   (a) afebrile
   (b) afebril
   (c) atrail
   (d) atrial

2. Variation from the normal rhythm of the heartbeat:
   (a) arhythmia
   (b) bruit
   (c) arrhythmia
   (d) bruite

3. Diagnostic procedure using ultrasound to study heart structure and motion:
   (a) syncope
   (b) echocardiogram
   (c) synscope
   (d) dysrrhythmia

4. Surgical procedure done to clear a blocked artery:
   (a) cholecystectomy
   (b) endartertomy
   (c) cholcystectomy
   (d) endarterectomy

5. Slowness of the heartbeat:
   (a) tachycardia
   (b) tachicardia
   (c) bradicardia
   (d) bradycardia

6. The presence of an abnormally large amount of cholesterol in the cells and plasma of the blood:
   (a) hypercholesterolemia
   (b) hypertensive
   (c) hypocholesterolemia
   (d) hypotensive

7. The narrowing or contraction of a body passage:
   (a) stensis
   (b) stenosis
   (c) amarosis
   (d) amaurosis

8. Hardening of an artery from plaque deposits within the vessel:
   (a) atherosclerotic
   (b) atheriosclerotic
   (c) normocephalic
   (d) normiocephalic

9. Loss of sight without an apparent lesion of the eye:
   (a) stensis
   (b) stenosis
   (c) amarosis
   (d) amaurosis

10. Formation of a blood clot within the vascular system:
    (a) myocardial
    (b) myocardal
    (c) thromosis
    (d) thrombosis

11. The center for ossification of the proximal and distal ends of a long bone:
    (a) hemptysis
    (b) hemoptysis
    (c) epiphysis
    (d) epiphtysis

12. A disease process of the heart muscle:
    (a) cardiomyopathy
    (b) cardioverter
    (c) cardomyopathy
    (d) cardoverter

13. Temporary suspension of consciousness; fainting:
    (a) syncope
    (b) echocardiogram
    (c) synscope
    (d) echocardogram

14. Surgical removal of the gallbladder:
    (a) cholecystectomy
    (b) endartertomy
    (c) cholcystectomy
    (d) endarterectomy

CHECK YOUR PROGRESS *(cont'd)*

15. Sudden recurrence or increase in intensity of symptoms; spasm or seizure:
    (a) paroxysm
    (b) paroxism
    (c) aneurism
    (d) aneurysm

16. Sudden insufficiency of arterial or venous blood supply:
    (a) heparin
    (b) heperin
    (c) infarction
    (d) infartion

17. Coughing or spitting of blood from the respiratory tract:
    (a) hemptysis
    (b) hemoptysis
    (c) epiphysis
    (d) epiphtysis

18. A secondary or accessory blood pathway:
    (a) collateral
    (b) inferolateral
    (c) coleratal
    (d) inferlateral

19. Serous membrane investing the lungs and lining the walls of the thoracic cavity:
    (a) polycythemia
    (b) pleura
    (c) polycyemia
    (d) pleuria

20. Pertaining to the principal artery of the neck:
    (a) pedal
    (b) padel
    (c) carotid
    (d) cariotid

21. Pertaining to the inner coat of a vessel:
    (a) intimal
    (b) intomal
    (c) doudenal
    (d) duodenal

22. Pertaining to the ilium:
    (a) pitting
    (b) iliac
    (c) piting
    (d) ilac

23. Pertaining to the duodenum, the first division of the small intestine:
    (a) intimal
    (b) intomal
    (c) doudenal
    (d) duodenal

24. Pertaining to exhalation:
    (a) expiratory
    (b) expiratery
    (c) hemblock
    (d) hemiblock

25. Redness of the skin due to capillary dilatation:
    (a) erythemia
    (b) erythema
    (c) ischema
    (d) ischemia

26. Radiographic visualization of blood vessels after injection of a contrast agent:
    (a) angiography
    (b) angography
    (c) artheriography
    (d) atherography

27. Radiographic visualization of an artery after injection of a contrast agent:
    (a) arthrography
    (b) artherography
    (c) arteriography
    (d) artrography

28. Pertains to the veins:
    (a) mediastinum
    (b) venous
    (c) medastinum
    (d) veinous

29. Pertains to the muscular tissue of the heart:
    (a) myocardial
    (b) myocardal
    (c) thromosis
    (d) thrombosis

30. Pertains to the foot or feet:
    (a) pedal
    (b) padel
    (c) carotid
    (d) cariotid

CHECK YOUR PROGRESS (cont'd)

31. Pertains to the chest or breast:
    (a) pectoralis
    (b) rhonchus
    (c) pectalis
    (d) rhionchus

32. Pertains to the atrium:
    (a) afebrile
    (b) afebril
    (c) atrail
    (d) atrial

33. Pertains to a location situated below and to the side:
    (a) colleratal
    (b) inferolateral
    (c) coleratal
    (d) inferlatral

34. Perspiration:
    (a) cyanosis
    (b) diaphoresis
    (c) cysainosis
    (d) diaphorsis

35. Having a normal-sized head; mesocephalic:
    (a) atherosclerotic
    (b) atheriosclerotic
    (c) normocephalic
    (d) normiocephalic

36. Mass of tissues and organs separating the sternum in front and the vertebral column behind:
    (a) mediastinum
    (b) venous
    (c) medastinum
    (d) veinous

37. Decreased supply of oxygenated blood to a body part:
    (a) erythemia
    (b) erythema
    (c) ischema
    (d) ischemia

38. Pertaining to the force of muscular contractions:
    (a) idiopathic
    (b) inotropic
    (c) idipathic
    (d) intropic

39. Greater than normal concentration of potassium ions in the blood:
    (a) hypolipidemia
    (b) hyperlipidemia
    (c) hypokalemia
    (d) hyperkalemia

40. Formation of a small depression:
    (a) pitting
    (b) iliac
    (c) piting
    (d) ilac

41. Failure to conduct an impulse down one division of the left bundle branch:
    (a) expiratory
    (b) expiratery
    (c) hemblock
    (d) hemiblock

42. Exceedingly rapid contractions of muscular fibrils:
    (a) caudication
    (b) claudication
    (c) fibrilation
    (d) fibrillation

43. Disorder associated with an inborn error of uric acid metabolism that increases production or interferes with the excretion of uric acid:
    (a) guot
    (b) sinus
    (c) gout
    (d) sinnus

44. Disease of unknown cause:
    (a) idiopathic
    (b) inotropic
    (c) idipathic
    (d) intropic

45. Device used to administer electrical shocks to the heart:
    (a) cardiomyopathy
    (b) cardioverter
    (c) cardomyopathy
    (d) cardoverter

TERMINOLOGY

CHECK YOUR PROGRESS (cont'd)

46. Defective rhythm:
    (a) rhonchus
    (b) dysrhythmia
    (c) ronchus
    (d) dysrrhythmia

47. Dark bluish or purplish coloration of the skin due to deficient oxygenation of the blood:
    (a) cyanosis
    (b) diaphoresis
    (c) cyainosis
    (d) diaphorsis

48. Cramp-like pains in the calf; limping:
    (a) caudication
    (b) claudication
    (c) fibrilation
    (d) fibrillation

49. Continuous dry rattling in the throat or bronchial tube due to a partial obstruction, heard on auscultation:
    (a) pectoralis
    (b) rhonchus
    (c) pectalis
    (d) rhionchus

50. Characterized by low blood pressure or causing a reduction in blood pressure:
    (a) hypercholesterolemia
    (b) hypertensive
    (c) hypocholesterolemia
    (d) hypotensive

51. Cavity or channel:
    (a) guot
    (b) sinus
    (c) gout
    (d) sinnus

52. An increase in total red cell mass of blood:
    (a) polycythemia
    (b) pleura
    (c) polycyemia
    (d) pleuria

53. Generic name for an antidepressant:
    (a) quindine
    (b) quinidine
    (c) nortrityline
    (d) nortriptyline

54. Generic name for an anticoagulant:
    (a) heparin
    (b) heperin
    (c) paroxysm
    (d) parxysim

55. Generic name for an antiarrhythmic agent used to treat atrial flutter, atrial fibrillation, premature ventricular contractions, and tachycardia:
    (a) quindine
    (b) quinidine
    (c) nortrityline
    (d) nortriptyline

56. An abnormally rapid heart rate:
    (a) tachycardia
    (b) tachicardia
    (c) bradicardia
    (d) bradycardia

57. A triple cadence to the heart sounds:
    (a) gallop
    (b) galop
    (c) bruit
    (d) briut

58. A sound or murmur heard in auscultation:
    (a) digoxin
    (b) digixin
    (c) bruit
    (d) briut

59. Localized abnormal dilatation of the wall of a blood vessel:
    (a) paroxysm
    (b) paroxism
    (c) aneurism
    (d) aneurysm

60. Generic name for a coronary vasodilator:
    (a) fibrilla
    (b) verapamil
    (c) fabrille
    (d) verpamil

CHECK YOUR PROGRESS *(cont'd)*

61. Generic name for a coronary vasodilator:
    (a) dobutamine
    (b) dobitamine
    (c) diltiazem
    (d) diltazem

62. A condition of elevated lipid levels in the blood:
    (a) hypolipidemia
    (b) hyperlipidemia
    (c) hypokalemia
    (d) hyperkalemia

63. Generic name for a cardiotonic:
    (a) digixin
    (b) paroxysm
    (c) digoxin
    (d) paroxism

64. Generic name for a cardiotonic agent:
    (a) dobutamine
    (b) dobitamine
    (c) cardiolite
    (d) cardialite

65. Trade name for an antihypertensive:
    (a) Capoten
    (b) Capatin
    (c) Zyloprim
    (d) Zylaprim

66. Trade name for myocardial perfusion agent for cardiac SPECT imaging:
    (a) Cardolite
    (b) Xanax
    (c) Cardiolite
    (d) Xanix

67. Trade name for a calcium channel blocker for atrial fibrillation:
    (a) Vasotec
    (b) Vasotic
    (c) Cardisem
    (d) Cardizem

68. Trade name for an anticoagulant:
    (a) Coumadim
    (b) Coumadin
    (c) Trentil
    (d) Trental

69. Trade name for a nonsteroidal anti-inflammatory drug (NSAID) used to prevent gastric ulcers:
    (a) Cycotec
    (b) Terramycin
    (c) Cytotec
    (d) Teramycin

70. Trade name for an analgesic, anti-inflammatory:
    (a) Ecotrin
    (b) Icotrin
    (c) Lasix
    (d) Laxis

71. Trade name for an NSAID:
    (a) Indocin
    (b) Endocin
    (c) Lotensin
    (d) Lotinsen

72. Trade name for an antianginal:
    (a) Lescol
    (b) Lescil
    (c) Isordol
    (d) Isordil

73. Trade name for a potassium supplement:
    (a) Theo-Dur
    (b) K-Dur
    (c) T-Dur
    (d) Kheo-Dur

74. Trade name for an antiarrhythmic, cardiotonic used to increase cardiac output:
    (a) Lanoxin
    (b) Lanozin
    (c) Tenormin
    (d) Tenorrmin

75. Trade name for a diuretic:
    (a) Ecotrin
    (b) Icotrin
    (c) Lasix
    (d) Laxis

76. Trade name for a reductase inhibitor for hypercholesterolemia:
    (a) Lescol
    (b) Lescil
    (c) Isordol
    (d) Isordil

TERMINOLOGY

NAME _____   DATE _____

CHECK YOUR PROGRESS (cont'd)

77. Trade name for an antihypertensive:
    (a) Indocin
    (b) Endocin
    (c) Lotensin
    (d) Lotinsen

78. Trade name for a reductase inhibitor for hypercholesterolemia:
    (a) Metavor
    (b) Mevacor
    (c) Synthroid
    (d) Syntoid

79. Trade name for a coronary vasodilator:
    (a) Persantine
    (b) Reglan
    (c) Presantine
    (d) Relan

80. Trade name for estrogen replacement therapy:
    (a) Provera
    (b) Prevera
    (c) Permarin
    (d) Premarin

81. Trade name for progestin for secondary amenorrhea and abnormal uterine bleeding:
    (a) Provera
    (b) Prevera
    (c) Permarin
    (d) Premarin

82. Trade name for an antiarrhythmic:
    (a) Quinidex
    (b) Senekot
    (c) Quindez
    (d) Senokot

83. Trade name for a gastrointestinal stimulant, antiemetic:
    (a) Persantine
    (b) Reglan
    (c) Presantine
    (d) Relan

84. Trade name for a laxative:
    (a) Quinidex
    (b) Senekot
    (c) Quindez
    (d) Senokot

85. Trade name for a thyroid hormone:
    (a) Metavor
    (b) Mevacor
    (c) Synthroid
    (d) Syntoid

86. Trade name for a beta blocker, antihypertensive agent:
    (a) Lanoxin
    (b) Lanozin
    (c) Tenormin
    (d) Tenorrmin

87. Trade name for an antibiotic:
    (a) Cycotec
    (b) Terramycin
    (c) Cytotec
    (d) Teramycin

88. Trade name for a bronchodilator:
    (a) Theo-Dur
    (b) K-Dur
    (c) T-Dur
    (d) Kheo-Dur

89. Trade name for an oral hemorheologic drug:
    (a) Xanax
    (b) Zanax
    (c) Trentil
    (d) Trental

90. Trade name for an antihypertensive agent:
    (a) Vasotec
    (b) Vasotic
    (c) Zyloprim
    (d) Zyloprime

91. Trade name for an antianxiety agent:
    (a) Cardolite
    (b) Xanax
    (c) Cardiolite
    (d) Xanix

92. Trade name for an antigout agent:
    (a) Capoten
    (b) Capatin
    (c) Zyloprim
    (d) Zylaprim

Professional transcriptionists proofread their own work. Can you?

WORD PROCESSING USERS

Open your word processing package.

Insert the appropriate audiocassette in your transcribing machine and find dictation *10T-2*.

Transcribe and proofread dictation *10T-2*, using the formatting guidelines established in Chapter 2.

Identify and correct all errors.

Save your work on your student disk.

After completing the transcription, refer to the answer key.

Manually complete the error analysis chart.

Manually complete the Production for Pay summary.

SOFTWARE USERS

Click on *Chapter 10, Proofreading Pretest (10T-2)*, and follow the directions.

PROOFREADING

Finding your own errors and correcting them is not easy, but it is an essential skill for your success as a medical transcriptionist. The worksheets in this activity will help you to develop your proofreading skills.

TEXTBOOK USERS

Proofread and correct errors in the medical documents shown in *Activities 10-4* and *10-5*.
Refer to the answer key (Appendix E) for immediate feedback.
Manually complete the error analysis chart for each document.

SOFTWARE USERS

Click on *Chapter 10, Activity 10-4*, and follow the directions.
Follow the same process for *Chapter 10, Activity 10-5*.

ACTIVITY 10-4
Proofreading Worksheet

Directions: Proofread this medical document, which contains multiple errors. Use open punctuation and all other formatting guidelines established in this textbook.

Current date

Charles P. Davis, MD
FedDes Wellness Center
Family Practice Division, Suite 300
101 Wellness Way Drive
New York, NY 10036
Re: George Niehls
Date of Birth: January 16, 19xx

Dear Dr. Davis

George Niehls is a 62 year old man who was admitted for a cystectomy because of carcinoma of the bladder. She has a history of intermitent visual bluring. A routine physical examination revealed a right carotid bruit. A carotid sonagram was obtained which suggested high grade stenosis of the left internal carotid. He is a long time cigarette smoker and has moderate exertional dispnea. There has been no definite angina pectis nor definite symptoms related to his right carotide lession. There is a long history of hypotension but drug therapy was discontinued in 1990.

Physical examination show a blood pressure of 180 over 100 and a pulse of 80 and regular. Venous pulses are unremarkable. There is a long left carotid bruitt. Ocassional rhonchus are present in the chest and there is a moderately slightly prolonged expiratery phrase. The heart is not inlarged. hier are no significant murmur or gallops. The adbomen contains no mases and no bruits. There is no periferal edema.

Mr. Neihls would appear to have high grade carotid artery stensis. With contemplated major surgery this should presumably be repaired pre-operatively despite it's essentially assymptomatic state. In addition combined coronary arterography with cerebral angography would be apropriate. With his long history of hypertension it would seem reasonable to also perform a renal arterogram during the same procedure.

ACTIVITY 10-4 *(cont'd)*

George Niehls
Current date
Page 2

We will arrange these studies and subsequent recomendations will be based on the results of the diagnostic findings. We appreciate the opportunity to participate in her car.

Sincerely,

Lucas Site MD

xx

ACTIVITY 10-5
Proofreading Worksheet

Directions: Proofread this medical document, which contains multiple errors. Use open punctuation and all other formatting guidelines established in this textbook.

HISTORY AND PHYSICAL EXAMINATION REPORT

Patient Name: Rolf, Nathan
File Number: 59025
Date of Birth: February 21, 19xx
Examination Date: *current date*

Physician: Adam Valence, MD

HISTORY

CHIEF COMPLAINT
Shortness of breathe.

HISTORY OF PRESENT ILLNESS
Nathan Rolfe is a 35 year old male with documented idopathic cardiomypathy. She became symptomatic in 1995 and a subsequent cardiac catheterization was performed in 1997 at which time an ejection faction of 25 was documented. His symptoms have progressed and she was recently hospitalized several weeks ago for intravenous Dobutamine therapy. He symptomatically improvedbut in the past week he developed increasing dispnea and orthipnea.

PHYSICAL EXAMINATION
VITAL SIGNS: Physical examination shows a blood pressure of one hundred thirty
    overseventy three and a pulse of 112 and irregular.
NECK: Jugular venus pulse is slightly prominent.
CHEST: The chest is fairly clear.
HEART: The heart is moderate inlarged with an S three gallop. No significant murmurs.

IMPRESSION
Mr. Rolf has severe cardiomyopathy. Parental enotropic agents will again be employ. Presumably his gastrointestinal symptoms is also indicative of congestive heart failure but a complicating factors needs to be included as well.

Plan
Admit to University's Hospital due to her increasing dispnea and orthipnea. He will again be assesed for a possible cardiac transplantation.

Adam Valence

av:xx D: current date T: current date

Now you are ready to make the transition from simply proofreading printed material to both transcribing and proofreading dictated material.

WORD PROCESSING USERS

Open your word processing package.

Insert the appropriate audiocassette in your transcribing machine and find dictation *10T-3.*

Step 1: Listen to the entire dictation to gain an understanding of the medical concepts and terms involved in the report. Rewind the tape to the beginning of the dictation and transcribe what you hear. Do not worry about formatting, style, or speed. Simply type what you hear being dictated, using correct punctuation, capitalization, and spelling. Stop as needed to look up words you do not understand or cannot spell. Adjust the speed control of the transcriber to a comfortable level, starting slowly to ensure no dictated words are missed, and increase the speed as your accuracy improves.

Step 2: Rewind the tape and transcribe dictation *10T-3* again, including correct spacing and formatting. Proofread the report. Identify and correct all errors. Save your work on your student disk. Refer to the answer key, and manually complete the error analysis chart and Production for Pay summary.

Follow the same process for dictation *10T-4.*

SOFTWARE USERS

Click on *Chapter 10, Activity 10-6 (10T-3), Step 1,* and follow the directions. When you feel comfortable with the dictation, click on *Chapter 10, Activity 10-6 (10T-3), Step 2,* and follow the directions.

Follow the same process for *Chapter 10, Activity 10-7 (10T-4), Step 1* and *Chapter 10, Activity 10-7 (10T-4), Step 2.*

Let's pause a minute and see how well you are doing. This section allows you to evaluate your success at transcribing and proofreading cardiology reports.

WORD PROCESSING USERS

Open your word processing package.

Insert the appropriate audiocassette in your transcribing machine and find dictation *10T-2*.

Transcribe and proofread dictation *10T-2*, using the formatting guidelines established in Chapter 2.

Identify and correct all errors.

Save your work on your student disk.

After completing the transcription, refer to the answer key.

Manually complete the error analysis chart.

Manually complete the Production for Pay summary.

SOFTWARE USERS

Click on *Chapter 10, Proofreading Check Your Progress (10T-2)*, and follow the directions.

PROOFREADING

Professional transcriptionists can transcribe and proofread their own work. Can you?

WORD PROCESSING USERS

Open your word processing package.

Insert the appropriate audiocassette in your transcribing machine and find dictation *10T-5*.

Transcribe and proofread dictation *10T-5*, using the formatting guidelines established in Chapter 2.

Identify and correct all errors.

Save your work on your student disk.

After completing the transcriptions, refer to the answer key.

Manually complete the error analysis chart.

Manually complete the Production for Pay summary.

Follow the same process for dictation *10T-6*.

SOFTWARE USERS

Click on *Chapter 10, Transcription Pretest (10T-5)*, and follow the directions.

Follow the same process for *Chapter 10, Transcription Pretest (10T-6)*.

CARDIOLOGY TRANSCRIPTION AT FEDDES WELLNESS CENTER

You have been hired as a transcriptionist at FedDes Wellness Center in the Cardiology Division. Your supervisor has asked you to transcribe today's dictation.

WORD PROCESSING USERS

Open your word processing package.

Insert the appropriate audiocassette in your transcribing machine and find dictation *10T-7*.

Create or use your existing templates as necessary for the six types of reports (chart note, chart note using history and physical format, history and physical examination, x-ray report, procedure report, consultation letter).

Transcribe and proofread dictation *10T-7*, using formatting guidelines established in Chapter 2.

Identify and correct all errors.

Save your work on your student disk.

After completing the transcriptions, refer to the answer key.

Manually complete the error analysis chart.

Manually complete the Production for Pay summary.

Follow the same process for dictations *10T-8* through *10T-12*.

SOFTWARE USERS

Click on *Chapter 10, Transcription at FedDes Wellness Center, Dictation 10T-7*, and follow the directions.

Follow the same process for each of the remaining dictations (*10T-8* through *10T-12*).

TRANSCRIPTION

Remember to follow the guidelines pertaining to capitalization, numbers, punctuation, abbreviations, measurements, symbols, and use of templates. This material is reviewed in Unit I.

10T-7

Consultation Report
Patient's Name: Naomi Isiaba
Requesting Physician: Izzy Sertoli, MD
Physician: Adam Valence, MD

Transcription Tips

- A hyphen is used between numbers and *year old*.
    You hear the dictator say: Naomi Isiaba is a 19 year old Asian female.
    You transcribe as: Naomi Isiaba is a 19-year-old Asian female.
- The following abbreviations are dictated in this report:
    DVT: deep vein thrombosis
    IV: intravenous
- The following test is dictated in this report:
    Doppler study: an ultrasound flowmeter used in assessing intermittent claudication, thrombus obstruction of deep veins, and several other abnormalities of blood flow in the major arteries and veins

- Figures are used for age, weight, height, blood pressure, pulse, and respiration. The diagonal (/) is used to indicate the word *over* in blood pressure.
    You hear the dictator say: B P one hundred over sixty.
    You transcribe as: BP 100/60.
- Capital letters are used for electrocardiographic (ECG) leads, waves, and segments. Chest leads are indicated with a *V* for the central terminal, an Arabic number for the chest electrode, and a letter for right or left arm or foot. The ECG leads are *V1* through *V6* and *aVL*, *aVR*, and *aVF*. Waves include P, Q, R, S, T, and U and their combinations.
    You hear the dictator say: peaked tees laterally.
    You transcribe as: peaked Ts laterally.
- Roman numerals are used for standard leads and intercostal space positions.
    You hear the dictator say: There is reciprocal depression in leads one and two.
    You transcribe as: There is reciprocal depression in leads I and II.
- A period is used to replace the word *point*.
    You hear the dictator say: WBC twenty point two hemoglobin fifteen point two.
    You transcribe as: WBC 20.2, hemoglobin 15.2.
- The following laboratory test is dictated in this report:
    GUSTO trial: global utilization of streptokinase and tissue plasminogen activator for occluded coronary arteries
- Words beginning with *non, re, pre,* and *post* are not hyphenated: nontender.

10T-8

History and Physical Examination Report
Patient's Name: Samuel Whitehead
Physician: Adam Valence, MD

Transcription Tips

- Capitalize the name of specific departments or sections in a hospital or institution.
    You hear the dictator say: He presented to the university hospital emergency room.
    You transcribe as: He presented to the University Hospital Emergency Room.
- The following abbreviations are dictated in this report:
    ECG: electrocardiogram
    WBC: white blood count

10T-9

History and Physical Examination Report
Patient's Name: Clifford Gallette
Physician: A. B. Doner, MD

Transcription Tips

- The following drugs are dictated in this report:
    Lotensin: trade name for an antihypertensive
    Terramycin: trade name for an antibiotic
    beta blockers: generic name for drugs that block the action of epinephrine at beta-adrenergic receptors on the cells of effector organs; used to treat angina pectoralis, hypertension, and cardiac arrhythmias
    aspirin: generic name for an analgesic, antipyretic, anti-inflammatory, antirheumatic

heparin: generic name for an anticoagulant
- Capital letters are used for electrocardiographic (ECG) leads, waves, and segments. Chest leads are indicated with a *V* for the central terminal, an Arabic number for the chest electrode, and a letter for the right or left arm or foot. The ECG leads are *V1* through *V6* and *aVL*, *aVR*, and *aVF*. Waves include P, Q, R, S, T, and U and their combinations.
    - You hear the dictator say: There is one millimeter of s t segment depression in leads two three and a v f.
    - You transcribe as: There is 1 mm of ST segment depression in leads II, III, and aVF.
- The diagonal (/) is used to indicate the word *per* in laboratory values and respirations or the word *over* in blood pressure.
    - You hear the dictator say: his blood pressure is one hundred forty four over eighty eight with a pulse of eighty respiratory rate is sixteen per minute.
    - You transcribe as: His blood pressure is 144/88 with a pulse of 80. Respiratory rate is 16/min.
- Words beginning with *non, re, pre*, or *post* are not hyphenated: nonsmoker, nondrinker, noncontributory.

10T-10

History and Physical Examination Report
Patient's Name: Lorraine Sosa
Physician: Erica Purkinje, MD

Transcription Tips
- The following abbreviations are dictated in this report:
    ICU: intensive care unit
    MI: myocardial infarction
    COPD: chronic obstructive pulmonary disease
- A hyphen is used to join two or more words when used as an adjective that precedes a noun. The following word pairs are dictated in this report: two-month, two-pack-a-day.
- Quotation marks are used to indicate a direct quote.
    - You hear the dictator say: She describes as an ache in her left upper chest.
    - You transcribe this sentence as follows: She describes as "an ache in her left upper chest."
- The following drugs are dictated in this report:
    Vasotec: trade name for an angiotensin-converting enzyme inhibitor
    diltiazem: generic name for a coronary vasodilator
    Pepcid: trade name for an acid controller for heartburn and acid indigestion
    Lasix: trade name for a diuretic

- The degree (°) sign is not used in describing temperature if the word *degree* is not dictated or not represented on the keyboard.
    - You hear the dictator say: There is no visible neck vein distention at forty five degrees.
    - You transcribe as: There is no visible neck vein distention at 45 degrees.
- Figures and capital letters are used with electrocardiographic waves.
    - You hear the dictator say: heart reveals a regular rhythm with an s four.
    - You transcribe as: heart reveals a regular rhythm with an S4.
- Figures are used with the + or − symbols.
    - You hear the dictator say: She has four plus pitting edema of her lower extremities.
    - You transcribe as: She has 4+ pitting edema of her lower extremities.
- Words beginning with *non, re, pre*, or *post* are not hyphenated: nontender.

10T-11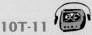

History and Physical Examination Report
Patient's Name: Michael Fellows
Physician: Lucas Site, MD

Transcription Tips
- The following drugs are dictated in this report:
    vitamin E: vitamin E supplement; topical emollient
    vitamin C: ascorbic acid, antiscorbutic, urinary acidifier
    Trental: trade name for an oral hemorheologic drug
    beta carotene: ultraviolet screen; vitamin A precursor
    Centrum Silver: trade name for a geriatric vitamin and mineral supplement
    Zyloprim: trade name for a xanthine oxidase inhibitor
    heparin: generic name for an anticoagulant
    Coumadin: trade name for an anticoagulant
- Plurals of double-digit numbers are formed by adding the letter *s*.
    - You hear the dictator say: His heart rate is in the seventies and regular.
    - You transcribe as: His heart rate is in the 70s and regular.
- The following abbreviation is dictated in this report:
    PERRLA: pupils equal, round, reactive to light and accommodation
- Words beginning with *non, re, pre*, and *post* are not hyphenated: nonfocal.

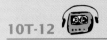

10T-12

Consultation Letter
Patient's Name: Marie Monyet
Requesting Physician: J. Thomas Geiger, MD
Physician: Erica Purkinje, MD

Transcription Tips

- The following abbreviations are dictated in this report:
    MRI: magnetic resonance imaging
    ECG: electrocardiogram
    HEENT: head, eyes, ears, nose, throat
- The percent sign (%) is used with words and figures.
    You hear the dictator say: a recent M R I angiogram showing a fifty percent right internal carotid artery stenosis.
    You transcribe as: a recent MRI angiogram showing a 50% right internal carotid artery stenosis.
- Capital letters are used for electrocardiographic leads, waves, and segments. Waves include P, Q, R, S, T, and U and their combinations.
    You hear the dictator say: abnormal electrocardiogram with anterior t wave abnormalities and a q wave in lead three.

You transcribe as: abnormal electrocardiogram with anterior T-wave abnormalities and a Q-wave in lead III.
- The following diagnostic tests are dictated in this report:
    dobutamine stress test: generic name for a synthetic catecholamine administered parenterally for inotropic support in short-term treatment of adults with cardiac decompensation
    liver function tests: a series of laboratory procedures that measure some aspect of liver functions, including serum protein electrophoresis and one-stage prothrombin time
- A hyphen is used between two "like" vowels: anti-inflammatories.
- The following drugs are dictated in this report:
    Tenormin: trade name for a beta blocker
    Indocin: trade name for nonsteroidal anti-inflammatory drug (NSAID)
    Cytotec: trade name for a protectant used to prevent NSAID-induced gastric ulcers
- Words beginning with *non*, *re*, *pre*, or *post* are not hyphenated: nonocclusive, nonsteroidal.

Check Your Progress (*10T-5* and *10T-6*)

Professional transcriptionists can transcribe and proofread their own work with speed and accuracy. Have you mastered the cardiology transcription rotation at FedDes Wellness Center?

WORD PROCESSING USERS

Open your word processing package.

Insert the appropriate audiocassette in your transcribing machine and find dictation *10T-5*.

Transcribe and proofread dictation *10T-5*, using the formatting guidelines established in Chapter 2.

Identify and correct all errors.

Save your work on your student disk.

After completing the transcription, refer to the answer key.

Manually complete the error analysis chart.

Manually complete the Production for Pay summary.

Follow the same process for dictation *10T-6*.

SOFTWARE USERS

Click on *Chapter 10, Transcription Check Your Progress (10T-5)*, and follow the directions.

Follow the same process for *Chapter 10, Transcription Check Your Progress (10T-6)*.

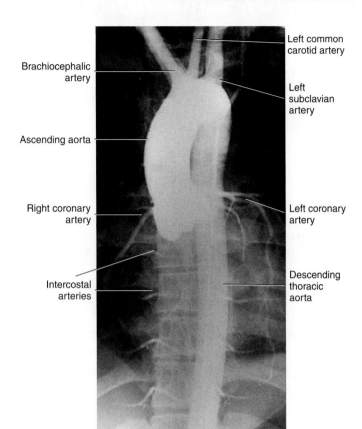

Brachiocephalic artery

Ascending aorta

Right coronary artery

Intercostal arteries

Left common carotid artery

Left subclavian artery

Left coronary artery

Descending thoracic aorta

Figure 10-1 Anteroposterior (AP) radiographic view of thoracic aorta that also demonstrates right and left coronary arteries. *(From Ballinger PW, Frank ED:* Merrill's atlas of radiographic positions and radiologic procedures, *ed 10, St Louis, 2003, Mosby.)*

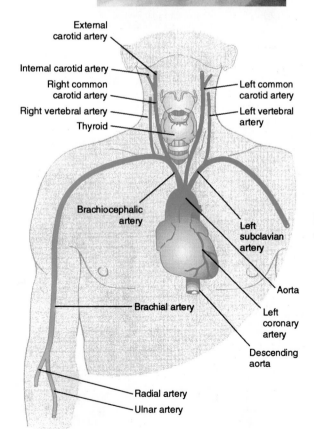

External carotid artery

Internal carotid artery

Right common carotid artery

Right vertebral artery

Thyroid

Left common carotid artery

Left vertebral artery

Brachiocephalic artery

Left subclavian artery

Aorta

Brachial artery

Left coronary artery

Descending aorta

Radial artery

Ulnar artery

Figure 10-2 Major arteries of the upper chest, neck, and arm.

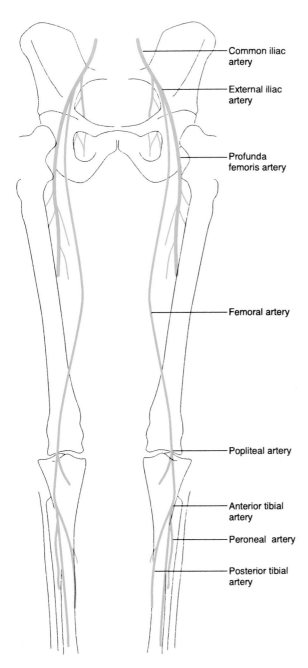

Figure 10-3 Arteries of the lower extremities.

Common iliac
artery

External iliac
artery

Profunda
femoris artery

Femoral artery

Popliteal artery

Anterior tibial
artery

Peroneal artery

Posterior tibial
artery

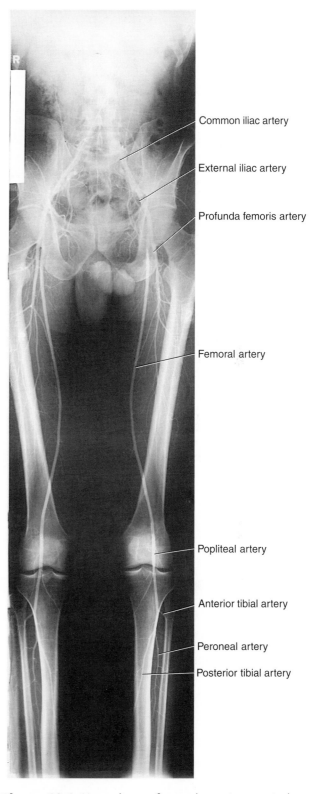

Common iliac artery

External iliac artery

Profunda femoris artery

Femoral artery

Popliteal artery

Anterior tibial artery

Peroneal artery

Posterior tibial artery

Figure 10-4 Normal aortofemoral arteriogram in late arterial phase. *(From Ballinger PW, Frank ED:* Merrill's atlas of radiographic positions and radiologic procedures, *ed 10, St Louis, 2003, Mosby.)*

Chapter 11

Office Medical Transcription from the Diagnostic Imaging Practice

OBJECTIVES

At the completion of Chapter 11, you should be able to do the following:

1. Match medical terms associated with the diagnostic imaging specialty with their definitions.
2. Spell medical terms associated with the diagnostic imaging specialty.
3. Transcribe medical terms in sentence structure.
4. Proofread, edit, and correct medical documents associated with the diagnostic imaging specialty that contain various errors.
5. Transcribe and proofread authentic medical documents associated with the diagnostic imaging specialty.

INTRODUCTION TO THE DIAGNOSTIC IMAGING ROTATION

Terminology
Pretest
Activities
    11-1: Keyboarding Medical Terms and Definitions
    11-2: Spelling Medical Terms
    11-3: Transcribing Medical Sentences, *11T-1*
Check Your Progress

Proofreading
Pretest, *11T-2*
Activities
    11-4: Proofreading Worksheet
    11-5: Proofreading Worksheet
    11-6: Proofreading Transcription Exercise, *11T-3*
    11-7: Proofreading Transcription Exercise, *11T-4*
Check Your Progress, *11T-2*

Transcription
Pretest, *11T-5* and *11T-6*
Diagnostic Imaging Transcription at FedDes Wellness Center
Index of Dictations and Associated Transcription Tips, *11T-7* through *11T-19*
Check Your Progress, *11T-5* and *11T-6*

Anatomical Illustrations and Medical Images

What's Ahead

The FedDes Wellness Center has four radiologists, or specialists in diagnostic radiology, on staff. Diagnostic radiology is the field of medicine concerned with the use of roentgen rays and other forms of energy in the diagnosis and treatment of diseases. The diagnostic radiologist uses a variety of techniques, including x-rays (radiographs), computed tomography (CT), magnetic resonance imaging (MRI), ultrasound, and nuclear medicine, to evaluate the anatomy of interest. Patients are often referred to a hospital or diagnostic imaging center for their medical imaging studies. A contracted or staff radiologist associated with the facility interprets the images and may also perform the exam with the assistance of a registered radiologic technologist.

The physicians in FedDes Diagnostic and Imaging Division perform and interpret sophisticated imaging such as MR images, CT scans, ultrasounds, positron emission tomography (PET) scans, digital subtraction angiography (DSA) scans, and nuclear medicine studies. Transcribed reports may be sent back to the referring physician in a letter format or in a more informal x-ray report format. Radiologists often dictate in the present tense because they are interpreting the findings as they view the films. As a general rule, the history is past tense and the findings are present tense.

In this unit, you assume the role of a medical transcriptionist employed at the Diagnostic Imaging Division of the FedDes Wellness Center. **Please remember to follow the guidelines pertaining to capitalization, numbers, punctuation, abbreviations, measurements, symbols, and use of templates to create medical reports at FedDes Wellness Center.** This material is reviewed in Unit I. The transcription exercises list the type of report, patient's name, and physician(s) as well as the associated transcription tips.

You will work with the textbook and CD-ROM or accompanying audiocassettes. Your mastery of diagnostic imaging transcription is assessed through worksheets, timed transcription exercises, the error analysis chart, and the Production for Pay summary.

All the answer keys are found in the textbook and CD-ROM, providing immediate feedback. After transcribing a report, you will proofread your work and correct any errors. Then you will compare your proofread work against a master transcript, categorize all errors, and tabulate the errors on the error analysis chart. The Production for Pay summary correlates your production to the FedDes Wellness Center pay scale. The scale is also linked to your grade. This system allows you to assess your mastery of transcription skills in a real-world scenario.

Let's find out if you can define and spell selected terminology and drugs of the diagnostic imaging specialty that are included in this chapter.

TEXTBOOK USERS

Select the correctly spelled term that matches its definition.
Refer to the answer key (Appendix E) for immediate feedback.

SOFTWARE USERS

Click on *Chapter 11, Terminology Pretest*, and follow the directions.

TERMINOLOGY

PRETEST

Directions: Select the correctly spelled term that matches its definition.

1. Set limits or boundaries:
   (a) demarcated
   (b) structure
   (c) demacated
   (d) stricture

2. Stone:
   (a) calulus
   (b) calculus
   (c) amorphous
   (d) amorphus

3. Pertaining to the cricoid cartilage and the pharynx:
   (a) cricoidpharyngeal
   (b) Pasavant's cushion
   (c) cricopharyngeal
   (d) Passavant's cushion

4. A ridge appearing on the posterior wall of the pharynx during swallowing due to contraction of the palatopharyngeal sphincter:
   (a) cricoidpharyngeal
   (b) Pasavant's cushion
   (c) cricopharyngeal
   (d) Passavant's cushion

5. Herniation of an abdominal organ through the esophageal opening of the diaphragm:
   (a) haitus hernai
   (b) hiatus hernia
   (c) hydronephrosis
   (d) hydronphrosis

6. Backward flow:
   (a) reflux
   (b) refluxe
   (c) reflex
   (d) reflax

7. Articulation between the acromial process of the scapula and the clavicle:
   (a) perarticular
   (b) acromiocalvicular
   (c) acromioclavicular
   (d) periarticular

8. Abnormal forward tilting of an organ:
   (a) antiverted
   (b) adnixa
   (c) anteverted
   (d) adnexa

9. Abnormal narrowing of a duct or passage:
   (a) demarcated
   (b) structure
   (c) demacated
   (d) stricture

10. Pertaining to fluid around the gallbladder:
    (a) pericholecystic
    (b) periartecular
    (c) periarticular
    (d) pariochelecystic

11. Lacking similar form or relationship of parts:
    (a) asymmetry
    (b) asites
    (c) ascites
    (d) asymetry

12. Escape and accumulation of serous fluid in the abdominal cavity:
    (a) asymmetry
    (b) asites
    (c) ascites
    (d) asymetry

13. Partial dislocation:
    (a) infarction
    (b) infaction
    (c) sublixation
    (d) subluxation

14. Pharmaceutical given to the patient to allow radiographic visualization of a body structure:
    (a) centrum semiovale
    (b) contrast medium
    (c) contast medium
    (d) centram semvale

15. The functional elements of an organ as distinguished from its structure:
    (a) parenchyma
    (b) pareshyma
    (c) paresthesia
    (d) parenchyesia

PRETEST *(cont'd)*

16. Behind the peritoneum:
    (a) criopharyngeal
    (b) crioperitoneal
    (c) retroperitoneal
    (d) retraperitoneal

17. Joint spaces between the carpal and metacarpal bones:
    (a) carpametacarpal
    (b) carpocarpal
    (c) carpometacarpal
    (d) carpacarpeal

18. Situated around a joint:
    (a) pericholecystic
    (b) periartecular
    (c) periarticular
    (d) parichelecystic

19. A decrease in bone mass below the norm:
    (a) ischemic
    (b) osteopenia
    (c) iscemia
    (d) ostepenic

20. Disease of the lymph nodes:
    (a) lymphadenopathy
    (b) lymphadepathy
    (c) etiology
    (d) etoilogy

21. A device that translates one form of energy to another:
    (a) transducer
    (b) lacsnar
    (c) lacunar
    (d) transducar

22. Within the liver:
    (a) intrehepatic
    (b) ischemic
    (c) intrahepatic
    (d) ischamic

23. Distention of the renal pelvis and calyces with urine:
    (a) calculus
    (b) calulus
    (c) hydronephrosis
    (d) hydrophrosis

24. Second section of the small intestine:
    (a) jejunum
    (b) jejum
    (c) joint mouse
    (d) jont mose

25. The causes or origin of a disease or disorder:
    (a) lymphadenopathy
    (b) lymphadepathy
    (c) etiology
    (d) etoilogy

26. Having no definite form:
    (a) asymmetry
    (b) amorphous
    (c) asymetry
    (d) amorphus

27. A factor that makes it undesirable to treat a patient in the usual manner:
    (a) contraindication
    (b) contradicate
    (c) contradiction
    (d) contrandicate

28. Both sides:
    (a) bileteral
    (b) vertex
    (c) bilateral
    (d) vertix

29. A small cavity within or between other body structures:
    (a) transducer
    (b) lacsna
    (c) lacuna
    (d) transducar

30. Lack of blood in a body part:
    (a) intrehepatic
    (b) ischemia
    (c) intrahepatic
    (d) ischamic

31. Loose bodies in synovial joints:
    (a) jejunum joint
    (b) jejum jonte
    (c) joint mouse
    (d) jonte mose

TERMINOLOGY

PRETEST *(cont'd)*

32. The top or crown of the head:
    (a) centrum semiovale
    (b) vertex
    (c) vertix
    (d) centrum semivale

33. Formation of a blood clot:
    (a) thrombosis
    (b) thrombasis
    (c) hydronephrosis
    (d) hydronphrosis

34. The white matter of the cerebral hemispheres that has an almost oval shape:
    (a) centrum semiovale
    (b) vertex
    (c) vertix
    (d) centrum semivale

35. The death of tissue due to lack of blood flow to the area:
    (a) sublaxation
    (b) infartion
    (c) subluxation
    (d) infarction

36. Sensation of tingling and numbness:
    (a) osteopania
    (b) osteopenia
    (c) paresthesia
    (d) peresthesia

37. Trade name for a drug used in restoring hormonal balance:
    (a) Provera
    (b) Synthroid
    (c) Synthoid
    (d) Provira

38. Trade name for a drug used as a replacement in decreased or absent thyroid function:
    (a) Provera
    (b) Synthroid
    (c) Synthoid
    (d) Provira

39. Trade name for a drug that decreases LDL cholesterol:
    (a) Isovue
    (b) Isovae
    (c) Liscol
    (d) Lescol

40. Trade name for a drug used as a contrast medium:
    (a) Isovue
    (b) Isovae
    (c) Liscol
    (d) Lescol

Let's learn to spell and define selected terminology and drugs of the diagnostic imaging specialty that are included in this chapter. Keyboarding these terms is an effective way to improve your skills.

Word Processing Users

Open your word processing package.
Read and type each word and its definition as shown below.
Save your work on your student disk.

1. Acromioclavicular (<u>ah</u>-kro-me-o-klah-<u>vik</u>-u-lar) describes the articulation between the acromial process of the scapula and the clavicle.
2. Amorphous (ah-<u>mor</u>-fus) means having no definite form, or shapeless.
3. Anteversion (<u>an</u>-te-<u>ver</u>-shun) is the abnormal forward tilting of an organ.
4. Ascites (ah-<u>si</u>-teez) is the escape and accumulation of serous fluid in the abdominal cavity.
5. Asymmetry (a-<u>sim</u>-e-tre) means without symmetry, lacking similar form or relationship of parts.
6. Bilateral (bi-<u>lat</u>-er-al) means affecting both sides.
7. Calculus (<u>kal</u>-ku-lus) is a stone.
8. Carpometacarpal (<u>kar</u>-po-met-ah-<u>kar</u>-pal) is the joint spaces between the carpal and metacarpal bones.
9. Centrum semiovale (<u>sen</u>-trum <u>sem</u>-i-o-<u>val</u>) is the white matter of the cerebral hemispheres that has an almost oval shape.
10. Contraindication (kon-trah-<u>in</u>-di-<u>ka</u>-shun) is a factor that makes it undesirable to treat a patient in the usual manner.
11. Contrast medium (<u>kon</u>-trast <u>med</u>-e-um) is the pharmaceutical given to the patient to allow radiographic visualization of a body structure.
12. Cricopharyngeal (kri-ko-fah-<u>rin</u>-je-al) pertains to the cricoid cartilage and the pharynx.
13. Demarcated (de-mar-<u>ka</u>-ted) means set limits or boundaries.
14. Etiology (e-te-<u>ol</u>-oj-e) is concerned with the causes or origin of a disease or disorder.
15. Hiatus hernia (hi-<u>a</u>-tus <u>her</u>-ne-ah) is the herniation of an abdominal organ through the esophageal opening of the diaphragm; also called hiatal hernia.
16. Hydronephrosis (hi-dro-ne-<u>fro</u>-sis) is the distention of the renal pelvis and calyces with urine, often as a result of an obstructed ureter.
17. Infarction (in-<u>farkt</u>-shun) is the death of tissue due to lack of blood flow to the area.
18. Intrahepatic (in-trah-he-<u>pat</u>-ik) means within the liver.
19. Ischemia (is-<u>ke</u>-me-ah) is the lack of blood in a body part.
20. Jejunum (je-<u>joo</u>-num) is the second section of the small intestine.
21. Joint mouse (joint mows) is the loose body in synovial joints.
22. Lacuna (lah-<u>ku</u>-nah) is a small cavity within or between other body structures.
23. Lymphadenopathy (lim-fad-e-<u>nop</u>-ah-the) is a disease of the lymph nodes.
24. Osteopenia (os-te-o-<u>pe</u>-ne-ah) is the decrease in bone mass below the normal.
25. Parenchyma (pah-<u>reng</u>-ki-mah) is the general anatomical term to describe the functional elements of an organ, as distinguished from its structure.
26. Paresthesia (par-es-<u>the</u>-ze-ah) is the sensation of tingling and numbness.
27. Passavant's cushion (pas-a-vants koosh-un) is a ridge appearing on the posterior wall of the pharynx during swallowing due to contraction of the palatopharyngeal sphincter.
28. Periarticular (per-e-ar-<u>tic</u>-u-lar) means situated around a joint.
29. Pericholecystic (per-i-ko-le-sis-<u>tic</u>) fluid is a coined term, meaning fluid around the gallbladder.
30. Reflux (<u>re</u>-fluks) is backward flow.
31. Retroperitoneal (ret-ro-<u>per</u>-i-to-<u>ne</u>-al) means behind the peritoneum.
32. Stricture (<u>strik</u>-chor) is an abnormal narrowing of a duct or passage.
33. Subluxation (sub-luk-<u>sa</u>-shun) is a partial dislocation.
34. Thrombosis (throm-<u>bo</u>-sis) is the formation of a blood clot.
35. Transducer (trans-<u>doo</u>-ser) is a device that translates one form of energy to another; in sonography it transforms a sound wave into an electronically displayed image.
36. Vertex (<u>ver</u>-teks) is the top or crown of the head.
37. Isovue (is-<u>o</u>-vu) is the trade name for a drug used as a contrast medium.
38. Lescol (<u>les</u>-kol) is the trade name for a drug that decreases LDL cholesterol.
39. Provera (pro-<u>ver</u>-ah) is the trade name for a drug used in restoring hormonal balance.
40. Synthroid (<u>sin</u>-throid) is the trade name for a drug used as a replacement in decreased or absent thyroid function.

Do you remember back in school when you had to write each spelling word ten times? Because you had to physically write each word, your mind and body were focused on the assignment, and the method worked. Let's follow this successful method by reinforcing the spelling of selected terms and drugs found in the diagnostic imaging specialty through keyboarding drills.

Word Processing Users

Open your word processing package.
Read, mentally spell, and type each word in its sequence.
Save your work on your student disk.

1. acromioclavicular adnexa amorphous acromioclavicular adnexa amorphous acromioclavicular

2. anteverted ascites asymmetry anteverted ascites asymmetry anteverted ascites asymmetry

3. bilateral calculus carpometacarpal bilateral calculus carpometacarpal bilateral calculus

4. centrum semiovale contrast medium centrum semiovale contrast medium centrum semiovale

5. contraindicate cricopharyngeal demarcated contraindicate cricopharyngeal demarcated

6. etiology hiatus hernia hydronephrosis etiology hiatus hernia hydronephrosis etiology

7. infarction intrahepatic ischemic infarction intrahepatic ischemic infarction intrahepatic

8. jejunum joint mouse lacuna jejunum joint mouse lacuna jejunum joint mouse lacuna

9. lymphadenopathy parenchyma paresthesia lymphadenopathy parenchyma paresthesia

10. Passavant's cushion periarticular reflux Passavant's cushion periarticular reflux periarticular

11. pericholecystic fluid osteopenia pericholecystic fluid osteopenia pericholecystic fluid

12. retroperitoneal stricture subluxation retroperitoneal stricture subluxation retroperitoneal

13. thrombosis transducer vertex thrombosis transducer vertex thrombosis transducer vertex

14. Isovue Lescol Provera Synthroid Isovue Lescol Provera Synthroid Isovue Lescol Provera

Now you are ready to make the transition from keyboarding medical terms, which is a visual process, to transcribing medical terms, an aural process. You are going to use audiocassette tapes or your CD-ROM rather than printed material.

WORD PROCESSING USERS

Open your word processing software.

Insert the appropriate audiocassette in your transcribing machine and find dictation *11T-1*.

You will be transcribing spelling words in sentence structure.

Listen carefully to each sentence on the audiocassette before transcribing.

Rewind and type (transcribe) the sentences.

Save your work on your student disk.

Refer to the answer key (Appendix E) for immediate feedback.

SOFTWARE USERS

Click on *Chapter 11, Activity 11-3 (11T-1)*, and follow the directions.

Let's pause a minute and see how well you are doing. This section allows you to evaluate your mastery of keyboarding and spelling selected terms and drugs found in the diagnostic imaging specialty.

TEXTBOOK USERS

Select the correctly spelled term that matches its definition.
Refer to the answer key (Appendix E) for immediate feedback.

SOFTWARE USERS

Click on *Chapter 11, Terminology Check Your Progress*, and follow the directions.

NAME _____   DATE _____

CHECK YOUR PROGRESS

Directions: Select the correctly spelled term that matches its definition.

1. A decrease in the bone mass below the normal:
   (a) ischemia
   (b) osteopenia
   (c) iscemia
   (d) ostepenic

2. A device that translates one form of energy to another:
   (a) transducer
   (b) lacsna
   (c) lacuna
   (d) transducar

3. A factor that makes it undesirable to treat a patient in the usual manner:
   (a) contraindication
   (b) contradicate
   (c) contradiction
   (d) contrandicate

4. A small cavity within or between other body structures:
   (a) transducer
   (b) lacsna
   (c) lacuna
   (d) transducar

5. Abnormal narrowing of a duct or passage:
   (a) demarcated
   (b) structure
   (c) demacated
   (d) stricture

6. Both sides:
   (a) bileteral
   (b) vertex
   (c) bilateral
   (d) vertix

7. A ridge appearing on the posterior wall of the pharynx during swallowing due to contraction of the palatopharyngeal sphincter:
   (a) cricoidpharyngeal
   (b) Pasavant's cushion
   (c) cricopharyngeal
   (d) Passavant's cushion

8. Abnormal forward tilting of an organ:
   (a) antivertion
   (b) adnixa
   (c) anteversion
   (d) adnexa

9. Articulation between the acromial process of the scapula and the clavicle:
   (a) perarticular
   (b) acromiocalvicular
   (c) acromioclavicular
   (d) periarticular

10. Backward flow:
    (a) reflux
    (b) refluxe
    (c) reflex
    (d) reflax

11. Behind the peritoneum:
    (a) criopharyngeal
    (b) crioperitoneal
    (c) retroperitoneal
    (d) retraperitoneal

12. Disease of the lymph nodes:
    (a) lymphadenopathy
    (b) lymphadepathy
    (c) etiology
    (d) etoilogy

13. Distention of the renal pelvis and calyces with urine:
    (a) calculus
    (b) calulus
    (c) hydronephrosis
    (d) hydrophrosis

14. Pertaining to fluid around the gallbladder:
    (a) pericholecystic
    (b) periartecular
    (c) periarticular
    (d) parichelecystic

15. Formation of a blood clot:
    (a) thrombosis
    (b) thrombasis
    (c) hydronephrosis
    (d) hydronphrosis

CHECK YOUR PROGRESS *(cont'd)*

16. Having no definite form:
    (a) asymmetry
    (b) amorphous
    (c) asymetry
    (d) amorphus

17. Herniation of an abdominal organ through the esophageal opening of the diaphragm:
    (a) haitus hernai
    (b) hiatus hernia
    (c) hydronephrosis
    (d) hydronphrosis

18. Joint spaces between the carpal and metacarpal bones:
    (a) carpametacarpal
    (b) carpocarpal
    (c) carpometacarpal
    (d) carpacarpeal

19. Lack of blood in a body part:
    (a) intrehepatic
    (b) ischemia
    (c) intrahepatic
    (d) ischamia

20. Lacking similar form or relationship of parts:
    (a) asymmetry
    (b) asites
    (c) ascites
    (d) asymetry

21. Loose bodies in synovial joints:
    (a) jejunum joint
    (b) jejum jonte
    (c) joint mouse
    (d) jonte mose

22. Partial dislocation:
    (a) infarction
    (b) infaction
    (c) sublixation
    (d) subluxation

23. Pertaining to the cricoid cartilage and the pharynx:
    (a) cricoidpharyngeal
    (b) Pasavant's cushion
    (c) cricopharyngeal
    (d) Passavant's cushion

24. Pharmaceutical given to the patient to allow radiographic visualization of a body structure:
    (a) centrum semiovale
    (b) contrast medium
    (c) contast medium
    (d) centram semvale

25. Second section of the small intestine:
    (a) jejunum
    (b) jejum
    (c) joint mouse
    (d) jont mose

26. Sensation of tingling and numbness:
    (a) osteopania
    (b) osteopenia
    (c) paresthesia
    (d) peresthesia

27. Set limits or boundaries:
    (a) demarcated
    (b) structure
    (c) demacated
    (d) stricture

28. Situated around a joint:
    (a) pericholecystic
    (b) periartecular
    (c) periarticular
    (d) parichelecystic

29. Stone:
    (a) calulus
    (b) calculus
    (c) amorphous
    (d) amorphus

30. The causes or origin of a disease or disorder:
    (a) lymphadenopathy
    (b) lymphadepathy
    (c) etiology
    (d) etoilogy

31. The death of tissue due to lack of blood flow to the area:
    (a) sublaxation
    (b) infartion
    (c) subluxation
    (d) infarction

CHECK YOUR PROGRESS *(cont'd)*

32. Escape and accumulation of serous fluid in the abdominal cavity:
    (a) asymmetry
    (b) asites
    (c) ascites
    (d) asymetry

33. The functional elements of an organ, as distinguished from its structure:
    (a) parenchyma
    (b) pareshyma
    (c) paresthesia
    (d) parenchyesia

34. The top or crown of the head:
    (a) centrum semiovale
    (b) vertex
    (c) vertix
    (d) centrum semivale

35. The white matter of the cerebral hemispheres that has an almost oval shape:
    (a) centrum semiovale
    (b) vertex
    (c) vertix
    (d) centrum semivale

36. Within the liver:
    (a) intrehepatic
    (b) ischemic
    (c) intrahepatic
    (d) ischamic

37. Trade name for a drug that decreases LDL cholesterol:
    (a) Isovue
    (b) Isovae
    (c) Liscol
    (d) Lescol

38. Trade name for a drug used as a contrast medium:
    (a) Isovue
    (b) Isovae
    (c) Liscol
    (d) Lescol

39. Trade name for a drug used as a replacement in decreased or absent thyroid function:
    (a) Provera
    (b) Synthroid
    (c) Synthoid
    (d) Provira

40. Trade name for a drug used in restoring hormonal balance:
    (a) Provera
    (b) Synthroid
    (c) Synthoid
    (d) Provira

Professional transcriptionists proofread their own work. Can you?

WORD PROCESSING USERS

Open your word processing package.

Insert the appropriate audiocassette in your transcribing machine and find dictation *11T-2*.

Transcribe and proofread dictation *11T-2*, using the formatting guidelines established in Chapter 2.

Identify and correct all errors.

Save your work on your student disk.

After completing the transcription, refer to the answer key.

Manually complete the error analysis chart.

Manually complete the Production for Pay summary.

SOFTWARE USERS

Click on *Chapter 11, Proofreading Pretest (11T-2)*, and follow the directions.

Finding your own errors and correcting them is not easy, but it is an essential skill for your success as a medical transcriptionist. The worksheets in this activity will help you to develop your proofreading skills.

TEXTBOOK USERS

Proofread and correct errors in the medical documents shown in *Activities 11-4* and *11-5*.

Refer to the answer key (Appendix E) for immediate feedback.

Manually complete the error analysis chart for each document.

SOFTWARE USERS

Click on *Chapter 11, Activity 11-4*, and follow the directions.

Follow the same process for *Chapter 11, Activity 11-5*.

ACTIVITY 11-4
Proofreading Worksheet

Directions: Proofread this medical document, which contains multiple errors. Use open punctuation and all other formatting guidelines established in this textbook.

current date

P.H. Waters, MD
FedDes Wellness Center
Family Practice Division, Suite 300
101 Wellness Way Drive
New York, NY 10036

RE: Robin Hatherode
Date of Birth: 12/19/53
Examination: LEFT WRIST ARITHROGRAM

Dear Dr. Waters

Scout films are unremarkable.

Following appropriate preparation of the skin a 22 gage needle was inserted into the radioavicular joint and 2 mL. of iodinated contast media was injected. Films were then obtained after minimal manipulation of the wrist. A additional group of films was obtained following further manipulation of the wrist. Contrast is present in the distal radioulnar joint indicating a tear of triangular fibrocartilage.

There is no evidence of contrast in the midcarpal joints to suggest the presence of a ligamentus tear. No additional findings of significence are seen.

IMPRESSION: Findings consistent with a tear of the triangular fibrocartilage.
Thank you for referring this patient to us.

Yours Truly,

Hounsfield T. Scanner, MD
hts: cd

ACTIVITY 11-5
Proofreading Worksheet

Directions: Proofread this medical document, which contains multiple errors. Use open punctuation and all other formatting guidelines established in this textbook.

current date
Ida Gundrum, MD
Railroad Station Health Center
321 Trainmaster Boulevard
Reading, PA 19604

RE: Tonya Guerrero
Date of Birth: 5/24/81
Examination: CT ADBOMEN AND PELVIS
Dear Dr. Gundrun

Computerized tomography was performed from the diafragm to the symphysis pubus with the use of oral and intravenous contast medium.

The liver and spleen are normal. I see no visible gallstones or pericholecystic fluid. There is no pancreatic mast or calcifications. The kidneys are both functional and inobstructed. There is no retropertoneal lymphadenpathy or pelvic lymphadenpathy. The uterus is mid line. There is some slight fullness in the right adnuxa. An ultrasound was performed on June 9 20xx that showed no adnuxal pathology. Asymetry is therefore probably due to the supine position of unopacified bowl over the adnexa. No other pelvic abnormality is seen.

IMPRESSION: Negative exam.

Thank you for refering this patient to us.

Yours Truly,

Hounsfield T. Scanner, MD

xx

Activities 11-6 and 11-7

Proofreading Transcription Exercises (11T-3 and 11T-4)

Now you are ready to make the transition from simply proofreading printed material to both transcribing and proofreading dictated material. This is the time to concentrate on building your medical vocabulary, which ultimately will improve your speed and accuracy.

WORD PROCESSING USERS

Open your word processing package.

Insert the appropriate audiocassette in your transcribing machine and find dictation *11T-3*.

Step 1: Listen to the entire dictation to gain an understanding of the medical concepts and terms involved in the report. Rewind the tape to the beginning of the dictation and transcribe what you hear. Do not worry about formatting, style, or speed. Simply type what you hear being dictated, using correct punctuation, capitalization, and spelling. Stop as needed to look up words you do not understand or cannot spell. Adjust the speed control of the transcriber to a comfortable level, starting slowly to ensure no dictated words are missed, and increase the speed as your accuracy improves.

Step 2: Rewind the tape and transcribe dictation *11T-3* again, including correct spacing and formatting. Proofread the report. Identify and correct all errors. Save your work on your student disk. Refer to the answer key, and manually complete the error analysis chart and the Production for Pay summary.

Follow the same process for dictation *11T-4*.

SOFTWARE USERS

Click on *Chapter 11, Activity 11-6 (11T-3), Step 1,* and follow the directions. When you feel comfortable with the dictation, click on *Chapter 11, Activity 11-6 (11T-3), Step 2,* and follow the directions.

Follow the same process for *Chapter 11, Activity 11-7 (11T-4), Step 1* and *Chapter 11, Activity 11-7 (11T-4), Step 2.*

Let's pause a minute and see how well you are doing. This section allows you to evaluate your success at transcribing and proofreading diagnostic imaging reports.

WORD PROCESSING USERS

Open your word processing package.

Insert the appropriate audiocassette in your transcribing machine and find dictation *11T-2*.

Transcribe and proofread dictation *11T-2*, using the formatting guidelines established in Chapter 2.

Identify and correct all errors.

Save your work on your student disk.

After completing the transcription, refer to the answer key.

Manually complete the error analysis chart.

Manually complete the Production for Pay summary.

SOFTWARE USERS

Click on *Chapter 11, Proofreading Check Your Progress (11T-2)*, and follow the directions.

Professional transcriptionists can transcribe and proofread their own work. Can you?

WORD PROCESSING USERS

Open your word processing package.

Insert the appropriate audiocassette in your transcribing machine and find dictation *11T-5*.

Transcribe and proofread dictation *11T-5*, using the formatting guidelines established in Chapter 2.

Identify and correct all errors.

Save your work on your student disk.

After completing the transcription, refer to the answer key.

Manually complete the error analysis chart.

Manually complete the Production for Pay summary.

Follow the same process for dictation *11T-6*.

SOFTWARE USERS

Click on *Chapter 11, Transcription Pretest (11T-5)*, and follow the directions.

Follow the same process for *Chapter 11, Transcription Pretest (11T-6)*.

TRANSCRIPTION

You have been hired as a transcriptionist at FedDes Wellness Center in the Diagnostic Imaging Division. Your supervisor has asked you to transcribe today's dictation.

WORD PROCESSING USERS

Open your word processing package.

Insert the appropriate audiocassette in your transcribing machine and find dictation *11T-7*.

Create or use your existing templates as necessary for the six types of reports (chart note, chart note using history and physical format, history and physical examination report, x-ray report, procedure report, consultation letter).

Transcribe and proofread dictation *11T-7*, using the formatting guidelines established in Chapter 2.

Identify and correct all errors.

Save your work on your student disk.

After completing the transcription, refer to the answer key.

Manually complete the error analysis chart.

Manually complete the Production for Pay summary.

Follow the same process for dictations *11T-8* through *11T-19*.

SOFTWARE USERS

Click on *Chapter 11, Transcription at FedDes Wellness Center, Dictation 11T-7*, and follow the directions.

Follow the same process for each of the remaining dictations (*11T-8* through *11T-19*).

Remember to follow the guidelines pertaining to capitalization, numbers, punctuation, abbreviations, measurements, symbols, and use of templates. This material is reviewed in Unit I. All documents are formatted as medical letters.

Radiologists often dictate in the present tense because they are interpreting the findings as they view the films. As a general rule, the history is past tense, and the findings are present tense.

11T-7

Right Breast Sonogram
Patient's Name: Stephanie D. Vaughn
Referring Physician: David Campella, MD
Physician: William C. Roentgen, MD

Transcription Tips

- The letter *x* is used to abbreviate the words *by* and *times* when it precedes a number or another abbreviation.

    You hear the dictator say: Eighteen by eight by twenty millimeters.
    You transcribe as: 18 x 8 x 20 mm.

- The expression *o'clock* is used to refer to points on a circular surface.

    You hear the dictator say: ten o'clock position.
    You transcribe as: 10 o'clock position.

- The hyphen is used to take the place of the word *to* or *through* to identify ranges.

    You hear the dictator say: breast projecting six to seven millimeters from the nipple.
    You transcribe as: breast projecting 6-7 mm from the nipple.

- A hyphen is used when two or more words are viewed as a single word: well-demarcated.

11T-8

IVP
Patient's Name: Helen MacBride
Referring Physician: J. Thomas Geiger, MD
Physician: William C. Roentgen, MD

Transcription Tips

- The plural form of the word calculus is *calculi*.
- Words beginning with *pre*, *re*, *post*, and *non* are generally not hyphenated: nonobstructing, postvoid, prevoid.
- The following studies are dictated in this report:

    Postvoid film: a film of the bladder area taken after the patient has emptied the bladder
    Prevoid film: a film of the bladder area taken before the patient has emptied the bladder

- Figures with capital letters are used to refer to the vertebral column and spinal nerves.

    You hear the dictator say: slight ureteral narrowing is noted at the L three level.
    You transcribe as: slight ureteral narrowing is noted at the L3 level.

- The following abbreviation is dictated in this report:
    IVP: intravenous pyelogram

11T-9

Video Esophagram and GI Series; Flat Plate of the Abdomen
Patient's Name: Elizabeth Nicholas
Referring Physician: Matthew D. Sponch, MD
Physician: William C. Roentgen, MD

Transcription Tips

- The following abbreviation is dictated in this report:
    GI: gastrointestinal
- A hyphen is used to join two or more words when used as an adjective that precedes a noun. The following word pairs are dictated in this report: stop-frame, pharyngeal-prevertebral.
- The following are new terms: nasopharynx, epiglottis, diverticulum, esophagogastric, mucosal.
- Quotation marks indicate a direct quote.

    You hear the dictator say: elderly patient who complains of food getting stuck in her throat when she eats and difficulty swallowing.
    You transcribe as: elderly patient who complains of food "getting stuck in her throat" when she eats and "difficulty swallowing."

TRANSCRIPTION

11T-10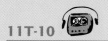

Bilateral Hands and Wrist
Patient's Name: Terresa Rosario
Referring Physician: J. Thomas Geiger, MD
Physician: Scott E. Film, MD
Copy to Leslie Albert, MD, Orchard Hills Rheumatology
  Associates

Transcription Tip

- Ordinal numbers are used to indicate order or position in a series rather than quantity. As with all numbers in medical reports, AAMT recommends using numerals (figures): 1st, 2nd, 3rd, etc.
  You hear the dictator say: degenerative changes at the first carpometacarpal joints bilaterally.
  You transcribe as: degenerative changes at the 1st carpometacarpal joints bilaterally.

11T-11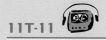

Bone Density Scan
Patient's Name: Cathy Evanson
Referring Physician: Matthew D. Sponch, MD
Physician: Scott E. Film, MD

Transcription Tips

- Hyphens are used between numbers and *year old*.
  You hear the dictator say: The patient is a seventy three year old postmenopausal white female.
  You transcribe as: The patient is a 73-year-old postmenopausal white female.
- Words beginning with *pre*, *re*, *post*, and *non* are generally not hyphenated: postmenopausal.
- A hyphen is used with words beginning with *ex* and *self*: self-history.
- The following drugs are dictated in this report:
  Synthroid: trade name for a drug used as a replacement in decreased or absent thyroid function; classification as a thyroid hormone
  Lescol: trade name for a drug that decreases low-density lipoprotein (LDL) cholesterol; classification as an antihyperlipoproteinemic
- The percent sign (%) is used with words and figures.
  You hear the dictator say: a total bone mineral density of ninety nine percent.
  You transcribe as: a total bone mineral density of 99%.

- The phrase "young normals" is dictated in this report, meaning normal readings in young subjects. Bone density is measured by several methods to determine bone mass loss. The bone mass loss is expressed as a percentage of the standard deviation, such as 99%.
  You hear the dictator say: a total bone mineral density of ninety nine percent compared to young normals which is zero point one three standard deviation below the mean.
  You transcribe as: a total bone mineral density of 99% compared to young normals, which is 0.13 standard deviation below the mean.
- The following standard deviations below the mean also are dictated in this report:
  Dictated: one point three two. Transcribed: 1.32.
  Dictated: two point one nine. Transcribed: 2.19.
  Dictated: one point zero to two point five. Transcribed: 1.0-2.5.
- Figures with capital letters are used to refer to the vertebral column and spinal nerves.
  You hear the dictator say: It is noted that L one and L two were eliminated from analysis.
  You transcribe this sentence as: It is noted that L1 and L2 were eliminated from analysis.

11T-12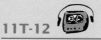

Pelvic Sonogram
Patient's Name: Nancy Spangler
Referring Physician: Ms. Pamela S. Barthonin, MA, RN, CRNP
Physician: Potter T. Bucky, MD

Transcription Tips

- The following diagnostic test is dictated in this report:
  Real-time ultrasound: rapid imaging system that produces a video display of organ motion
- The following abbreviation is dictated in this report:
  AP: anterior-posterior (anteroposterior)

11T-13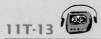

Bone Density Scan
Patient's Name: Eileen Bunny
Referring Physician: Charles P. Davis, MD
Physician: William C. Roentgen, MD

Transcription Tips

- A dangerous abbreviation is dictated within this transcript:

  You will hear the dictator say: 400-800 IU of vitamin D per day

  You should transcribe as: 400-800 international units of vitamin D per day

- Words beginning with *pre*, *re*, *post*, and *non* are generally not hyphenated: postmenopausal.

- A hyphen is used with words beginning with *ex* and *self*: self-history.

- Capitalize words that express the name of a particular people: Caucasian.

- The following drugs are dictated in this report:

  Estrace: trade name of an estrogen; classification as an antineoplastic

  Provera: trade name for a drug used in restoring hormonal balance; classification as a progestin, antineoplastic

- The percent sign (%) is used with words and figures.

  You hear the dictator say: a total bone mineral density of seventy one percent.

  You transcribe as: a total bone mineral density of 71%.

- The following standard deviations below the mean are dictated in this report.

  Dictated: two point seven nine. Transcribed: 2.79.

  Dictated: three point zero nine. Transcribed: 3.09.

- A hyphen is used to join two or more words when used as an adjective that precedes a noun. The following word pair is dictated in this report: follow-up.

- A hyphen is used to take the place of the word *to* or *through* to identify ranges.

  You hear the dictator say: placing the patient on one thousand to fifteen hundred milligrams of calcium and four hundred to eight hundred IU of vitamin D per day.

  You transcribe as: placing the patient on 1000-1500 mg of calcium and 400-800 international units of vitamin D per day.

11T-14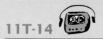

Abdominal Sonogram (Real-Time Imaging)
Patient's Name: Donald Nathan Helix
Referring Physician: Matthew D. Sponch, MD
Physician: Potter T. Bucky, MD

Transcription Tips

- A hyphen is used when two or more words are viewed as a single word: real-time.

- A hyphen is used between two "like" vowels: intra-abdominal.

11T-15

Mammography
Patient's Name: Laura Dobbins
Referring Physician: Charles P. Davis, MD
Physician: Potter T. Bucky, MD

Transcription Tips

- For mammography sonograms, the radiologists at FedDes Wellness Center include two paragraphs before closing sentence. These paragraphs should be transcribed in all capitals as shown.

  NOTE: IT SHOULD BE NOTED THAT THERE IS A 10% FALSE-NEGATIVE RATE IN MAMMOGRAPHIC DETECTION OF BREAST CARCINOMA. MANAGEMENT OF A PALPABLE ABNORMALITY SHOULD BE BASED ON CLINICAL GROUNDS.

  A NEGATIVE REPORT SHOULD NOT DELAY BIOPSY IF A CLINICALLY PALPABLE OR SUSPICIOUS MASS IS PRESENT.

- The mammography section at FedDes Wellness Center is accredited by the American College of Radiology. The statement below is included after the "false-negative" disclaimer and before the closing sentence:

  Our mammography facilities are accredited by the American College of Radiology.

11T-16

Upper GI Series
Patient's Name: Allison Lapinski
Referring Physician: Kate Cobalamin, MD
Physician: Hounsfield T. Scanner, MD

Transcription Tip

- A hyphen is used in the dictation to take the place of the words *to* or *through* to identify ranges.

  You hear the dictator say: After an interval of approximately twenty to twenty five minutes the stomach emptied in normal fashion.

  You should transcribe this sentence as follows: After an interval of approximately 20-25 minutes, the stomach emptied in normal fashion.

11T-17

Upper GI Series; Flat Plate of the Abdomen
Patient's Name: Timothy Lavage
Referring Physician: Anna Bolism, MD
Physician: Scott E. Film, MD

Transcription Tips

- The following abbreviation is dictated in this report:
    GI: gastrointestinal
- Ordinal numbers are used to indicate order or position in a series rather than quantity. As with all numbers in medical reports, AAMT recommends using numerals (figures).

    You hear the dictator say: The second third and fourth portions of the duodenum.

    You transcribe as: The 2nd, 3rd, and 4th portions of the duodenum.

11T-18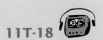

Barium Enema; KUB
Patient's Name: Barbara Whitefelter
Referring Physician: Gwenn Maltase, MD
Physician: Scott E. Film, MD

Transcription Tips

- Figures are used to express metric measurements. No period follows metric abbreviations unless the abbreviation ends a sentence.

    You hear the dictator say: two point three by zero point eight centimeters.

    You transcribe as: 2.3 x 0.8 cm.
- Words beginning with *pre*, *re*, *post*, and *non* are generally not hyphenated: postevacuation.
- The following abbreviation is dictated in this report:
    KUB: kidneys, ureters, bladder.

11T-19

Doppler Study of the Deep Veins of the Right Leg
Patient's Name: Sarah Fleb
Referring Physician: Charles P. Davis, MD
Physician: Scott E. Film, MD

Transcription Tips

- The following procedure is dictated in this report:
    Doppler scanning: technique used in sonography to image and analyze the behavior of a moving substance, such as blood flow or a beating heart
- A hyphen is used when two or more words are viewed as a single word: real-time, color-flow.

Professional transcriptionists can transcribe and proofread their own work with speed and accuracy. Have you mastered the diagnostic imaging transcription rotation at FedDes Wellness Center?

WORD PROCESSING USERS

Open your word processing package.

Insert the appropriate audiocassette in your transcribing machine and find dictation *11T-5*.

Transcribe and proofread dictation *11T-5* using the formatting guidelines established in Chapter 2.

Identify and correct all errors.

Save your work on your student disk.

After completing the transcription, refer to the answer key.

Manually complete the error analysis chart.

Manually complete the Production for Pay summary.

Follow the same process for dictation *11T-6*.

SOFTWARE USERS

Click on *Chapter 11, Transcription Check Your Progress (11T-5)*, and follow the directions.

Follow the same process for *Chapter 11, Transcription Check Your Progress (11T-6)*.

Muscular System

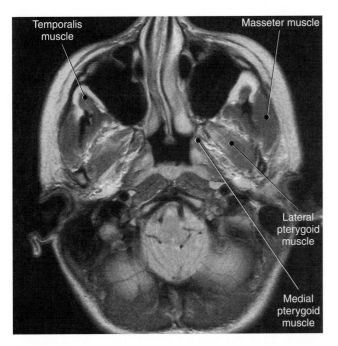

Figure 11-1 Axial magnetic resonance (MR) scan of neck with muscles of mastication. *(From Kelley LL, Petersen CM: Sectional anatomy for imaging professionals, St Louis, 1996, Mosby.)*

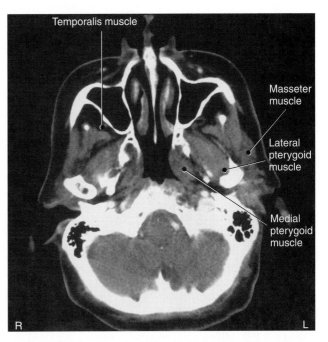

Figure 11-2 Axial computed tomography (CT) scan of neck with muscles of mastication. *(From Kelley LL, Petersen CM: Sectional anatomy for imaging professionals, St. Louis, 1996. Mosby).*

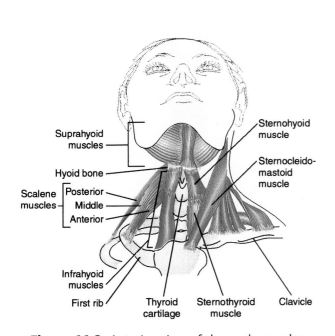

Figure 11-3 Anterior view of the neck muscles.

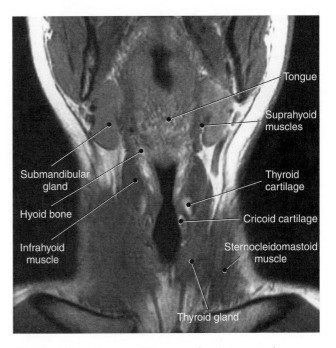

Figure 11-4 Coronal MR scan of anterior neck muscles. *(From Kelley LL, Petersen CM: Sectional anatomy for imaging professionals, St Louis, 1996, Mosby.)*

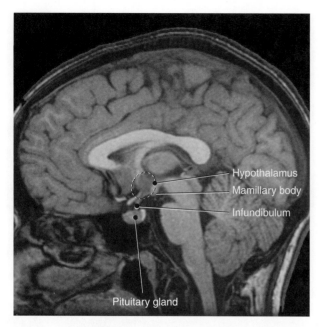

Figure 11-5 Midsagittal magnetic resonance (MR) scan of hypothalamus. *(From Kelley LL, Petersen CM: Sectional anatomy for imaging professionals, St Louis, 1996, Mosby.)*

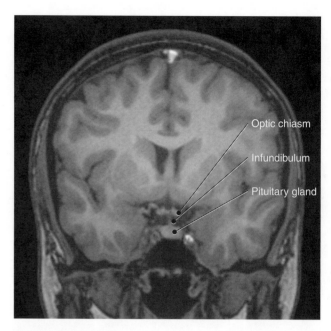

Figure 11-6 Coronal MR scan of pituitary gland and optic chiasm. *(From Kelley LL, Petersen CM: Sectional anatomy for imaging professionals, St Louis, 1996, Mosby.)*

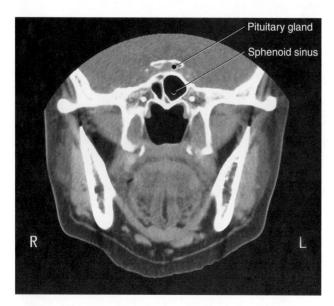

Figure 11-7 Coronal computed tomography (CT) scan of pituitary gland. *(From Kelley LL, Petersen CM: Sectional anatomy for imaging professionals, St Louis, 1996, Mosby.)*

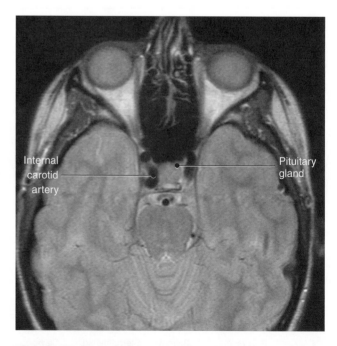

Figure 11-8 Axial MR scan of pituitary gland. *(From Kelley LL, Petersen CM: Sectional anatomy for imaging professionals, St Louis, 1996, Mosby.)*

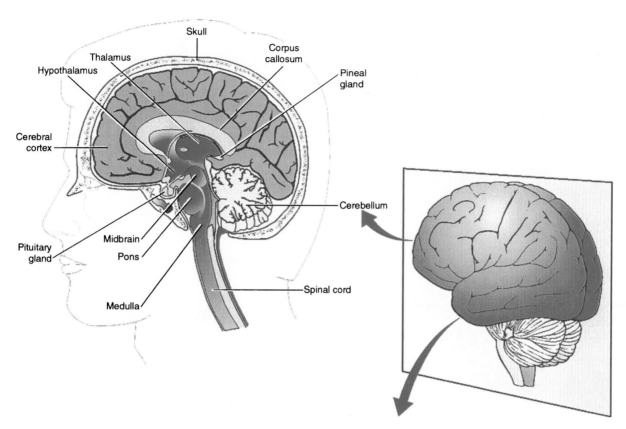

Figure 11-9a Sagittal section of brain and spinal cord.

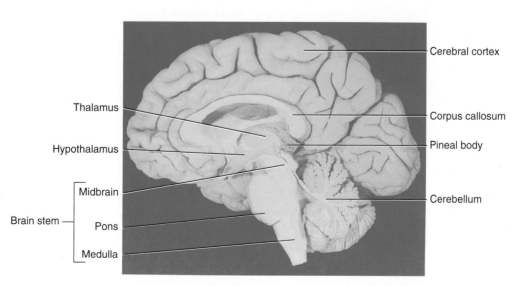

Figure 11-9b Cadaver section of brain. *(From Thibodeau GA, Patton KT:* The human body in health and disease, *ed 3, St Louis, 2002, Mosby.)*

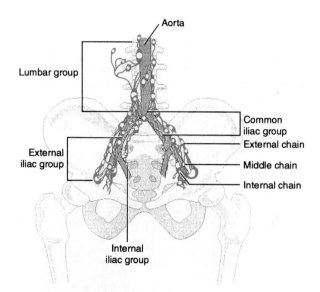

Figure 11-10 Iliopelvic-aortic lymphatic system (anterior projection).

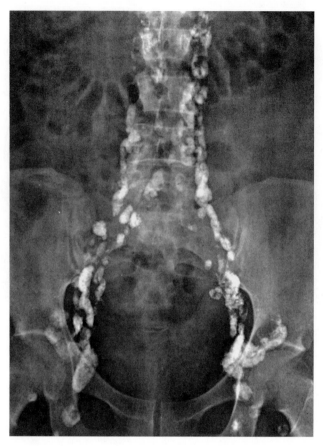

Figure 11-11 Anteroposterior (AP) x-ray view of iliopelvic-abdominoaortic lymph nodes. *(From Ballinger PW, Frank ED:* Merrill's atlas of radiographic positions and radiologic procedures, *ed 10, St Louis, 2003, Mosby.)*

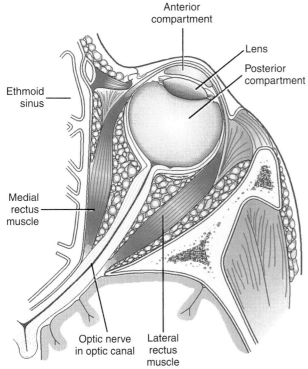

Figure labels: Anterior compartment, Lens, Posterior compartment, Ethmoid sinus, Medial rectus muscle, Optic nerve in optic canal, Lateral rectus muscle

Figure 11-12 Axial view of orbit.

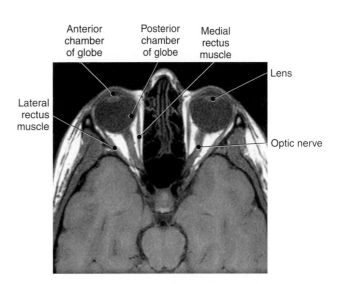

Figure labels: Anterior chamber of globe, Posterior chamber of globe, Medial rectus muscle, Lateral rectus muscle, Lens, Optic nerve

Figure 11-13 Axial magnetic resonance (MR) scan of orbit. *(From Kelley LL, Petersen CM: Sectional anatomy for imaging professionals, St Louis, 1996, Mosby.)*

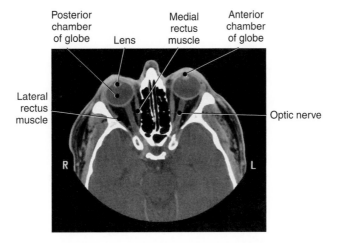

Figure labels: Posterior chamber of globe, Lens, Medial rectus muscle, Anterior chamber of globe, Lateral rectus muscle, Optic nerve, R, L

Figure 11-14 Axial computed tomography (CT) scan of orbit. *(From Kelley LL, Petersen CM: Sectional anatomy for imaging professionals, St Louis, 1996, Mosby.)*

Appendix A

Error Analysis Chart

The error analysis chart was developed as a tool to categorize and track undetected errors. A transcription error analysis chart for each document will help you and your instructor prescribe a remedy for each error. Observing the occurrence of repeated mistakes through charting will improve your transcription skills.

The chart is divided into two major categories, Medical Language and English Language, as shown below. The medical language errors have a higher "error value" than English language errors. Because medication and allergy errors and incorrect patient identification adversely affect patient care, medical transcriptionists are heavily penalized if such errors are found during quality assurance audits. Some institutions strip incentive pay no matter when the error is discovered—even if it is discovered weeks later. An error follows you!

NAME _____   DOCUMENT NO. _____

TYPE OF ERROR	ERROR VALUE	NUMBER OF ERRORS	TOTAL ERROR VALUE*
Medical Language			
Add/omit word(s)			
Misspelled word(s)			
Incorrect date(s) or number(s)			
Total Medical Language Errors	3 ×	=	
English Language			
Add/omit word(s)			
Misspelled word(s)			
Grammatical error(s)			
Punctuation error(s)			
Total English Language Errors	1 ×	=	
Total Language Errors			

*To compute total error value, multiply the number of errors by the error value (number of errors × error value = total error value).

Appendix B

Production for Pay Summary

In medical transcription, the transcriber's salary is often based on the amount of work produced rather than a regular monthly salary. The character is the preferred method of measuring productivity and has been supported by several national allied health organizations. A character is any letter, number, symbol, or function key necessary for the final appearance and content of a document, including the space bar, enter key, underscore, bold, and any character contained within a macro, header, or footer. Typically, the industry calculates five characters as one word.

The Production for Pay Summary demonstrates the way a transcriber's wage is determined for documents transcribed in this textbook. The summary includes the total number of words produced, total production time, and total number of errors to compute the net production pay. A $0.15 per minute per net production word rate is used to compute wages.

Document No.	
Total Word Count	
Total Production Time	
Words per Minute (Total Word Count ÷ Total Production Time)	
Total Error Value (Error Analysis Chart)	
Net Production (Words per Minute − Total Error Value)	
Production for Pay ($ 0.15 × Net Production)	

Figures C-1 through C-10 are cited and discussed in Chapter 2.

↕ **top margin 1″ (line 6)**

↔ **left margin 1″** CHART NOTE
      ↕ **double space**
Patient Name: Felter, Michael
Date of Birth: July 3, 1954
Examination Date: *current date*
      ↕ **double space**
SUBJECTIVE
Patient complains of right elbow pain for past 3 months. He has been playing tennis once a week over the summer with gradually worsening pain.
      ↕ **double space**
OBJECTIVE
Tenderness over right medial epicondyle. Pain radiates to the forearm and back of the hand with flexion and supination.
      ↕ **double space**
ASSESSMENT
Epicondylitis.
      ↕ **double space**
PLAN
Advised patient to stop playing tennis for 3 weeks and rest elbow until inflammation subsides. Prescribed Motrin 200 mg p.o. q.i.d. Urged the patient to wear an elastic strap for support when playing tennis in the future.
      ↕ **quadruple space**

Harry A. Medulla MD
Harry A. Medulla, MD
      ↕ **double space**
ham:cd
D: *current date*
T: *current date*

Figure C-1 Formatting a sample chart note using the SOAP note style.

↔ left margin 1″ CHART NOTE
↕ double space
Patient Name: Schaeffer, Carolyn
Date of Birth: April 18, 19xx
Examination Date: *current date*
↕ double space
CHIEF COMPLAINT
Chest pain.
↕ double space
HISTORY OF PRESENT ILLNESS
Carolyn is a 52-year-old white female who experienced chest pressure, palpitations, heart racing, numbness, and weakness in her right arm while at church services this morning. This episode lasted approximately 4 minutes. She also felt somewhat nauseated and clammy. Patient's cardiac risk factors include tobacco abuse, hyperlipidemia, and obesity. She is currently under therapy for hypothyroidism.
↕ double space
PAST MEDICAL HISTORY
1. Vaginal hysterectomy in 1975 for excessive bleeding.
2. Hyperlipidemia with triglycerides in the 350 range and cholesterol over 300. While taking Lopid, cholesterol fell to approximately 252 and triglycerides were 183.
3. Obesity.
4. Tobacco abuse.
5. Hypothyroidism.
↕ double space
PHYSICAL EXAMINATION
GENERAL: She is a very pleasant and cooperative patient in no acute distress.
HEENT: She is wearing corrective lenses. Sclerae anicteric. Tympanic membranes clear. Nose clear. Throat normal. She has a normal gag reflex. She has multiple filled caries.
NECK: Supple without thyromegaly or lymphadenopathy. Carotids 2+ bilaterally without bruits.
CHEST: Clear to auscultation anteriorly and posteriorly.
HEART: Regular rate and rhythm with a grade 1/6 systolic murmur heard best at the aortic region.
ABDOMEN: Mildly obese. Normoactive bowel sounds. Nontender, no organomegaly.
BREASTS/PELVIC/RECTAL: Deferred as these were done at the office 1 month ago and were normal.

continued

Figure C-2 Formatting a chart note using the history and physical style.

↔ left margin 1″   CHART NOTE
Patient's Name: Schaeffer, Carolyn
Date of Birth: April 18, 19xx
Page 2
↕ double space
EXTREMITIES: Without clubbing, cyanosis, or edema. Pulses 2+ in the upper and lower extremities.
NEUROLOGICAL: No focal neurologic deficits.
↕ double space
ASSESSMENT
1. Chest pain.
2. Hypothyroidism.
3. Obesity.
4. Tobacco abuse.
↕ double space
PLAN
1. Obtain serial ECGs and cardiac enzymes to rule out myocardial infarction.
2. Obtain stress thallium test.
3. Use nitroglycerin paste to the chest wall. Avoid any other cardiac medications unless there is an indication for them. Her symptoms are not clearly cardiac in nature.
↕ quadruple space

Adam Valence MD
Adam Valence, MD
↕ double space
av:cd
D: *current date*
T: *current date*

Figure C-2 *(cont'd)* Formatting a chart note using the history and physical style.

↔ left margin 1″ HISTORY AND PHYSICAL EXAMINATION REPORT

↕ double space

Patient Name: Rouf, Andrea
File Number: 2348901
Date of Birth: April 10, 19xx
Examination Date: *current date*
Physician: Gwenn Maltase, MD

↕ double space

HISTORY

↕ double space

CHIEF COMPLAINT
Abdominal pain, right lower quadrant for 3 days.

↕ double space

HISTORY OF PRESENT ILLNESS
The patient is a 27-year-old legal secretary, who first noted the onset of colicky lower abdominal pain situated slightly to the right of midline, below the umbilicus and above the pubic bone, 3 days ago. The pain has been getting worse and is associated for the past 36 hours with anorexia and nausea. She has vomited 4-5 times in the past 24 hours, mostly a bile-colored, watery liquid. The pain is not affected by positional change or ingestion of food. There is no radiation of pain. She denies fever, chills, hematemesis, or change in bowel habits.

↕ double space

PAST HISTORY
The patient had varicella at age 2 and the mumps at age 4. She had a tonsillectomy and adenoidectomy at age 11. There is no family history of diabetes.

↕ double space

REVIEW OF SYSTEMS

↕ double space

GENITOURINARY: Gravida 2, para 2, AB 0. No frequency, hematuria, or nocturia.

↕ double space

footer *continued*

Figure C-3 Formatting a sample history and physical examination report.

header   HISTORY AND PHYSICAL EXAMINATION REPORT
Patient Name: Rouf, Andrea
File Number: 2348901
Page 2

PHYSICAL EXAMINATION
GENERAL: The patient is alert, oriented and in moderate distress.
BP 120/80, pulse 106 and regular, temperature 37.2 C, respirations 14/min.
HEENT: Mild upper respiratory infection 2 weeks prior to present illness manifested by rhinitis and sore throat.
LUNGS: Clear to P&A.
HEART: Normal sinus rhythm, no cardiomegaly, no murmurs, gallops, or thrills.
ABDOMEN: Flat. Tenderness with muscle guarding in right lower quadrant. Rebound tenderness was present. Bowel sounds are normal. No organomegaly.
PELVIC: Bartholins, urethral, and Skene's gland normal. Adnexa normal. Uterus not enlarged.
EXTREMITIES: Within normal limits. No edema. Good range of motion.
NEUROLOGICAL: Grossly intact.
       ↕ double space
IMPRESSION
1. Acute appendicitis.
2. Rule out ureteral calculus.
       ↕ double space
PLAN
1. Refer to John Smithson, MD for surgical consult.
2. Patient to be admitted to General Hospital.
3. White blood count and IVP ordered upon admission.
       ↕ quadruple space

Gwenn Maltase MD
Gwenn Maltase MD
       ↕ double space
gm:cd
D: *current date*
T: *current date*

Figure C-3 *(cont'd)* Formatting a sample history and physical examination report.

↔ left margin 1″ X-RAY REPORT

↕ double space

Patient Name: Farley, Cassandra
File Number: 5690341
Date of Birth: February 1, 19xx
Examination Date: *current date*
Ordering Physician: Izzy Sertoli, MD

↕ double space

EXAMINATION
PA and Lateral Chest X-Ray.

↕ double space

HISTORY
This is a 57-year-old female with a history of lung cancer and increased shortness of breath for 1 week.

↕ double space

FINDINGS
CHEST: There is mild fibrotic change at both lung bases, over the left lung apex, and along the left chest wall laterally. There is some deformity to the left rib cage, apparently reflecting several old, healed rib fractures. There are some increased markings at the left lung base.

↕ double space

IMPRESSION
Early pneumonia, superimposed upon the underlying fibrotic changes. The heart size is normal.

↕ quadruple space

Adam Valence, MD
Adam Valence, MD

↕ double space

av:cd
D: *current date*
T: *current date*

Figure C-4 Formatting a sample x-ray report.

current date
↕ **quadruple space**

Charles P. Davis, MD
FedDes Wellness Center
Family Practice Division, Suite 300
101 Wellness Way Drive
New York, NY 10036
↕ **double space**
Re: Betty McWilliams
    Date of Birth: February 2, 1949
↕ **double space**
Dear Dr. Davis
↕ **double space**
Comparison is made to the prior mammogram dated January 25, 20xx. An 18 × 8 × 20 mm well-demarcated simple cyst is demonstrated within the central 12 o'clock position of the right breast corresponding to the well-demarcated density noted on mammography in this region. The cyst exhibits posterior wall enhancement and sound through transmission.
↕ **double space**
A second cyst measuring 6.1 × 7.1 × 4.4 mm is present in the approximate 10 o'clock position of the breast projecting 6-7 mm from the nipple corresponding to the density noted on mammography in this region.
↕ **double space**
No additional lesions are identified.
↕ **double space**
IMPRESSION: The two densities noted in the right breast on the recent mammogram correspond to simple cysts as described.
↕ **double space**
Thank you for the opportunity to participate in the care of this patient.
↕ **double space**
Sincerely yours
↕ **quadruple space**

Potter T. Bucky, MD
Potter T. Bucky, MD
↕ **double space**
xx

Figure C-5 Formatting a sample diagnostic imaging letter with typical letterhead style. Diagnostic imaging letters are usually typed on letterhead.

↔ left margin 1″   PROCEDURE REPORT
              ↕ double space
Patient Name: Shauback, Ann
File Number: 200-00-2000
Date of Birth: July 3, 1955
Examination Date: *current date*
Ordering Physician: Charles P. Davis, MD
              ↕ double space
PROCEDURE
Exercise Stress Test.
              ↕ double space
Baseline electrocardiogram, normal sinus rhythm, normal active
intervals, no baseline ST segment abnormalities.
              ↕ double space
The patient was exercised according to standard Bruce protocol,
exercised for 9 minutes, achieving 10 mets. Reached a maximum
heart rate of 186, which was 101% of predicted. Reached a peak blood
pressure of 140/110. There was no chest pain with exercise. There were
no arrhythmias observed.
              ↕ double space
IMPRESSION
1. Negative for ECG evidence for ischemia.
2. No chest pain with exercise.
3. No hypertensive response to exercise.
4. No arrhythmia with exercise.
5. Normal functional aerobic capacity.
              ↕ quadruple space

Potter T. Bucky, MD
Potter T. Bucky, MD
              ↕ double space
ptb:cd
D: *current date*
T: *current date*

Figure C-6 Formatting a sample procedure report.

↕ top margin 1″ (line 6)

↔ left margin 1″   OPERATIVE REPORT
↕ double space
Patient Name: Samuelson, Jack
File Number: 203798
Date of Birth: July 13, 1946
Operation Date: *current date*
↕ double space
PREOPERATIVE DIAGNOSIS
Microscopic hematuria.
↕ double space
POSTOPERATIVE DIAGNOSIS
Normal cystoscopy.
↕ double space
OPERATION
Cystoscopy.
↕ double space
PROCEDURE
The patient was placed in the supine position and draped in the usual
fashion. The penis was prepped with Betadine. A local anesthetic of
10 mL of 2% lidocaine jelly was injected into the urethra.
↕ double space
The flexible cystourethroscope was advanced through the urethra to the
level of the verumontanum. No strictures were noted within the urethra.
The prostate was not obstructed. Once entrance was obtained into the
bladder, the mucosa was examined in a circumferential fashion and
found normal. The orifices were normal. The scope was removed.
↕ double space
The patient tolerated the procedure well. There were no complications.
↕ double space
IMPRESSION
Normal examination.
↕ quadruple space

Theodore Trigone, MD
Theodore Trigone, MD
↕ double space
tt:cd
D: *current date*
T: *current date*

Figure C-7 Formatting a sample operative report.

↔ left margin 1″   CONSULTATION REPORT
↕ double space
Patient Name: McWilliams, Betty
File Number: 5678123
Date of Birth: February 2, 1949
Examination Date: *current date*
Requesting Physician: Charles P. Davis, MD
↕ double space
HISTORY OF PRESENT ILLNESS
Ms. McWilliams appears to be more stable with the supportive measures already instituted. The respiratory rate is still rapid, but her color is better. There are no signs of congestive heart failure.
↕ double space
IMPRESSION/RECOMMENDATIONS
Review of the clinical picture, chest x-ray, and lung scan point definitely toward a pulmonary embolus. I would recommend checking the blood gases, maintaining the oxygen and supportive measures, and starting her on anticoagulation with heparin. She should be maintained on the ECG monitor.
↕ double space
I feel she also has evidence of thrombophlebitis of the left leg and should be treated with elevation and soaks to this extremity. Thank you. I will follow.
↕ quadruple space

Adam Valence, MD
Adam Valence, MD
↕ double space
av:cd
D: *current date*
T: *current date*
↕ double space
c: June Smith, MD

Figure C-8 Formatting a sample consultation report (informal style with headings).

↔ left margin 1″   *current date*
↕ quadruple space

Charles P. Davis, MD
FedDes Wellness Center
Family Practice Division, Suite 300
101 Wellness Way Drive
New York, NY 10036
↕ double space
Re: Betty McWilliams
     Date of Birth: February 2, 1949
↕ double space
Dear Dr. Davis
↕ double space
Ms. McWilliams appears to be more stable with the supportive measures
already instituted. The respiratory rate is still rapid, but her color is better.
There are no signs of congestive heart failure.
↕ double space
Review of the clinical picture, chest x-ray, and lung scan point definitely
toward a pulmonary embolus. I would recommend checking the blood
gases, maintaining the oxygen and supportive measures, and starting
her on anticoagulation with heparin. She should be maintained on the
ECG monitor.
↕ double space
I feel she also has evidence of thrombophlebitis of the left leg and should
be treated with elevation and soaks to this extremity. Thank you. I will
follow.
↕ double space
Sincerely yours
↕ quadruple space

Adam Valence, MD
Adam Valence, MD
↕ double space
xx
↕ double space
c: June Smith, MD

Figure C-9 Formatting a sample business and consultation letter (formal style
without headings).

‡ top margin 2″

↔ left margin 1″   *current date*
                        ‡ quadruple space

Mr. James McCleary
Savory Supplied Inc.
467 Montgomery Street
New York, NY 10013
                ‡ double space
Re: Invoice No. 7231
                ‡ double space
Dear Mr. McCleary
                ‡ double space
Today I received the twenty boxes of latex gloves that I ordered last
week.
                ‡ double space
On your Invoice No. 7231, which I am enclosing, I notice that you have
charged me $12.50 per box for these gloves. This charge must be a
mistake. I have your price list, which gives the price as $10.50 per box.
                ‡ double space
Please send me a corrected invoice.
                ‡ double space
Sincerely yours
                ‡ quadruple space

Adam Valence, MD
Adam Valence, MD
                ‡ double space
xx
                ‡ double space
Enclosure

Figure C-10 Formatting a sample business letter.

FedDes Wellness Center Physician Directory

The FedDes Wellness Center is located at 101 Wellness Way Drive, New York, NY 10036. Providers on site include 24 physicians, a physical therapist, and a certified nurse practitioner.

Family Practice Division, Suite 300

Charles P. Davis, MD
J. Thomas Geiger, MD
Matthew D. Sponch, MD
Izzy Sertoli, MD
P. H. Waters, MD
Melissa A. Anconeus, MS, PT
Pamela S. Barthonin, MA, RN, CRNP

Orthopedic Division, Suite 133

David Treppe, MD
James P. Osseous, MD
Harry A. Medulla, MD

Urology Division, Suite 237

Helen Loop, MD
Theodore Trigone, MD
Benjamin Keytone, MD

Pulmonary Medicine Division, Suite 451

Allan Bolus, MD
Neal Alveoli, MD
Douglas Sputum, MD

Gastroenterology Division, Suite 279

Gwenn Maltase, MD
Kate Cobalamin, MD
Anna Bolism, MD

Cardiology Division, Suite 413

Erica Purkinje, MD
Lucas Site, MD
A. B. Doner, MD
Adam Valence, MD

Diagnostic Imaging Division, Suite 157

William C. Roentgen, MD
Hounsfield T. Scanner, MD
Potter T. Bucky, MD
Scott E. Film, MD

Formatting Guidelines

FedDes Wellness Center has its own format and guidelines for transcribing physicians' dictation. All the rules and guidelines presented in Chapters 2 and 3, as well as those described here and in Chapter 4, apply to the medical documents that are transcribed at FedDes Wellness Center. To research extensive technical questions, FedDes Wellness Center complies with *AAMT Book of Style for Medical Transcription*, 2nd edition.

1. All medical reports use the block style format with 1-inch margins. No tabulation appears in the document. Letters are formatted with a 2-inch first-page top margin and 1-inch second-page top margin.
2. Lowercase letters for both sets of initials, with a colon between them and no periods, are used for the dictator and transcriptionist initials placed at the end of a medical report.
3. All medical letters use open punctuation. No punctuation marks follow the salutation and complimentary closing.
4. The complete headings, sections/topics, and subheadings are always used. These are keyed in all capital letters.
5. The dictated words current date must be transcribed as the actual month, day, and year. The dictated words yesterday's date should be transcribed as the day before the actual date the document is transcribed.
6. Identifying statistical data must be included on medical reports.

Example
CHART NOTE
Patient Name: Felter, Michael
Date of Birth: July 3, 1954
Examination Date: *current date*

Example
HISTORY AND PHYSICAL EXAMINATION REPORT
Patient Name: Doe, Jane
File Number: 1235678
Date of Birth: January 3, 1950
Examination Date: *current date*
Physician: Charles P. Davis, MD

Example
X-RAY REPORT
Patient Name: Doe, Jane
File Number: 1235678
Date of Birth: January 3, 1950
Examination Date: *current date*
Ordering Physician: Izzy Sertoli, MD

Example
PROCEDURE REPORT
Patient Name: Doe, Jane
File Number: 1235678
Date of Birth: January 3, 1950
Examination Date: *current date*
Ordering Physician: Izzy Sertoli, MD

Example
CONSULTATION REPORT
Patient Name: Doe, Jane
File Number: 1235678
Date of Birth: January 3, 1950
Examination Date: *current date*
Requesting Physician: Izzy Sertoli, MD

7. All medical documents formatted as a letter should include a reference line above the salutation line.

Example
Re: Betty Williams
Date of Birth: February 2, 1949
Examination: RIGHT BREAST SONOGRAM
Dear Dr. Davis

8. When a medical report is longer than one page, the name of the report, patient's name, file number, and page number are keyed in the header pane on each printed page.

Example
HISTORY AND PHYSICAL EXAMINATION REPORT
Patient Name: Doe, Jane
File Number: 1235678
Page 2

9. For multiple-page letters, the header includes the patient's name, date, and page number beginning at the 1-inch top margin.

Example
Patient Name
Date
Page 2

10. When a medical report is longer than one page, the word "continued" is keyed in the footer pane on each printed page before the last page. A medical letter does not have a footer.

11. Do not carry a single line of a report or letter onto a continuation page.

12. Do not allow a continuation page to include only the signature block and the data following it.

13. The signature line includes the physician's or dictator's name and title entered four lines below the final line of text, flush left. The dictator and transcriptionist initials are placed at the end of each report. Enter the initials flush left and two lines below the physician's name. Use all lowercase letters for both sets of initials with a colon or diagonal between them, without the use of periods. The date of the dictation, indicated by the letter D, and date the document was transcribed, indicated by the letter T, are entered flush left below the initials of the dictator and transcriptionist.

Example
(4 lines)
Potter T. Bucky, MD
(2 lines)
ptb:cd
D: 11/20/xx (date the report was dictated)
T: 11/21/xx (date the report was transcribed)

14. Keep the numeral and unit of measure together at line breaks. This is important when transcribing a drug and its corresponding dosage.
Example: The specimen measured 3 cm in diameter. Erythromycin 250 mg t.i.d. was prescribed.

Usage Guidelines

1. When the age of the patient is mentioned within the body of the transcript, the patient's year of birth is not provided, and the student will need to calculate this date.

2. All dates are spelled out in medical documents regardless of where the date appears on a report or letter.
Example: The patient was seen in this office on Monday, January 12, 20xx.

3. A comma separates each vital sign.
Example: BP 108/72, pulse 78 and regular, respirations 20/min.

4. Drug allergies are typed in all capitals.
Example
ALLERGIES: TETRACYCLINE.

5. Drug dosages are expressed in Latin abbreviations and transcribed in lowercase letters with periods and no internal spaces.
Example: The patient was started on Keflex, 250 mg q.i.d.

6. Measurements of tumors are expressed in metric terms.
Example: The tumor measured 12 x 12 x 6 mm.

7. Place a zero before a decimal that lacks a whole number.
Example: The lesion measured 0.75 x 1 cm.

8. Mixed numbers are transcribed in figures (Arabic numerals).
Example: The 5½-year-old female was seen at 1 p.m.

9. Figures are used almost exclusively as opposed to spelled-out numbers to improve clarity and avoid potential mistakes. There are always exceptions, and judgment and discretion are needed when deciding whether to use numerals or to spell out numbers.
Examples
Mrs. Jones is widowed, but she resides with one of her three children.
Patient complains of right elbow pain for the past 3 weeks.
The patient smokes 2 packs per day and has done so for 24 years.

10. Figures are used in lists.
Example
IMPRESSION
1. Acute appendicitis.
2. Rule out ureteral calculus.

11. Figures are used to indicate the patient's weight, height, blood pressure (BP), pulse, and respiration. Figures are used to indicate patient's age, except at the beginning of a sentence.
Examples
This is the second admission for this 2-year-old.
Two-year-old patient was admitted for the second time.
Her physical findings are: Weight 25 pounds, height 21 inches, BP 142/72, pulse 117, respirations 20/min.

12. Figures and the number sign are used for suture materials.
Example: The subcutaneous tissues were closed with interrupted #3-0 plain catgut.

13. Figures are used for ranges and ratios.
Example: She has vomited 4-5 times in the past 24 hours, and the vomit is mostly a bile-colored, watery liquid.

14. Figures are used to refer to grade, phase, and pregnancy and delivery.
Examples
She was diagnosed with grade 3/6 holosystolic murmur.
The patient is gravida 1, para 1.

15. The plurals of single-digit numbers, letters, and symbols are formed by adding s.

16. The plurals of double-digit numbers and all-capital abbreviations are formed by adding the letter s.
Example: The patient's blood pressure has been relatively well controlled, with systolic pressures running 140-150s.

17. Roman numerals are generally used to express stages and clotting factors.
Example: She was diagnosed with stage IV decubitus ulcer.
Prothrombin time is a test to measure the activity of factors I, II, V, VII, and X, which participate in the extrinsic pathway of coagulation.

18. Roman numerals are used for standard leads and intercostal space positions.
Example: There is reciprocal depression in leads I and II.

19. Ordinal numbers are used to indicate order or position in a series rather than quantity. As with all numbers in medical reports, AAMT recommends using numerals (figures): 1st, 2nd, 3rd, etc.
Example: On the 3rd day, the baby's temperature was normal.

20. Do not use superscripts and subscripts when expressing electrocardiographic leads, vertebral columns, chemical compounds, and so on.
Examples
The leads are V1 through V6.
We used distilled H2O.

21. Do not use the degree symbol when expressing temperature. The word degree is included only if dictated. Fahrenheit or Celsius is included only if dictated, and is expressed as a capital letter, F or C.
Example: Her temperature was 98.6 F.

22. The letter x is used to abbreviate by and times when it precedes a number or another abbreviation.
Examples
The lesion on her leg is 1.5 x 1 cm.
The patient was prescribed Augmentin, 500 mg p.o. t.i.d. x 2 weeks.

23. A hyphen is used between numbers and year old.
Example: The patient was a 26-year-old female.

24. A hyphen is used between two "like" vowels.
Example: We will plan to see the patient in 3 weeks for re-evaluation.

25. A hyphen is used to take the place of the word to or through to identify ranges.
Example: The last time he vomited was 4-5 hours ago.

26. Hyphens are used to form compound adjectives.
Example: Although the stated age of this patient is 45, his speech is child-like.

27. A diagonal or virgule (/) is used to indicate the word per in laboratory values and respirations or the word over in blood pressure.
Example: BP 120/80, pulse 106 and regular, temperature 37.2 C, respirations 14/min.

28. The number or pound (#) symbol is used to abbreviate the word number when followed by a medical instrument or apparatus.
Example: The small piece of metal was removed with a #25-gauge needle.

29. Do not use an abbreviation for common non-metric units of measure to express weight, depth, distance, height, length, and width, except in tables.
Example: The patient was 5 feet 3 inches and weighed 105 pounds.

30. One space follows end-of-sentence punctuation.
Example: The patient is a 45-year-old computer programmer. He presents with a sinus headache.

31. One space follows commas, semicolons, and colons.
Examples
She denies associated fever, chills, or hematemesis.
Pupils are constricted and midline; they react to light.

32. Space once after a period that ends an abbreviation.
Example: Dr. Smith was called for the consultation.

33. No spaces are used after a period within an abbreviation.
Example: Her medication was ordered t.i.d. by her doctor.

34. No spaces are used before or after a hyphen, apostrophe, or diagonal.
Example: The patient was a well-developed, well-nourished 29-year-old in mild distress.

35. No spaces are used between symbol and referent.
Example: Her temperature was 98.6°.

FedDes Wellness Center Approved Abbreviation List

AB	abortion
ABG	arterial blood gas
ACTH	adrenocorticotropic hormone
A&D	ascending and descending
ADL	activities of daily living
AP	anteroposterior, apical pulse
A&P	auscultation and percussion
ARD	acute respiratory distress
ASAP	as soon as possible
ASCVD	atherosclerotic cardiovascular disease
AV	atrioventricular
BCC	basal cell carcinoma
BE	barium enema
BLE	both lower extremities
BLT	bilateral tubal ligation
BM	bowel movement
BP	blood pressure
BPH	benign prostatic hypertrophy
BS	blood sugar, bowel sounds
BUN	blood urea nitrogen
BUS	Bartholin, urethral, and Skene (glands)
CABG	coronary artery bypass graft surgery
CAD	coronary artery disease
CBC	complete blood count
CHF	congestive heart failure
CNS	central nervous system
COPD	chronic obstructive pulmonary disease
CPR	cardiopulmonary resuscitation
CR	cardiorespiratory
C&S	culture and sensitivity
CT	computed tomography
CVA	cerebrovascular accident
D&C	dilation and curettage
DJD	degenerative joint disease
DOE	dyspnea on exertion
DPT	diphtheria-pertussis-tetanus
DTR	deep tendon reflexes
DVT	deep vein thrombosis
EAC	external auditory canal
ECG	electrocardiogram
EGD	esophagogastroduodenoscopy
EKG	electrocardiogram
EOM	extraocular movements
EOMI	extraocular movements intact
ER	emergency room
ESR	erythrocyte sedimentation rate
FB	foreign body
FBS	fasting blood sugar
FUO	fever of unknown origin
GB	gallbladder
GI	gastrointestinal
GYN	gynecology/gynecologist
HCG	human chorionic gonadotropin
H&P	history and physical
HPI	history of present illness
I&D	incision and drainage
IM	intramuscular
INR	International Normalized Ratio
IV	intravenous
IVP	intravenous pyelogram
KUB	kidneys, ureters, bladder
L&A	light and accommodation
LLQ	left lower quadrant
LMP	last menstrual period
LUQ	left upper quadrant
MI	myocardial infarction
MM	mucous membrane
NKA	no known allergies
NOS	not otherwise specified
NPH	no previous history
NSAID	nonsteroidal anti-inflammatory drug
NSR	normal sinus rhythm

NTP	normal temperature and pressure	STD	sexually transmitted disease
OB-GYN	obstetrics and gynecology	T&A	tonsillectomy and adenoidectomy
PA	posteroanterior	TAB	therapeutic abortion
P&A	percussion and auscultation	TM	tympanic membrane
PERL	pupils equal and reactive to light	TPR	temperature, pulse, respirations
PERLA	pupils equal and reactive to light and accommodation	TUR	transurethral resection
		TURP	transurethral resection of the prostate
PERRLA	pupils equal, round, reactive to light and accommodation	UA	urinalysis
		URI	upper respiratory infection
PID	pelvic inflammatory disease	UTI	urinary tract infection
PIP	proximal interphalangeal	UV	ultraviolet
PSA	prostate-specific antigen	VPB	ventricular premature beat
RBC	red blood cell (count)	VS	vital signs
RLQ	right lower quadrant	V&T	volume and tension
ROM	range of motion	WBC	white blood cell (count)
RUQ	right upper quadrant	WF	white female
SGOT	serum glutamic-oxaloacetic transaminase	WM	white male
SOB	shortness of breath	WNL	within normal limits

Appendix E

Answer Key

CHAPTER 2 / PRETEST

1. F: Four parts
2. T
3. T
4. T
5. T
6. F: templates are frequently used
7. T
8. F: high-frequency
9. F: four paragraphs
10. T
11. T
12. T
13. F: initials to be avoided
14. T
15. T
16. F: sentence fragments
17. F: two sections
18. T
19. F: "Social history"
20. T
21. F: History of Present Illness
22. F: includes type of examination
23. F
24. F: two projections
25. T
26. d
27. b
28. c
29. c
30. b
31. a
32. b
33. c
34. d
35. b
36. d
37. d
38. c
39. d
40. c
41. a
42. b
43. a
44. a
45. d
46. c
47. a
48. a
49. a
50. b

CHAPTER 2 / ACTIVITY 2-1

1. T
2. T
3. T
4. F: "Neurological" topic
5. F: outpatient services
6. T
7. T
8. F: abbreviations/phrases are used
9. F: statistical data appear on all pages
10. T
11. T
12. T
13. F: can include many headings
14. T
15. T
16. F:Past Medical History
17. T
18. F: "History of present illness" topic
19. T
20. T
21. T
22. T
23. T
24. F: months spelled out
25. T
26. c
27. d
28. b
29. a
30. b
31. c
32. b
33. c
34. d
35. a

CHAPTER 2 / ACTIVITY 2-2

1. F: subjective
2. F: more than
3. T
4. T
5. T
6. T
7. F
8. T
9. F: high-frequency
10. T
11. F: not all the time
12. T
13. T
14. T
15. T
16. T
17. T
18. T
19. F
20. T
21. T
22. T
23. T
24. T
25. F: "Chest" topic
26. b
27. a
28. b
29. d
30. a
31. d
32. c
33. d
34. b
35. c

CHAPTER 2 / ACTIVITY 2-3

CHART NOTE

Patient Name: Felter, Michael
Date of Birth: July 3, 1954
Examination Date: *current date*

SUBJECTIVE
Patient complains of right elbow pain for past 3 months. He has been playing tennis once a week over the summer with gradually worsening pain.

OBJECTIVE
Tenderness over right medial epicondyle. Pain radiates to the forearm and back of the hand with flexion and supination.

ASSESSMENT
Epicondylitis.

PLAN
Advised patient to stop playing tennis for 3 weeks and rest elbow until inflammation subsides. Prescribed Motrin 200 mg p.o. q.i.d. Urged the patient to wear an elastic strap for support when playing tennis in the future.

_____

Harry A. Medulla, MD

ham:cd
D: *current date*
T: *current date*

HISTORY AND PHYSICAL EXAMINATION REPORT

Patient Name: Rouf, Andrea
File Number: 2348901
Date of Birth: April 10, 19xx
Examination Date: *current date*
Physician: Gwenn Maltase, MD

HISTORY

CHIEF COMPLAINT
Abdominal pain, right lower quadrant for 3 days.

HISTORY OF PRESENT ILLNESS
The patient is a 27-year-old legal secretary, who first noted the onset of colicky lower abdominal pain situated slightly to the right of midline, below the umbilicus and above the pubic bone, 3 days ago. The pain has been getting worse and is associated for the past 36 hours with anorexia and nausea. She has vomited 4-5 times in the past 24 hours, mostly a bile-colored, watery liquid. The pain is not affected by positional change or ingestion of food. There is no radiation of pain. She denies fever, chills, hematemesis, or change in bowel habits.

PAST HISTORY
The patient had varicella at age 2 and the mumps at age 4. She had a tonsillectomy and adenoidectomy at age 11. There is no family history of diabetes.

REVIEW OF SYSTEMS

GENITOURINARY
Gravida 2, para 2, AB 0. No frequency, hematuria, or nocturia.

PHYSICAL EXAMINATION
GENERAL: The patient is alert, oriented and in moderate distress. BP 120/80, pulse 106 and regular, temperature 37.2 C, respirations 14/min.
HEENT: Mild upper respiratory infection 2 weeks prior to present illness manifested by rhinitis and sore throat.
LUNGS: Clear to P&A.
HEART: Normal sinus rhythm, no cardiomegaly, no murmurs, gallops, or thrills.
ABDOMEN: Flat. Tenderness with muscle guarding in right lower quadrant. Rebound tenderness was present. Bowel sounds are normal. No organomegaly.
PELVIC: Bartholin's, urethral, and Skene's gland normal. Adnexa normal. Uterus not enlarged.
EXTREMITIES: Within normal limits. No edema. Good range of motion.
NEUROLOGICAL: Grossly intact.

continued

HISTORY AND PHYSICAL EXAMINATION REPORT
Patient Name: Rouf, Andrea
File Number: 2348901
Page 2

IMPRESSION
1. Acute appendicitis.
2. Rule out ureteral calculus.

PLAN
1. Refer to John Smithson, MD, for surgical consult.
2. Patient to be admitted to General Hospital.
3. WBC and IVP ordered upon admission.

_____

Gwenn Maltase, MD
gm:xx
D: *current date*
T: *current date*

current date

Charles P. Davis, MD
FedDes Wellness Center
Family Practice Division, Suite 300
101 Wellness Way Drive
New York, NY 10036

Re: Betty McWilliams
    Date of Birth: February 2, 1949

Dear Dr. Davis

Comparison is made to the prior mammogram dated January 25, 20xx. An 18 x 8 x 20 mm well-demarcated simple cyst is demonstrated within the central 12 o'clock position of the right breast, corresponding to the well-demarcated density noted on mammography in this region. The cyst exhibits posterior wall enhancement and sound through transmission.

A second cyst measuring 6.1 x 7.1 x 4.4 mm is present in the approximate 10 o'clock position of the breast projecting 6-7 mm from the nipple, corresponding to the density noted on mammography in this region.

No additional lesions are identified.

IMPRESSION: The two densities noted in the right breast on the recent mammogram correspond to simple cysts as described.

Thank you for the opportunity to participate in the care of this patient.

Sincerely yours

_____

Potter T. Bucky, MD

xx

CHAPTER 2 / CHECK YOUR PROGRESS

1. T	13. T	24. F: low	37. c
2. T	14. F: plan	levels	38. b
3. T	15. T	25. T	39. c
4. F	16. F: more	26. T	40. c
5. F: easy	negative	27. T	41. d
process	17. T	28. T	42. b
6. T	18. F: "Neck"	29. F	43. d
7. T	topic	30. T	44. d
8. T	19. F: above	31. T	45. b
9. T	20. F: below	32. T	46. c
10. F	21. T	33. T	47. b
11. T	22. T	34. b	48. a
12. F: narrow	23. T	35. c	49. b
margins		36. c	50. c

CHAPTER 3: PRETEST (3-1, 3-2, AND 3-3)

See Check Your Progress (3-1, 3-2, and 3-3).

Errors are indicated in **bold italic**. Margins are formatted at 1 inch.

CHART NOTE

Double space

Patient Name: Bernshaw, Sue
Date of ***Birth***: ***September 12, 1965***
Examination Date: ***Current date***

SUBJECTIVE
Removal of sutures placed 10 days ago.

OBJECTIVE
The wound on the lateral ***aspect*** of the left knee ***looks*** well healed. The #***5-0*** nylon sutures were removed without difficulty.

ASSESSMENT
Laceration of ***left*** knee, well healed.

PLAN
Advised applying vitamin ***E*** to the area.

Quadruple space

_____
Harry A. Medulla, MD

ham:xx
D: *current date*
T: *current date*

Errors are indicated in **bold italic**. Margins are formatted at 1 inch.

CHART NOTE

Double space

Patient Name: Gapolli, Rachi
Date of ***Birth***: ***February 3, 1969***
Examination Date: *current date*

SUBJECTIVE
Patient complains of sensitive ***pimple-like*** bump on right posterior ***shoulder*** area.

OBJECTIVE
A mole, approximately ***1 cm*** in diameter***,*** is visible. It is uniformly brown in color with ***no irregular*** borders. Patient denies pain or discharge***, although*** she does ***admit*** that the area ***has been*** quite sensitive for the ***past*** 3 days.

ASSESSMENT
Nevus.

PLAN
I am referring the patient to a dermatologist for ***its*** removal and biopsy.

Quadruple space

_____
Charles Davis, MD

cd:***xx***
D: *current date*
T: *current date*

Errors are indicated in **bold italic**. Margins are formatted at 1 inch.

CHART NOTE

Double space

Patient Name: Brodrick, Heather
Date of Birth: April 19, 1989
Examination Date: current date

SUBJECTIVE
Patient complains of ***warts*** on palm of ***right hand*** that ***are*** becoming ***bothersome***.

OBJECTIVE
Examination ***of both*** hands reveals a ***3 mm*** growth over the dorsum of the distal 4th and 5th ***metacarpals*** of the ***right*** hand.

ASSESSMENT
Verruca.

PLAN
(Start new line) The ***warts*** were ***frozen*** with liquid ***nitrogen*** without incident. Recheck in ***2-3*** weeks if problem not resolved.

_____
Charles ***Davis,*** MD

cd:xx
D: *current date*
T: *current date*

Errors are indicated in **bold italic**. Margins are formatted at 1 inch.

CHART NOTE

Double space

Patient Name: ***Wright, Nathan***
Date of Birth: ***November 30, 1983***
Examination Date: ***current date***

SUBJECTIVE
Patient presents with typical ***flu-like*** symptoms of fever, muscular aches and pains, shaking chills, headache, and weakness.

OBJECTIVE
Bilateral tympanic membranes are clear. ***Oropharynx*** is not ***injected***. ***No*** neck nodes detected. Chest is clear to ***percussion*** and auscultation. Temperature ***102.3 F.***

ASSESSMENT
Influenza.

PLAN
Symptomatic therapy. ***Acetaminophen p.r.n.*** for fever and pain. ***Recheck*** in ***5-12*** days if not improving.

_____
Charles Davis, MD

cd:xx
D: *current date*
T: *current date*

Errors are indicated in **bold italic**. Margins are formatted at 1 inch.

HISTORY AND PHYSICAL EXAMINATION REPORT

Patient Name: **Monahan, Esther**
File Number: 2348901
Date of Birth: September 10, 19xx
Examination Date: *current date*
Physician: Harry A. Medulla, MD

HISTORY

HISTORY OF PRESENT ILLNESS
This **88-year-old** lady was admitted to a nursing home with an **extensive cellulitis** involving the right side of the **abdomen** and the chest. She had been living at home with her daughter, but had become increasingly unable to eat. She developed **hyponatremia** and dehydration along with the cellulitis. The cause of the cellulitis was never clearly determined. It was felt ultimately to be **due** to cracks in the skin from her poor condition and then **an** infection starting. She received **6** days of **Ancef**, was put on **Keflex** for **follow-up.** There is some suggestion of possible alcohol use involved, and she did receive some thiamine.

PAST MEDICAL HISTORY
Otherwise fairly benign. Dr. Peebody had provided most of her care.

SOCIAL HISTORY
No pertinent data.

FAMILY HISTORY
As above.

REVIEW OF SYSTEMS
Left hip has bothered her from a hip fracture **12** years ago with **pinning**. Other medical problems include GI bleed, which occurred back in February. Decision was made by the daughter and the patient not to investigate further. She had been on **aspirin** at the time, and it was stopped. It sounds like it was a lower GI bleed rather than an upper at that time.

PHYSICAL EXAMINATION
GENERAL: Elderly woman who is a little **hard of hearing**. Her vision is poor. Vital signs are good.
HEENT: No jaundice. Mouth and **pharynx** are unremarkable.
NECK: Supple. Carotids are equal. No **JVD**.
LUNGS: Clear to **percussion** and auscultation.
HEART: Regular rhythm. No murmurs, no gallops.
BREASTS: Atrophic.
ABDOMEN: Soft **without** organomegaly. The right side of the abdomen and chest, particularly underneath the breast, is still a bit irritated and red, but clearly much better than had been previously described.
EXTREMITIES: Ankles show **3**+ edema up to the knee.

continued

HISTORY AND PHYSICAL EXAMINATION REPORT
Patient Name: Monahan, Esther
File Number: 2348901
Page 2

IMPRESSION
1. Resolving cellulitis of the right side of abdomen and chest. Continue antibiotics.
2. Ankle edema attributed to congestive heart failure. Prescribed **Lotensin**, 5 **mg** daily along with brief regimen of diuretics. Will monitor progress.
3. Right hip pain.
4. Questionable alcohol abuse versus dementia.

_____

Harry A. Medulla, MD

ham:xx
D: *current date*
T: *current date*

Errors are indicated in **bold italic**. Margins are formatted at 1 inch.

current date

Dr. Katherine Davis
Medical Practice Ltd.
312 Main Street
New York, **NY** 10010

Re: Kevin Schlitz
Date of Birth: October 29, 1936

Dear Dr. Davis

I had the opportunity to examine Mr. Schlitz in my office on *current date* in **regards to** his slow-healing ulceration of his right foot. The wound definitely looks improved from the last time I saw it. **He** has been doing a good job at not bearing weight upon his right foot.

At this point, I think it would be appropriate to place him in some extra-depth shoes or boots with **accommodative insoles** to help reduce pressure in the **forefoot** area. I am concerned that he has a very high potential for ulceration beneath the **3rd** metatarsal due to increased loading in this area.

I wrote a prescription and sent him to an orthotic specialist for new shoes and to have accommodative insoles constructed. I think the patient has an unrealistic outlook in regards to what type of insoles will be in his shoes. He is currently wearing a very rigid functional device. This is not the appropriate device to reduce pressure in the **forefoot** area. The prosthesis I am **recommending** should help cushion and distribute his weight evenly in the forefoot area as well as help maintain the rear foot in a better functioning position. Please feel free to contact me if you have any questions in regard to this matter.

Sincerely

_____

Harry A. Medulla, **MD**

xx

Errors are indicated in **bold italic**. Margins are formatted at 1 inch.

current date

Arthur Guttenberg, MD
5723 North Front Street
New York, **NY** 10010

Double space

Re: Martha Ultress
Date of **Birth: June 19, 1959**

Dear Dr. **Guttenberg**

Thank you for seeing **Martha** for her right rotator cuff tendinitis. She has **had** intermittent pain of the right shoulder during the past **2** months. Over the **past** few days**,** the pain has gotten very severe.

On examination**,** she could barely abduct past **30** degrees. **The x-ray** was notable for some calcific tendinitis. I injected the subacromial bursa with **steroids,** and obtained a rather dramatic improvement in her bursitis**,** only to have it return again **1 week** later. I started her on a **physical therapy** program and would appreciate **your** evaluation concerning the continuing care and treatment of this patient.

Very **truly yours**

_____

Harry A. Medulla, MD

xx

—————————————

CHAPTER 3 / CHECK YOUR PROGRESS 3-2

Errors are indicated in **bold italic**. Margins are formatted at 1 inch.

CHART NOTE

Patient Name: **Ramirez, Jose**
Date of Birth: May 23, 19xx
Examination Date: *current date*

HISTORY OF PRESENT ILLNESS
This **15-year-old** male is seen for a follow-up on his acne. He has been using **Clearasil Medicated Astringent** and **Oxy Wash** for about **2** months with no improvement. He is on no **oral** medications, denies any **allergies,** and is in good health.

PHYSICAL EXAMINATION
Today's exam **reveals** inflammatory **cystic** lesions along the jaw line and upper back. Some deep **cysts** are palpable on the chin and over the right shoulder area.

PLAN
He is to start E-Mycin **250 mg b.i.d.** and **10%** Benzac topically nightly after washing. He is to **continue** washing with **Oxy Wash x 3** a day as tolerated. He has been cautioned not to **pick** at the **lesions.** We discussed the need to keep **his** hands away from his face as much as possible and to stop leaning on his elbow with his chin in his hand. It is a bad habit that only promotes the spread of bacteria and should be **discontinued**. He will be seen again in **4-6** weeks.

Quadruple space

_____

Allan Pore, MD

ap:xx
D: *current date*
T: *current date*

—————————————

CHAPTER 3 / CHECK YOUR PROGRESS 3-3

Errors are indicated in **bold italic**. Margins are formatted at 1 inch.

CHART NOTE

Patient Name: Smithers, Linda
Date of Birth: August 13, 19xx
Examination Date: *current date*

CHIEF COMPLAINT
Itching and a rash.

SUBJECTIVE
The patient is a pleasant, **26-year-old** female who is **quite** cooperative and in no **acute** distress. She complains **of** a rash that began about 2 **weeks** ago. **She has** taken **Benadryl** at bedtime with no relief. Upon questioning, **she** admits to using a new, perfumed body lotion after her shower.

OBJECTIVE
Vital Signs: Temperature 98.6, **BP** 136/72, weight 165 **pounds**, height **5 feet 3 inches,** pulse 74, respirations **22/min.** Smooth, erythematous rash over neck extending over trunk and

back. On the upper extremities, she has **an** erythematous rash extending to her wrists.

ASSESSMENT
Contact **dermatitis,** secondary to allergy to perfume.

PLAN
1. **Discontinue** use of perfumed body lotion.
2. Wash all clothing and bed linen that were exposed to the perfumed lotion.
3. Take **Benadryl 25 mg q.6h.** x 3 days.

Quadruple Space

_____

Allan Pore, MD

ap:xx
D: *current date*
T: *current date*

—————————————

CHAPTER 4 / PRETEST

1. T	14. T	27. d	40. a
2. T	15. T	28. c	41. a
3. T	16. F	29. d	42. c
4. F	17. F	30. a	43. c and/or d
5. F	18. F	31. c	44. c
6. T	19. F	32. b	45. a
7. T	20. F	33. a	46. b
8. T	21. F	34. c	47. d
9. F	22. F	35. a	48. a
10. T	23. T	36. d	49. c
11. T	24. F	37. a	50. c
12. F	25. T	38. c	
13. T	26. a	39. d	

—————————————

CHAPTER 4 / ACTIVITY 4-1

1. a	10. d	19. d	28. b
2. d	11. d	20. c	29. c
3. d	12. a	21. d	30. a
4. d	13. d	22. a	31. b
5. a	14. d	23. b	32. c
6. d	15. a	24. a	33. d
7. b	16. c	25. b	34. a
8. a	17. c	26. c	35. c
9. c	18. a	27. a	

—————————————

CHAPTER 4 / ACTIVITY 4-2

1. d	10. d	19. b	28. b
2. d	11. d	20. a	29. d
3. b	12. a	21. c	30. a
4. d	13. c	22. b	31. c
5. a	14. d	23. a	32. b
6. d	15. a	24. a	33. a
7. b	16. c	25. d	34. a
8. a	17. a	26. a	35. d
9. c	18. b	27. c	

1. F	14. F	27. a	40. a
2. T	15. T	28. a	41. c
3. T	16. T	29. a	42. a
4. T	17. F	30. c	43. c
5. T	18. T	31. d	44. a
6. T	19. F	32. a	45. b
7. T	20. F	33. c	46. a
8. F	21. T	34. a	47. c
9. F	22. F	35. a	48. a
10. F	23. T	36. c	49. d
11. T	24. T	37. a	50. b
12. T	25. F	38. d	
13. T	26. d	39. a	

CHAPTER 5 / TERMINOLOGY PRETEST

1. a	24. c	47. d	70. a
2. c	25. a	48. a	71. a
3. a	26. b	49. c	72. c
4. b	27. c	50. b	73. b
5. d	28. a	51. a	74. c
6. c	29. a	52. c	75. b
7. a	30. c	53. b	76. a
8. b	31. c	54. a	77. b
9. c	32. b	55. a	78. b
10. d	33. a	56. c	79. c
11. a	34. a	57. c	80. c
12. a	35. d	58. a	81. d
13. b	36. c	59. b	82. b
14. c	37. a	60. b	83. a
15. a	38. a	61. c	84. c
16. b	39. c	62. a	85. d
17. c	40. c	63. b	86. b
18. a	41. a	64. c	87. c
19. d	42. a	65. d	88. a
20. b	43. a	66. c	89. a
21. b	44. b	67. a	90. a
22. d	45. a	68. c	
23. c	46. b	69. d	

CHAPTER 5 / ACTIVITY 5-3 (5T–1)

1. Adenoma is a benign tumor in which cells are derived from glandular epithelium.
   The patient had an adenomatous polyp.
2. Adenopathy is the enlargement of the glands, especially the lymph nodes.
   She has no cervical adenopathy.
3. Adnexa are the tissues or body parts that are near or next to one another.
   The adnexa are without masses or tenderness.
4. Aeration is the exchange of carbon dioxide for oxygen by the blood in the lungs.
   The lungs are clear to aeration.
5. Amenorrhea is the absence of the menses.
   She is 12 weeks amenorrheic with complaints of vaginal spotting.
6. Auscultation is the act of listening for sounds produced within the body with the unaided ear or with a stethoscope.
   The chest is clear to auscultation.
7. Bimanual is the use of both hands.
   Bimanual palpation was ineffective.
8. Blepharospasm is a spasm of the orbicular muscle of the eyelid.
   Renee has a history of blepharospasm.
9. Bleb is a bulla or blister.
   Using sterile procedure and raising a small bleb of lidocaine, a #22-gauge needle was introduced.
10. Bruit is a sound or murmur heard on auscultation.

No abdominal bruits were heard.
11. Buccal pertains to the cheek.
    Buccal mucosa is moist.
12. *Chlamydia* is a widespread genus of gram-negative, nonmotile bacteria.
    DNA probe for *Chlamydia* was obtained.
13. Cyanosis is the bluish discoloration of the skin and mucous membranes due to excessive concentration of reduced hemoglobin in the blood.
    The patient's extremities were without clubbing, cyanosis, or pedal edema.
14. Decubitus is the state of lying down.
    The patient was placed in the left lateral decubitus position, and a digital rectal exam was performed.
15. Distal is the farthest from any point of reference; remote.
    Distal pulses are intact.
16. Doxycycline is a generic name for a broad-spectrum antibiotic that is active against a wide range of gram-positive and gram-negative organisms.
    I will begin treatment with doxycycline.
17. Dysmenorrhea is painful menstruation.
    She presents with a 1-year history of dysmenorrhea that has worsened over the past 3 months.
18. Dyspnea is labored or difficult breathing.
    No chest pain, leg cramps, or exertional dyspnea was noted.
19. Dysuria is painful or difficult urination.
    She denies any dysuria.
20. Edema is the accumulation of excess fluid in the tissues of the body.
    Extremities show no edema.
21. Effusion is the escape of fluid from blood vessels because of rupture or seepage, usually into a body cavity.
    There is no evidence of effusion.
22. Erythema is redness of the skin.
    We are concerned about the erythema and associated warmth that is occurring after only minimal amounts of time on her feet.
23. Evert is to turn inside out.
    The eyelid was everted and examined.
24. Exacerbation is the increase in the severity of a disease or its symptoms.
    Mr. Franklin has had further exacerbation of multiple sclerosis.
25. Exudate is an accumulation of fluid in the tissues.
    The pharynx appears injected with some possible left anterior tonsillar exudates.
26. Flank is the side of the body between the ribs and ilium.
    The patient had no organomegaly or flank discomfort.
27. Fundus is the bottom or base of an organ.
    Fundi of the eyes were benign.
28. Gallop is an abnormal rhythm of the heart.
    The cardiac exam revealed heart regular in rate and rhythm without murmurs, rubs, or gallops appreciated.
29. Ganglion is a knot or knotlike mass.
    She has a history of a previous carpal tunnel release and ganglion cyst excision.
30. Granuloma is a small nodule, tumor, or growth.
    Calcified granuloma is noted in the right lung, laterally.
31. Guarding is a body defense method to prevent movement of an injured part.
    Normal bowel sounds with no masses or guarding.
32. Hemoptysis is the coughing and spitting of blood.
    No cough, hemoptysis, or SOB was noted.
33. Hepatosplenomegaly is the enlargement of the liver and spleen.
    No hepatosplenomegaly or masses were noted.
34. Hyperlipidemia is the elevated concentration of any or all lipids in the plasma.
    Her history is also notable for hyperlipidemia.
35. Labyrinthitis is the inflammation of the internal ear, otitis interna.
    The patient was assessed with probable acute labyrinthitis.
36. Lamina is a thin, flat layer.
    Mild lamina propria edema was noted of the mucosa.
37. Laparoscope is an endoscope for examining the peritoneal cavity.
    In 1988 she underwent a laparoscopy at Community Hospital that showed pelvic adhesions.
38. Lingula is a small, tongue-shaped anatomic structure.
    There is a questionable early lingular infiltrate on the left.

39. Meclizine is a generic name for an antiemetic especially effective for control of nausea and vomiting for motion sickness.
The patient will be treated with 25 mg of meclizine p.r.n.

40. Mucosa is the mucous membrane.
Nasal mucosa is clear.

41. Myalgia is muscular pain.
This 32-year-old white male presents with sore throat, nonproductive cough, nasal congestion, and myalgia for the past 4 days.

42. Myringotomy is an incision of the tympanic membrane.
She has had a myringotomy as a child.

43. Nystagmus is an involuntary rapid rhythmic movement of the eyeball.
No nystagmus was noted.

44. Orthopnea is the ability to breathe easily only in an upright position.
No chest pain, edema, orthopnea, leg cramps, or exertional dyspnea was noted.

45. Os is an opening, mouth, or bone.
Examination reveals a small amount of blood from the cervical os.

46. Palpitation is an unusually rapid, strong, or irregular heartbeat.
No chest pain, edema, palpitations, orthopnea, leg cramps, or exertional dyspnea was noted.

47. Penicillin is a generic name for any of a large group of natural or semisynthetic antibacterial antibiotics.
He is allergic to PENICILLIN.

48. Perirectal is around the rectum.
Her perirectal area appeared normal.

49. Polypoid resembles a polyp.
A small polypoid lesion was identified in the sigmoid colon.

50. Pruritus ani is the intense chronic itching in the anal region.
I am referring Ms. Biscuit to you for pruritus ani.

51. Rebound is a reversed response occurring upon withdrawal of a stimulus.
The abdomen was soft, nontender, without guarding or rebound.

52. Rhinitis is the inflammation of the mucous membrane of the nose.
Renee has a history of seasonal allergic rhinitis.

53. Rhonchus is an abnormal sound heard on chest auscultation due to an obstructed airway.
The lungs are clear to aeration, but positive to transient rhonchi in the mid and upper lung fields.

54. Sigmoidoscopy is the examination of the interior of the sigmoid colon.
Ms. Biscuit has had persistent rectal itching and was advised to have a sigmoidoscopy.

55. Sputum is the mucous secretion from the lungs, bronchi, and trachea that is ejected through the mouth.
No cough, sputum production, hemoptysis, or SOB was noted.

56. Sulfacetamide is a generic name for an ophthalmic antibiotic.
Two drops of sulfacetamide were placed in the eye.

57. Terpin is used as an expectorant.
We will treat the patient with terpin hydrate with codeine, 1-2 tsp at bedtime.

58. Thyromegaly is an enlargement of the thyroid gland.
There is no thyromegaly or mass.

59. Uvula is a small soft structure hanging from the free edge of the soft palate.
Tongue and uvula are midline.

60. Vulva is the external genital organs in the female.
She also had noticed some itching in the vulvar area.

61. Amoxil is the trade name for a preparation of amoxicillin, an antibiotic.
The patient was placed on Amoxil 500 mg p.o. t.i.d. x 10 days.

62. Augmentin is the trade name for a preparation of amoxicillin, an antibiotic.
The patient was placed on Augmentin 500 mg p.o. t.i.d. x 2 weeks.

63. Biaxin is the trade name for an antibiotic.
He was treated with Biaxin 500 mg b.i.d.

64. Botox is the trade name for a powder for extraocular muscle injection.
Renee has a history of blepharospasm, for which she receives Botox injections, as well as seasonal allergic rhinitis.

65. Claritin is the trade name for a nonsedating antihistamine.
Claritin is controlling her allergy symptoms.

66. Copolymer is the trade name for one of the immune-modulating drugs.
The disease has progressed to the point that it would be beneficial to place him on Copolymer.

67. Cytotec is the trade name for a drug used for the prevention of NSAID-induced gastric ulcers.
I have placed him on Cytotec 100 mg q.i.d.

68. Darvocet is the trade name for a fixed combination preparation of analgesic and an antipyretic.
The patient occasionally used Darvocet for pain.

69. Ditropan is the trade name for a urinary antispasmodic.
She states the Ditropan has worked wonders for her bladder.

70. E.E.S. is the trade name for an antibiotic.
We will treat the patient with E.E.S. 400 mg 1 q.i.d. and terpin hydrate with codeine 1-2 teaspoons at bedtime only.

71. Evista is the trade name for a selective estrogen receptor modulator (SERM) for the prevention of postmenopausal osteoporosis.
Her current medications include Evista 60 mg p.o. daily.

72. Indocin is the trade name for a nonsteroidal anti-inflammatory drug (NSAID).
I have placed him on Indocin 50 mg p.o. t.i.d.

73. Klonopin is the trade name for an anticonvulsant.
She attributes her improvement, in part, to her B-12 injections, and Klonopin.

74. Lipitor is the trade name for an antihyperlipidemic that reduces cholesterol synthesis.
She is also taking Lipitor 10 mg p.o. nightly.

75. Lo-Ovral is the trade name for an oral contraceptive.
She was on the Lo-Ovral for about 2 weeks but continued to have bleeding.

76. Melatonex is the trade name for a sleep aid.
Melatonex did not help her sleep; in fact, it made her insomnia worse.

77. Naprosyn is the trade name for a nonsteroidal anti-inflammatory drug (NSAID).
I have discontinued his Naprosyn and placed him on Indocin 50 mg p.o. t.i.d., which is in addition to his Cytotec 100 mg q.i.d.

78. Neosporin is the trade name for a topical antibiotic.
She is intolerant to NEOSPORIN.

79. Norvasc is the trade name for a calcium channel blocker, antihypertensive.
I am increasing the Norvasc to 5 mg b.i.d.

80. Ophthetic is the trade name for proparacaine hydrochloride; eye drops.
The eye was instilled with some Ophthetic eye drops.

81. Ortho Tri-Cyclen is the trade name for a triphasic oral contraceptive.
Milly has a 2-month history of persistent bleeding out of cycle while taking Ortho Tri-Cyclen.

82. Paxil is the trade name for an antidepressant.
She attributes her improvement, in part, to her B-12 injections, and the Paxil and Klonopin medications.

83. Persantine is the trade name for an antiplatelet agent.
He is allergic to PENICILLIN and PERSANTINE.

84. Phenergan is the trade name for an antihistamine, antiemetic.
He was given a prescription for Phenergan 25 mg p.o. b.i.d.

85. Prilosec is the trade name for a gastric acid secretion inhibitor.
He was treated with Prilosec 20 mg b.i.d.

86. Proctocream HC is the trade name for a topical corticosteroidal anti-inflammatory used as anorectal cream.
Ms. Biscuit had tried Proctocream HC several months prior to this appointment with no improvement noted.

87. Skelaxin is the trade name for a skeletal muscle relaxant.
I have prescribed Skelaxin 400 mg t.i.d. p.r.n.

88. Triamcinolone is a generic name for a corticosteroid.
She did have a vulvar dermatitis, which responded well to treatment with triamcinolone.

89. Vancenase is the trade name for a corticosteroid for bronchial asthma; pocket inhaler.
The patient was prescribed Vancenase AQ inhaler 1 puff each nostril t.i.d.

90. Xylocaine is the trade name for a preparation of lidocaine and is classified as an antiarrhythmic, anesthetic.
There is marked trigger point tenderness in the left rhomboid area, which had been treated with a 1% Xylocaine injection.

1. a	24. d	47. b	70. a
2. b	25. b	48. c	71. a
3. a	26. c	49. b	72. a
4. d	27. c	50. a	73. c
5. c	28. a	51. c	74. b
6. c	29. d	52. a	75. b
7. b	30. c	53. a	76. b
8. c	31. a	54. a	77. b
9. a	32. a	55. c	78. c
10. a	33. a	56. b	79. c
11. a	34. d	57. a	80. a
12. b	35. b	58. b	81. d
13. d	36. a	59. c	82. b
14. a	37. a	60. b	83. a
15. b	38. c	61. a	84. c
16. c	39. c	62. b	85. c
17. c	40. c	63. c	86. d
18. d	41. a	64. d	87. b
19. a	42. a	65. c	88. c
20. b	43. c	66. c	89. a
21. a	44. a	67. c	90. a
22. c	45. b	68. d	
23. b	46. d	69. a	

CHAPTER 5 / ACTIVITY 5–4

Errors are indicated in **bold italic**. Margins are formatted at 1 inch.

CHART NOTE

Patient Name: Harris, Donna
Date of Birth: **October 21, 1950**
Examination Date: *current date*

SUBJECTIVE
Donna comes in today for **a** follow-up**.** Her weight **has,** fortunately, stayed the same. She still feels weak. Her blood **work** looks good. X-ray demonstrates prominent markings in the **right** middle lobe and a questionable nodular density in the **right** apex. Her appetite remains about the same. Her living situation is unchanged**;** and**,** despite our best efforts**,** we have really not been able to help her significantly with this.

OBJECTIVE
Weight 92 **pounds,** BP 120/68. She has no cervical **adenopathy.** Lungs show decreased **breath** sounds. Cardiac exam **regular in rate and rhythm** without murmurs, rubs, or gallops appreciated. She has normal chest **wall** excursion. Abdomen is soft. She has some tenderness in the right rib cage.

ASSESSMENT
1. Chronic obstructive pulmonary disease.
2. Weight loss which at this point has stabilized.

PLAN
I am planning to check apical lordotic views of this abnormality in her lung and have them compared with previous films. I will continue to follow her weight loss. I doubt that she has lung cancer**;** but**,** just to make sure, I will **re-evaluate the** right upper lobe a little better. At this point**,** I plan to follow her rib pain as well. I really **was not** able to elicit much information today.

Charles P. Davis, MD

cpd:xx
D: *current date*
T: *current date*

CHAPTER 5 / ACTIVITY 5–5

Errors are indicated in **bold italic**. Margins are formatted at 1 inch.

Current date

J. Thomas Geiger, MD
Family Practice Division, Suite 300
101 Wellness Way Drive
New York, NY 10036

Double space
Re: Charlotte Mekola
Date of Birth: **October 19, 1958**
Examination: CHEST.

Dear Dr. Geiger

There is a substantial area of **alveolar** infiltrate that involves the superior segment of the right lower lobe. I do not identify a mass or any definite hilar **adenopathy**. The lungs are otherwise clear. There is probably an element of **COPD**. The heart is mildly **enlarged,** but the pulmonary vessels do not appear prominent. There is no **effusion**. The visualized bony thorax and soft tissues are remarkable for an accentuated kyphosis and probable osteoporosis.

IMPRESSION: Alveolar infiltrate in the superior segment of the **right** lower lobe. Simple pneumonia is the most likely diagnosis. A follow-up until clearing is **recommended**.

Thank you for **referring** this patient to us.

Yours **truly**

Potter T. Bucky, MD

xx

CHAPTER 6 / TERMINOLOGY PRETEST

1. a	21. d	41. c	61. b
2. b	22. a	42. a	62. a
3. c	23. c	43. d	63. d
4. d	24. a	44. b	64. a
5. d	25. c	45. a	65. d
6. a	26. a	46. a	66. b
7. a	27. b	47. d	67. b
8. d	28. a	48. b	68. c
9. b	29. a	49. b	69. b
10. c	30. c	50. c	70. a
11. a	31. c	51. b	71. a
12. c	32. d	52. a	72. b
13. a	33. b	53. d	73. b
14. d	34. a	54. d	74. c
15. a	35. c	55. b	75. a
16. a	36. b	56. a	76. b
17. c	37. a	57. a	77. c
18. c	38. c	58. c	78. d
19. b	39. c	59. a	
20. a	40. c	60. d	

1. Abduction is the movement of an extremity away from midline.
   Her strength is mildly diminished in external rotation, good in internal and abduction.
2. Acromion is a spinous projection off the scapula.
   A magnetic resonance imaging scan showed acromial spur, but no sign of a rotator cuff tear.
3. Adduction is the movement of an extremity toward the midline.
   She has pain with cross-chest adduction.
4. Apophysis is any outgrowth or swelling; a process or projection of a bone.
   X-rays show a fracture at the apophysis of the proximal 5th metatarsal that is displaced somewhat.
5. Arthroplasty is the reconstruction surgery to repair or reshape a diseased joint.
   As you know, she underwent hip arthroplasty in 1995 with an excellent result.
6. Arthroscopy is the examination of the interior of a joint with an arthroscope.
   We are going to proceed with arthroscopic subacromial decompression.
7. Aspirate is to draw in or out by suction.
   Her right knee was aspirated, and cortisone was injected today.
8. Asymptomatic is without symptoms.
   At this point, she is asymptomatic.
9. Avulsion is the tearing away forcibly of a part or structure.
   He is a 39-year-old, right hand-dominant male who injured his left 3rd finger yesterday at work and had an avulsion of the tip.
10. Bilateral means affecting or relating to two sides.
    She has well-healed carpal tunnel incisions bilaterally.
11. Calcaneus is the heel bone or os calcis.
    There are moderately sized posterior and plantar calcaneal spurs.
12. Callus is the new growth of bony tissue surrounding the bone ends in a fracture; part of the repair process of a fractured bone.
    X-ray examination shows no remarkable change in the position of the fragments, but I also do not see any remarkable callus formation yet.
13. Codeine is the generic name for an opioid analgesic.
    The patient is allergic TO CODEINE.
14. Contusion is commonly called a *bruise*, where there is trauma to the body part but there is no break in the skin surface.
    There is some increased signal in the rotator cuff, but I think this is more contusion.
15. Cortisone is the generic name for a corticosteroid used to treat inflammations.
    The patient received a cortisone injection to relieve the inflammation.
16. Crepitus is the grating sound of bone fragments rubbing together.
    He has had about a 3-month history of pain and crepitus around the shoulder.
17. Debridement is the removal of dead or damaged tissue.
    It was stated to him that if it does not show improvement over the next 2-3 months, wrist arthroscopy could be entertained with debridement of his TFCC.
18. Digit is a finger or toe.
    On my exam today, she is no longer painful with resisted wrist or digit extension.
19. Dorsiflexion is to bend the joint toward the posterior aspect of the body.
    Dorsiflexion is 10-15 degrees with plantar flexion to 25 degrees.
20. Ecchymosis is the black-and-blue appearance of the skin.
    There is considerable ecchymosis and a little bit of deformity of the wrist.
21. Effusion is the escape of fluid from blood vessels because of rupture or seepage, usually into a body cavity.
    He has no effusion and good motion.
22. Exostosis is an abnormal, benign growth on the surface of a bone, also called *hyperostosis*.
    Tom returns with a chief complaint that his right lower leg is still painful in the area where the exostosis was removed.
23. Fasciculations are the uncontrolled twitching of a group of muscle fibers.
    No paraspinal spasm or fasciculations were noted.
24. Flexion is the movement by a joint that decreases the angle between the two adjoining bones; the bending of a joint.
    Flexion was severely limited.
25. Fusiform is a spindle-shaped structure that is tapered at both ends.
    On examination today, she had 45 degrees of active flexion, fusiform swelling on the ulnar side of the PIP joint, and tenderness of the synovium.
26. Genu varum is the Latin term for *bowleg*.
    Patient's gait is genu varum.
27. Gluteus medius is one of the three muscles that form the buttocks; acts to abduct and rotate the thigh.
    I have reviewed with her what was done in therapy; unfortunately, they did not initiate a gluteus medius stretching and strengthening program as I had ordered.
28. Greater trochanter is the large projection at the proximal end of the femur.
    The patient continues to demonstrate significant weakness with pain over the greater trochanter.
29. Hypertrophy is an increase in the size of an organ or structure.
    She has a large hypertrophic callus over the PIP joint, with an ingrown corn.
30. Interarticular is between two joints.
    With his ulnar-sided wrist pain, recommendations today are an interarticular cortisone injection to help with his discomfort and a removable Futura wrist splint to wear intermittently when doing activities.
31. Interosseous is situated or occurring between bone.
    On examination, she had a deep, soft cystic mass in the area of the 1st dorsal interosseous, which was slightly tender to touch.
32. Lipoma is a benign tumor composed mostly of fat cells.
    I ordered an MRI of the hand to determine if it was indeed a cystic or lipomatous lesion.
33. Lymphadenopathy is the disease of the lymph nodes.
    He does have good sensation and good peripheral circulation with no edema or lymphadenopathy.
34. Lymphedema is edema due to obstruction of lymph vessels.
    There is no lymphedema.
35. Malleolus is either of the two rounded projections on either side of the ankle joint.
    Soft tissue swelling is present over both malleoli, particularly over the lateral malleolus.
36. Meniscectomy is the surgical removal of a meniscus.
    Tom returns 1 week status post arthroscopy and partial medial meniscectomy, right knee.
37. Meniscus is the crescent-shaped fibrocartilage in the knee joint.
    The lateral meniscus appears intact.
38. Metatarsus is any of the five long bones of the foot between the ankle and the toes.
    X-rays show a fracture at the apophysis of the proximal 5th metatarsal that is displaced somewhat.
39. Osteophyte is an outgrowth of bone that is usually found around a joint.
    His lumbar spine x-rays show only anterior osteophytes without disc space narrowing at the thoracolumbar junction, L2 and L4.
40. Paronychia is the inflammation involving the folds of tissue surrounding the nail.
    The nail bed on the right great toe is healing well following removal of the nail for paronychia infection.
41. Penicillin is the generic name of any of a large group of anti-bacterial antibiotics derived from strains of fungi of the genus *Penicillium*.
42. Peripheral is occurring away from the center.
    She can move her fingers okay and has good peripheral circulation and sensation.
43. Phalanx is the general term for any bone of a finger or toe.

On physical exam of his left 3rd finger, there is a tip avulsion of soft tissue with bare bony exposure of his distal phalanx.

44. Pisiform is a pea-shaped, smallest carpal bone.
The pisiform is nontender to palpation and compression.

45. Plantar relates to the sole of the foot.
Dorsiflexion is 10-15 degrees with plantar flexion to 25 degrees.

46. Purulence means containing pus.
The right great toe has significant nail bed infection, erythema, purulence, and tenderness, particularly on the lateral nail fold area.

47. Radiculitis is the inflammation of a spinal nerve root.
He does get some aches around the upper back and neck area, but no true radiculitis symptoms.

48. Spironolactone is the generic name for a diuretic.
His medications included spironolactone, Lopressor, and aspirin.

49. Symptomatology is the symptoms of a specific disease.
She has shown improvement within her left trochanteric symptomatology, but incomplete resolution of her problems.

50. Synovia is the lubricating fluid of joints.
On examination today, she had 45 degrees of active flexion, fusiform swelling on the ulnar side of the PIP joint, and tenderness of the synovium.

51. Tendinitis is the inflammation of a tendon.
He appears to have a chronic cuff tendinitis with a mild impingement syndrome.

52. Tetracycline is the generic name for an antibiotic.
The patient was given tetracycline for the infection.

53. Trapezius is the muscle of the back of the neck and shoulder.
He has tenderness of the lower cervical spine and over the left trapezius, but he has full range of motion of his C-spine.

54. Turgor is the normal resiliency of the skin.
His skin turgor is normal.

55. Ulna is the inner and larger bone of the forearm, on the side opposite the thumb.
She noted both pain and swelling primarily on the ulnar side of the PIP joint.

56. Volar pertains to the palm of the hand or sole of the foot.
Left 3rd fingertip amputation with exposed distal phalanx and loss of volar skin.

57. Biaxin is the trade name for an antibiotic.
The patient is allergic to BIAXIN.

58. Dolobid is the trade name for an analgesic, anti-inflammatory.
I have changed his prescription to Dolobid 500 mg to be taken on a b.i.d. basis.

59. Keflex is the trade name for an antibiotic.
I have started him on Keflex 250 mg q.i.d. and soaks 3x a day.

60. Lanoxin is the trade name for an antiarrhythmic, cardiotonic.
She is currently taking Lanoxin.

61. Lipitor is the trade name for an antihyperlipidemic.
Her medications included Lipitor, baby aspirin, and vitamin supplements.

62. Lopressor is the trade name for a beta-adrenergic blocker.
Her medications included Lopressor, Lipitor, Lanoxin, and baby aspirin.

63. Percocet is the trade name for an opioid analgesic.
I did renew a prescription for Percocet just to take at night as needed.

64. Vicodin is the trade name for a narcotic analgesic.
He is taking Vicodin as needed.

65. Vicoprofen is the trade name for a narcotic analgesic.
The patient was treated in February by Dr. Enrique Hernandez, who has had the patient on Vicoprofen.

66. Xylocaine is the trade name for an antiarrhythmic, anesthetic.
I have proceeded with reduction of the fracture with 1% Xylocaine local anesthesia.

CHAPTER 6 / TERMINOLOGY CHECK YOUR PROGRESS

1. a	17. a	33. b	49. d
2. d	18. c	34. a	50. b
3. a	19. a	35. d	51. b
4. d	20. b	36. b	52. c
5. b	21. a	37. a	53. b
6. c	22. c	38. d	54. a
7. c	23. c	39. d	55. a
8. a	24. d	40. b	56. b
9. d	25. b	41. a	57. b
10. a	26. a	42. a	58. c
11. a	27. b	43. c	59. a
12. c	28. a	44. a	60. b
13. a	29. c	45. d	61. c
14. d	30. c	46. b	62. d
15. a	31. c	47. d	
16. c	32. a	48. a	

CHAPTER 6 / ACTIVITY 6–4

Errors are indicated in **bold italic**. Margins are formatted at 1 inch.

HISTORY AND PHYSICAL EXAMINATION

Double space
Patient Name: Winster, Penny
File Number: 41390
Date of **Birth**: March 16, 19xx
Examination Date: *current date*
Physician: James P. Osseous, MD

HISTORY

HISTORY OF PRESENT ILLNESS
I had the pleasure of seeing Penny in the office today. This is a **43-year-old right-hand**–dominant woman who saw **Dr. Zart** for left rotator cuff tendinitis. She has **impingement. An** MRI **showed** acromial spur, no sign of a rotator cuff tear. **She** has an early **cyst** formation. She has undergone **2** injections. The first did not help. The second seemed to help her for a few days. She has had physical therapy for **3** months.

PAST MEDICAL HISTORY
Significant for cardiac **arrhythmia**.

MEDICATIONS
She is intermittently on **Lopressor**. She **has not** always been real compliant with that if she is not having any problems.

ALLERGIES
CODEINE.

REVIEW OF SYMPTOMS
She denies liver or kidney disease. She has had an ulcer in the remote past. She has not had any problems with it recently.

SOCIAL HISTORY
One-half pack per day smoker for **15** years.

PHYSICAL EXAMINATION
On examination, this is a **well-developed** woman in no **acute** distress. She has full**, painless** range of motion of her neck. Has **had** pain in the Neer and Hawkins **impingement** tests. Active **abduction** is 135 degrees. Forward flexion is 125 degrees. Passively, I could take her the rest of the way. Her strength is mildly diminished in external rotation, good in internal and abduction. She has a negative lift-off test. She is missing about **2** levels internal rotation up her back. She has pain with **cross-chest abduction**. There is no pain at the sternoclavicular or AC joint. No clavicular tenderness is noted. Neurovascularly, she is intact.

DIAGNOSTIC TESTS
I reviewed the MRI as above. We got an AP and outlet x-ray, which shows a type III **acromion.**

continued

HISTORY AND PHYSICAL EXAMINATION
Patient Name: Winster, Penny
File Number: 41390

Page 2

PLAN
Penny has chronic **impingement.** We discussed the options. We are going to **proceed** with **arthroscopic** subacromial **decompression.** We discussed the surgery and the risks involved**,** which she understands. All questions were answered**,** and an **instructional** booklet given. We will schedule this in a timely fashion after appropriate **preoperative** testing.

Quadruple space

James P. Osseous, MD

jpo:xx
D: current date
T: current date

CHAPTER 6 / ACTIVITY 6–5

Errors are indicated in **bold italic**. Margins are formatted at 1 inch.

CHART NOTE

Double space

Patient Name: Smith, Lucy
Date of Birth: February 28, 19xx
Examination Date: *current date*

SUBJECTIVE
Lucy is an **84-year-old** female who **fell** directly onto her right hand yesterday.

OBJECTIVE
She suffered a wrist fracture. She is **right-hand** dominant. **She** can move **her** fingers okay and has good **peripheral** circulation and sensation. **There** is considerable **ecchymosis** and a little bit of deformity of the wrist. **X-rays** show a reversed **Colles** or Smith fracture.

ASSESSMENT
Reversed **Colles** fracture, **right** wrist.

PLAN
I have proceeded with reduction of the fracture with 1% **Xylocaine** local anesthesia and have placed her in a sugar tong splint. Post reduction x-rays **show** essentially an anatomic reduction. I am going to plan to keep her immobilized for **6** weeks. I will have her return to the office in **1 week** for an x-ray **through** the cast.

Quadruple space

James P. Osseous, **MD**

jpo:xx
D: current date
T: current date

1. a	22. a	43. a	64. b
2. c	23. c	44. a	65. a
3. d	24. b	45. b	66. d
4. a	25. a	46. a	67. a
5. b	26. c	47. c	68. c
6. c	27. a	48. c	69. b
7. d	28. c	49. d	70. b
8. a	29. b	50. c	71. d
9. a	30. d	51. b	72. a
10. b	31. b	52. a	73. a
11. c	32. d	53. a	74. b
12. c	33. c	54. d	75. c
13. d	34. a	55. a	76. b
14. c	35. a	56. b	77. c
15. a	36. c	57. a	78. c
16. d	37. b	58. d	79. d
17. c	38. a	59. a	80. a
18. a	39. a	60. a	81. b
19. a	40. b	61. c	82. c
20. b	41. d	62. b	
21. c	42. a	63. a	

CHAPTER 7 / ACTIVITY 7-3 (7T–1)

1. Amoxicillin is a generic name for an antibiotic.
   At this point in time, we will use amoxicillin.
2. Arteriogram is a radiograph of an artery.
   The patient is admitted at this time for further evaluation that includes an arteriogram of the right collecting system.
3. Atrioventricular pertains to an atrium and the ventricle of the heart.
   Rule out atrioventricular malformation.
4. Bacitracin is a generic name for a bactericidal antibiotic.
   The wound was cleaned with bacitracin ointment, sterile fluff dressing, and a supporter.
5. Bradycardia is the slowness of the heartbeat.
   The patient's EKGs have been remarkable for the presence of left ventricular sinus bradycardia.
6. Calculus is an abnormal concretion; stone.
   The patient had a history of ureteral calculus.
7. Captopril is a generic name for an angiotensin-converting enzyme inhibitor.
   He is maintained on captopril 25 mg t.i.d.
8. Cholecystectomy is the removal of the gallbladder.
   She had a cholecystectomy.
9. Cholecystitis is the inflammation of the gallbladder.
   The etiology of the pain remains unclear, although possibilities would include a calculus cholecystitis or another ovarian cyst.
10. Coapt is to bring together, as suturing a laceration.
    With the Valsalva maneuver, the bladder neck was not well coapted.
11. Colporrhaphy is the suture of the vagina.
    The patient was scheduled for a vaginal hysterectomy, anterior colporrhaphy, and endoscopic urethral suspension.
12. Concomitant takes place at the same time.
    The patient was diagnosed with possible concomitant urinary tract infection.
13. Coudé is bent or elbowed.
    The existing catheter was removed and a #24 French coudé catheter was passed with little difficulty.
14. Creatinine is a normal alkaline constituent of urine and blood.
    Her creatinine is normal.
15. Cystitis is the inflammation of the urinary bladder.
    There is no history of cystitis.
16. Cystocele is the herniation of the urinary bladder into the vagina.
    Examination at that time demonstrated a marked cystocele and a positive Marshall test.
17. Cystometrography is the graphic record of the pressure in the bladder at varying stages of filling.
    Cystometrogram in my office revealed normal bladder compliance.

18. Cystoscope is an endoscope especially designed for passing through the urethra into the bladder to permit visual inspection of its interior.
    Subsequently, the rigid cystoscope was inserted, and the cystoscopy was performed.
19. Cystourethroscope is an instrument for examining the posterior urethra and bladder.
    The 23.5 cystourethroscope was assembled, lubricated, and advanced through the urethra and into the bladder.
20. Diuresis is an increased excretion of urine.
    A diuresis renogram was performed, and this study was normal, with no evidence of obstruction of either collecting system.
21. Diverticulum is a sac or pouch in the walls of a canal or organ.
    The patient had a history of hypertension, Crohn's disease, and diverticulitis.
22. Dyspnea is labored or difficult breathing.
    He currently presents in an acute anxiety state and is dyspneic.
23. Ecchymosis is a skin discoloration caused by a hemorrhage.
    No hematoma or ecchymosis is noted.
24. Extravasation is a discharge or escape of fluid from a vessel into the tissues.
    There is no sign of any extravasation.
25. Flank is the side of the body between the ribs and ilium.
    The patient is a 38-year-old male in mild distress secondary to right-sided flank discomfort.
26. Fossa is a hollow or depressed area.
    The prostatic fossa demonstrates grade 2/4 obstruction as viewed from the veru.
27. Fulguration is the destruction of living tissue by electric sparks generated by a high-frequency current.
    Fulguration of the lumens of both the cut ends was performed with electrocautery.
28. Genitourinary pertains to the genitalia and urinary organs.
    There is no previous history of urinary tract infections, stones, or genitourinary surgery.
29. Hematuria is the discharge of blood in the urine.
    An examination revealed microscopic hematuria.
30. Heme is the nonprotein, insoluble, iron constituent of hemoglobin.
    Urinalysis shows 3+ heme, which is greater than 30 per high-power field.
31. Hydrocele is an accumulation of fluid in a sac-like cavity.
    The right testicle is noteworthy for a moderate-sized hydrocele.
32. Hydrochlorothiazide is a generic name for a diuretic, antihypertensive agent.
    The patient was given hydrochlorothiazide 25 mg daily for hypertension.
33. Hydronephrosis is the distention of the renal pelvis and calyces with urine.
    This newborn has very mild, yet persistent hydronephrosis, with no evidence of progression.
34. Incontinence is the inability to control excretory functions.
    The patient's chief complaint was urinary incontinence.
35. Laminectomy is the surgical excision of the lamina.
    He is hypertensive, with a previous history of a laminectomy for a herniated disc.
36. Leukocytes are colorless blood corpuscles.
    Urinalysis shows 2+ leukocytes, which were greater than 10 per high-powered field, and 3+ heme, which is greater than 30 per high-powered field.
37. Lithotomy is an incision of a duct or organ for the removal of calculi.
    The patient was brought to the cytoscopy suite and placed in the dorsal lithotomy position.
38. Meatus is an opening.
    The penis is circumcised and the meatus adequate.
39. Meclizine is a generic name for an antiemetic, antihistamine, motion sickness relief.
    The patient was given meclizine on a p.r.n basis for dizziness.
40. Nephrectomy is the surgical removal of the kidney.
    The patient was admitted to University Hospital for a right nephrectomy.
41. Occlude is to close tight.
    Two clips were placed in opposing directions on both cut ends to further occlude the lumen.

42. Oophorectomy is the excision of one or both ovaries.
    She has had an oophorectomy but has her uterus.
43. Panendoscope is a cystoscope that gives a wide-angle view of the bladder.
    The panendoscopy was performed with a #16 French flexible panendoscope.
44. Parenchyma are the essential elements of an organ.
    No deformity to the parenchyma or fluid loss is noted.
45. Periumbilical is around the umbilicus.
    The pain appeared to start in the periumbilical area and then improved.
46. Pessary is an instrument placed in the vagina to support the uterus or rectum.
    Because of her age, I convinced her to try therapy with a pessary, and a 2-inch Gellhorn pessary was inserted.
47. Phallus is the penis.
    The phallus is uncircumcised, with normal full foreskin.
48. Pyelogram is an x-ray study of the renal pelvis and uterus.
    An intravenous pyelogram and voiding cystourethrogram were normal, as well as urine cytology and urine culture.
49. Pyelonephritis is the inflammation of the kidney and renal pelvis.
    The negative urinalysis would also mitigate against a pyelonephritis, and the pain is clearly abdominal rather than in the CVA region.
50. Pyuria is pus in the urine.
    She has a 3-month history of persistent pyuria.
51. Raphe is a seam or ridge noting the line of junction of halves of a part.
    The left vas was regrasped and brought into the median raphe.
52. Rectocele is a hernia protrusion of part of the rectum into the vagina.
    Upon removal of the pessary, there is a large cystocele and a small rectocele.
53. Resect is to cut off or cut out a portion of a tissue or organ.
    The patient underwent prostatic resection and hernia repair in 1998.
54. Staghorn is the calculus of the renal pelvis, usually extending into multiple calyces.
    X-rays reveal a large staghorn calculus with minimal obstruction.
55. Suprapubic is above the pubis.
    The abdomen is soft and tender in the suprapubic region.
56. Syncope is the temporary suspension of consciousness; fainting.
    The patient is free of any dizziness, lightheadedness, syncope, or near syncope.
57. Trabeculation is a small beam or supporting structure.
    The mucosa was examined in full circumferential fashion and was without tumors, trabeculation, or diverticula.
58. Trigone is a triangular area.
    The bladder showed a normal trigone with normal orifices bilaterally.
59. Urethrocele is the prolapse of the female urethra through the urinary meatus.
    GENITALIA: Moderate urethrocele.
60. Urethrotrigonitis is the inflammation of the urethra and trigone of the bladder.
    Cystoscopy revealed some mild changes of urethrotrigonitis, and stress incontinence was demonstrated.
61. Urogram is a diagnostic x-ray study of kidneys, ureters, and bladder.
    A recent urogram showed a filling defect of the left kidney.
62. Urosepsis is the poisoning from retained and absorbed urinary substances.
    The patient was seen and evaluated several years ago for a suspected urosepsis with an associated high fever, secondary to a staghorn calculus and chronic urinary infection.
63. Vas deferens is the excretory duct of the testis.
    The vas deferens was grasped and brought into the median raphe and anesthesia infiltrated.
64. Vasculature is the supply of vessels to a specific region.
    The patient is scheduled for an arteriogram later today to further define the vasculature of the left kidney and hopefully identify the bleeding site.
65. Verumontanum is the elevation on the floor of the prostatic portion of the urethra where the seminal ducts enter.

The flexible cystourethroscope was advanced through the urethra to the level of the verumontanum.

66. Aldactone is the trade name for a diuretic.
    The patient's medications included Aldactone.
67. Bactrim is the trade name for an antibiotic.
    Medications include a recent course of Bactrim, which has caused nausea and headache.
68. Betadine is the trade name for a topical antibacterial, antiseptic.
    The genitalia were prepped with a Betadine scrub and draped in a sterile fashion.
69. Calan is the trade name for an antianginal, antiarrhythmic, antihypertensive.
    His only medication was Calan SR 240 mg 1 p.o. daily.
70. Cardura is the trade name for an antihypertensive, antiadrenergic.
    His only medication is Cardura 3 mg at bedtime.
71. Cipro is the trade name for a fluoroquinolone antibiotic, antibacterial drug.
    Antibiotics in the form of Cipro were given.
72. Imodium is the trade name for an antidiarrheal.
    Her medications included Imodium.
73. Lopressor is the trade name for an antianginal, antihypertensive.
    Her medications included Aldactone, Imodium, and Lopressor.
74. Maxaquin is the trade name for a fluoroquinolone antibiotic, antibacterial.
    The patient was started on Maxaquin 400 mg p.o. daily for a 7-day course.
75. Neptazane is the trade name for a diuretic, antiglaucoma agent.
    He takes one aspirin a day and is maintained on Neptazane 1 b.i.d.
76. Noroxin is the trade name for an antibacterial, urinary tract anti-infective.
    I have placed her on Noroxin 400 mg p.o. b.i.d. for 5 days.
77. Propine is the trade name for an antiglaucoma agent, eye drops.
    He also uses Propine eye drops.
78. Timoptic is the trade name for a topical antiglaucoma agent.
    He also uses Propine and Timoptic eye drops.
79. Tolinase is the trade name for an antidiabetic agent.
    He is maintained on Tolinase 250 mg p.o. daily, as well as captopril 25 mg t.i.d.
80. Toradol is the trade name for a nonsteroidal anti-inflammatory analgesic drug for acute, moderately severe pain.
    His pain is quite severe but was relieved with intravenous Toradol.
81. Trimpex is the trade name for an antibacterial, antibiotic.
    After he finishes the Bactrim, I will place him on Trimpex 100 mg daily.
82. Xylocaine is the trade name for an anesthetic, antiarrhythmic.
    Xylocaine jelly was injected into the urethra.

CHAPTER 7 / TERMINOLOGY CHECK YOUR PROGRESS

See Terminology Pretest.

CHAPTER 7 / ACTIVITY 7–4

Errors are indicated in *bold italic*. Margins are formatted at 1 inch.

CONSULTATION REPORT

Patient Name: Barnes, Franklyn
File Number: 003416
Date of Birth: February 13, 19xx
Examination Date: *current date*
Requesting Physician: Izzy Sertoli, MD

HISTORY OF PRESENT ILLNESS
This *22-year-old* gentleman fell approximately *27 feet* off a scaffold. He landed on a stack of concrete blocks and sustained *an* abrasion of his right flank. The patient informs me that he did not have much pain immediately after the fall and*, therefore,* did not come to see you for evaluation until later in the day. A urine *analysis* performed in your office showed 20-50 *RBCs*. Due to your concern about *right* flank trauma*,* I was asked to evaluate the patient.

The patient is *alert* and oriented. There is no tenderness over the abdomen. There is a *right* flank abrasion measuring about 4 *cm*. No *hematoma* or *ecchymosis is* noted. The left flank area is smooth and *unremarkable*. There is no tenderness in the lower abdomen. The testicles are normal. The prostate is 1+, smooth and nontender. His *hemoglobin* is *14*.

Double space

An IVP was performed that showed a large *gas* pattern over the entire *abdomen*. The left kidney functions *promptly* and is smooth. The right kidney shows good function in both the upper and lower poles. There is some decreased *filling* of the renal *pelvis,* but there is good *excretion* of *contrast*. The renal pelvis does not really fill out *well* in the entire *midline* area*,* which I think is consistent with a renal *contusion*. *There* is no sign of any *extravasation*.

Double space

A renal *sonogram* also shows the kidney to be totally *intact*. No deformity to the *parenchyma* or fluid loss is noted. It is essentially a *normal-appearing* kidney.

Double space

IMPRESSION
Right renal contusion. No signs of any *extravasation*.

Double space

PLAN
The patient will be admitted to *University Hospital* and placed on *bed rest* with observation. I will order a urine culture and sensitivity test. He will be started on IV antibiotics*,* and I will follow along with you in his care. Thank you for *referring* this patient to us.

Quadruple space

Benjamin Keytone, MD

Double space

bk:xx
D: *current date*
T: *current date*

Errors are indicated in **bold italic**. Margins are fomatted at 1 inch.

OPERATIVE REPORT

Patient Name: Cruise, Jason
File Number: 0045612
Date of Birth: March 16, 1967

Operation Date: *current date*

PREOPERATIVE DIAGNOSIS
Carcinoma of the prostate.

Double space

POSTOPERATIVE DIAGNOSIS
Carcinoma of the prostate.

OPERATION
Flexible cystoscopy.

Double space

PROCEDURE
Flexible cystoscopy.
The patient was identified by me**,** prepped**,** and draped in the usual fashion. The **panendoscopy** was performed with a **#16 French** flexible panendoscope. The anterior urethra was unremarkable. The membranous urethra is **intact**. There is no evidence of any **stricture**.

The **prostatic fossa** demonstrates grade **2/6** obstruction as viewed from the **veru**. This probably represents **15-20 gm** of resectable adenoma. **There** is no evidence of tumor within the **prostatic fossa**. The bladder neck anatomy is unremarkable. The bladder mucosa is healthy **throughout**. There were no stones, tumors, or diverticula identified.

Right and left ureteral orifices were in normal position and normal configuration. Clear **efflux** is seen bilaterally. The bladder neck anatomy **is unremarkable** as noted from a retroflex position. There is no evidence of any tumor **invasion** into the bladder base. The scope was withdrawn. The patient tolerated the procedure well.

PLAN
Trimpex 100 **mg b.i.d**. Schedule a **follow-up** appointment in 2 weeks to discuss treatment options for carcinoma of the **prostate**.

_____

Theodore Trigone, MD

Double Space

tt:xx
D: *current date*
T: *current date*

1. a	26. a	51. a	76. a
2. a	27. a	52. c	77. a
3. a	28. d	53. b	78. c
4. b	29. a	54. b	79. c
5. b	30. c	55. d	80. b
6. c	31. a	56. d	81. b
7. a	32. d	57. c	82. c
8. d	33. c	58. a	83. a
9. b	34. a	59. d	84. b
10. d	35. d	60. b	85. d
11. c	36. a	61. b	86. a
12. b	37. b	62. a	87. c
13. b	38. b	63. d	88. a
14. d	39. c	64. b	89. b
15. c	40. d	65. c	90. c
16. b	41. a	66. a	91. a
17. b	42. b	67. c	92. c
18. c	43. c	68. a	93. d
19. c	44. c	69. c	94. a
20. a	45. b	70. a	95. b
21. a	46. b	71. a	96. a
22. a	47. d	72. a	97. d
23. c	48. a	73. b	98. c
24. b	49. d	74. a	
25. b	50. b	75. c	

CHAPTER 8 / ACTIVITY 8–3 (8T–1)

1. Adenocarcinoma is a malignant tumor of the glands.
   She is status post abdominal surgery for adenocarcinoma of uterus in 1990.
2. Adenopathy is the enlargement of the glands, especially the lymph nodes.
   The neck was bull-like without adenopathy or venous distention.
3. Afebrile is without fever.
   The patient has been afebrile.
4. Amoxicillin is the generic name for an aminopenicillin antibiotic.
   She was also started on another antibiotic, which may have been amoxicillin.
5. Aneurysm is a localized dilatation of the wall of a blood vessel.
   He is 6 weeks status post aortic aneurysm repair.
6. Arteriogram is the radiographic visualization of an artery after injection of a contrast medium.
   Previous assessment includes a carotid arteriogram.
7. Ascites is the accumulation of fluid in the peritoneal cavity.
   The abdomen is distended, and there may be ascites.
8. Atelectasis is the collapse of a portion of the lung.
   Chest x-ray showed atelectasis in the right upper lobe.
9. Auscultation is the act of listening for sounds produced within the body with an unaided ear or with a stethoscope.
   The chest is clear to auscultation.
10. Bilateral is affecting both sides.
    He had a bilateral hernia repair 3 years ago.
11. Bronchodilator is any drug that has the capability of increasing the capacity of the pulmonary air passages and improve ventilation to the lungs.
    After his hospital course, we will try to get him to stop smoking and start him on an inhaled bronchodilator program for his obstructive lung disease.
12. Bruit is a sound or murmur heard on auscultation.
    There is a short right carotid bruit.
13. Caries is the condition of decay and destruction of a tooth.
    Periodontal disease and caries were noted in various stages.
14. Cephalosporin is a generic name for any of the large group of broad-spectrum antibiotics.
    A first-generation cephalosporin would cover his staph aureus.

15. Claudication is cramping pains of the calves caused by poor circulation to the leg muscles.
He does not have symptoms of claudication.
16. Continent is the ability to control urination and defecation urges.
He does have bladder spasms and remains partially continent.
17. Cor pulmonale is an abnormal heart condition characterized by the increased size of the right ventricle.
The patient exhibited cor pulmonale, severe emphysema, and hypertension.
18. Cyanosis is the bluish purple discoloration of the skin due to lack of oxygenated blood.
No clubbing or cyanosis was noted in the extremities.
19. Dentition refers to the position and condition of the teeth.
There was poor dentition with some periodontal disease noted and caries in various stages.
20. Diuresis is the increased excretion of urine.
We will have an answer if the next chest x-ray results show improvement with diuresis.
21. Diuretic is a substance that promotes the excretion of urine.
Diuretics have already been ordered.
22. Doxepin is the generic name for an antidepressant.
Her current medication included doxepin 1 tablet t.i.d.
23. Dyspnea is the labored or difficult breathing.
The dyspnea is worse on exertion, especially when climbing stairs and doing his job as a janitor.
24. Dysrhythmia is a disordered rhythm.
Heather Williams is a 78-year-old lady with a long history of hypertension and recurrent supraventricular dysrhythmia.
25. Echocardiogram is a diagnostic procedure using ultrasound to study heart structure and motion.
Previous assessment includes a carotid arteriogram and an echocardiogram for left ventricular function that was normal.
26. Edema is the accumulation of excess fluid in the tissues of the body.
There was no edema noted in the extremities.
27. Effusion is the escape of fluid into a body cavity.
The patient's past history was remarkable for a hospital admission 2 months ago for a large pleural effusion and mass.
28. Embolus is a mass that is brought by the blood from another vessel that obstructs blood circulation.
I suspect there is a substantial chance this may yet be a pulmonary embolus.
29. Emesis is vomit.
She was starting to spike fevers of 102 and felt toxic with coughing and emesis.
30. Empiric is treating a disease based upon observation and experience rather than reasoning alone.
I would empirically proceed with pulmonary angiography.
31. Erythema is redness of the skin.
Over the past 2-3 months, she has noticed increasing pedal edema, although there has been no erythema, inflammation, or calf tenderness.
32. Erythromycin is a generic name for a broad-spectrum antibiotic.
The patient was seen a couple of weeks ago and was started on erythromycin.
33. Fibrillation is the uncoordinated twitching of muscle fibers.
This is a 49-year-old white male admitted with new onset of atrial fibrillation.
34. Flora are normally occurring microorganisms that live within the body that provide natural immunity against certain organisms.
A first-generation cephalosporin would cover both his normal flora and staph aureus.
35. Gallop is an abnormal heart rhythm.
The heartbeat was regular without murmur, gallop, or rub.
36. Hemoptysis is the coughing or spitting up of blood from the respiratory tract.
She has had some mild pleuritic pain, but no hemoptysis.
37. Heparin is the generic name for an anticoagulant.
He was treated initially with intravenous nitroglycerin and intravenous heparin.
38. Homans' sign is calf pain with dorsiflexion of foot.
No clubbing, cyanosis, edema or Homans' sign was noted in the extremities.

39. Hydrate is a compound containing water molecules.
We will also gently hydrate her over the next 24 hours and get a follow-up chest x-ray.
40. Infiltrate is when fluid, cells, or other substances pass into tissue spaces.
Chest x-ray shows left lower lobe infiltrate.
41. Intrauterine means within the uterus.
Her last normal menstrual period was approximately 1 month ago, but she denies the possibility of intrauterine pregnancy.
42. Ischemia is a decreased supply of oxygenated blood to a body part.
Perhaps a dobutamine MUGA scan will also be required at some point to exclude myocardial ischemia.
43. Isosorbide is the generic name for a nitrate-based antianginal agent.
Her medications included isosorbide 10 mg p.o. q.i.d.
44. Lorazepam is a generic antianxiety drug.
She is taking lorazepam 1 mg t.i.d. p.r.n.
45. Metastasis is the transfer of disease from one organ or part to another not directly connected with it.
My impression is that we are dealing with a man with a known mass in his right lung with probable metastasis to his brain.
46. Nebulization is a treatment by a spray.
The patient was placed on nebulization p.r.n.
47. Nifedipine is a generic calcium channel blocker drug.
He is taking nifedipine 1 tablet t.i.d.
48. Nitroglycerin is a generic name for a coronary vasodilator, antianginal.
The patient's medications include nitroglycerin spray p.r.n.
49. Nocturnal is something that occurs at night.
We will arrange a nocturnal oxygen saturation test along with a chest x-ray, pulmonary function tests, and a room-air arterial blood gas.
50. Nystagmus is the involuntary, rapid, rhythmic movement of the eyeball.
Extraocular movements were intact without nystagmus.
51. Occlusion is the act of closure or state of being closed.
Previous assessment includes a carotid arteriogram that showed a right carotid occlusion and an echocardiogram for left ventricular function that was normal.
52. Pedal is a term relating to the foot.
Over the past 2-3 months, she has noticed increasing pedal edema, although there has been no erythema, inflammation, or calf tenderness.
53. Pneumonectomy is the surgical removal of all or a segment of the lung.
A pneumonectomy was recommended because of evidence of cancer.
54. Pneumothorax is the presence of air or gas in the pleural cavity.
Chest x-ray showed no evidence of pneumothorax with some hyperinflation and chronic obstructive pulmonary disease changes.
55. Prednisone is a generic corticosteroid drug.
We will admit, treat with IV antibiotics, oral prednisone, and aerosol bronchodilators.
56. Pulmonary toilet is the cleansing of the trachea and bronchial tree.
The patient was admitted to the hospital and placed on intravenous antibiotic therapy with pulmonary toilet.
57. Purulent means containing pus.
She denies fever, sweats, chills, purulent sputum, hemoptysis, or chest pain.
58. Rale is an abnormal crackle sound heard on chest auscultation.
Chest exam showed decreased breath sounds and wheezes without local rales.
59. Rhonchus is an abnormal sound heard on chest auscultation due to an obstructed airway.
Lung exam demonstrated scattered expiratory wheezes and rhonchi, but fair air excursion.
60. Rub is a sound caused by the rubbing together of two surfaces.
There was no cardiac rub.
61. Saphenous pertains to the two main superficial veins of the lower leg.
He has no history of ankle edema or deep vein thrombosis, although he has had coronary artery bypass grafting and a saphenous vein harvest on the left side.

62. Sequela is any abnormal condition that follows and is the result of a disease, treatment, or injury.
He also has a history of a right hip fracture, with residual pain, an appendectomy, a myocardial infarction, and a small CVA with no sequelae.

63. Somnolence is drowsiness.
He denies any significant daytime somnolence.

64. Sputum is the material coughed up from the lungs and ejected through the mouth.
She has had some mild pleuritic pain, scant sputum production, but no hemoptysis.

65. Stasis is an abnormal slowing or stopping of fluid flowing through a vessel.
Extremity evaluation reveals some stasis changes of the lower extremities, with almost absent pulses at the dorsalis pedis and posterior tibialis.

66. Supraventricular refers to situated or occurring above the ventricles.
Susan is a 65-year-old lady with a history of hypertension and recurrent supraventricular dysrhythmia.

67. Syncope is the act of fainting.
There has been no syncope.

68. Tachycardia is an abnormally fast heartbeat.
She had a sinus tachycardia of 110.

69. Theophylline is a generic name for a bronchodilator.
She was complaining of staggering gait and overall weakness, which was thought to be in part secondary to her theophylline level.

70. Thoracentesis is the aspiration of fluid from the chest cavity.
She underwent thoracentesis, closed needle biopsy, and bronchoscopy under general anesthesia, which resulted in no definitive diagnosis.

71. Thyromegaly is the enlargement of the thyroid gland.
No neck mass or thyromegaly was noted.

72. Ancef IV is the trade name for a cephalosporin antibiotic.
We will also place him on Ancef IV and erythromycin orally.

73. Ascriptin is the trade name for a preparation of aspirin with Maalox, an analgesic and anti-inflammatory.
Her medications included insulin NPH 30 units, regular 6 units in the morning, and Ascriptin 1 tablet a day.

74. Atrovent is the trade name for a nasal spray, bronchodilator.
Her current medications include Atrovent, 2 puffs q.i.d.

75. Azmacort is the trade name for a corticosteroid for the prevention or treatment of bronchial asthma.
His current medications include Azmacort 4 puffs b.i.d.

76. Bumex is the trade name for a loop diuretic.
The physician prescribed Bumex 2 mg q. a.m.

77. Cardizem is the trade name for a calcium channel blocker for atrial fibrillation.
Her medications included insulin NPH 30 units, regular 6 units in the morning, Cardizem 30 b.i.d., and Ascriptin 1 tablet a day.

78. Colace is the trade name for a stool softener.
Her medications included Cardizem 30 b.i.d., Ascriptin 1 tablet a day, and Colace.

79. Compazine is the trade name for a tranquilizer and antiemetic.
We will place him on Compazine for nausea.

80. Darvon is the trade name for a narcotic analgesic.
The patient was taking Darvon 1 p.o. q.6h. p.r.n.

81. Dilantin is the trade name for an anticonvulsant used in the treatment of epilepsy.
Her epilepsy was controlled with Dilantin 100 mg q.i.d.

82. Fibercon is the trade name for a bulk-forming laxative.
Her medications included insulin NPH 30 units, regular 6 units in the morning, Cardizem 30 b.i.d., Ascriptin 1 tablet a day, FiberCon, and Colace.

83. Lopressor is the trade name for an antihypertensive.
The patient's current medications include Lopressor 50 mg q. a.m., Bumex 2 mg q. a.m., and isosorbide 10 mg p.o. q.i.d.

84. Mevacor is the trade name for an antihyperlipidemic.
The patient's current medications include Lopressor 50 mg q. a.m., Bumex 2 mg q. a.m., isosorbide 10 mg p.o. q.i.d., and Mevacor 20 mg p.o. daily.

85. NPH (neutral protamine Hagedorn) insulin is the trade name for an insulin that decreases blood sugar.

He has added additional doses of regular insulin to his usual regimen of 30 units of NPH and 6 units of regular insulin in the morning.

86. Paxil is the trade name for an antidepressant.
The physician prescribed prednisone and Paxil.

87. Pepcid is the trade name for an acid controller for heartburn and acid indigestion.
The physician prescribed Pepcid, prednisone, and Paxil.

88. Procardia is the trade name for a coronary vasodilator.
The patient is taking Dilantin 100 mg q.i.d., Procardia 30 mg q. a.m., and Lopressor 50 mg q. a.m.

89. Proventil MDI is a trade name for a bronchodilator, metered-dose inhaler.
We will provide Proventil MDI on a p.r.n. basis.

90. Restoril is the trade name for a sedative-hypnotic.
The physician prescribed Pepcid, prednisone, Restoril, and Paxil.

91. Serevent is the trade name for an aerosol bronchodilator.
The patient was using several bronchodilators, including Serevent 2 puffs b.i.d. and Azmacort 4 puffs b.i.d.

92. Slo-bid is the trade name for an extended-release bronchodilator.
Her current medications are Slo-bid 300 mg p.o. b.i.d., lorazepam 1 mg t.i.d. p.r.n., Nitro-Derm patch 0.2 mg daily p.r.n., and oxygen 2 liters by nasal cannula 24 hours a day.

93. Theo-Dur is the trade name for a bronchodilator.
His current medications are potassium 2 tablets t.i.d., doxepin 1 tablet t.i.d., nifedipine 1 tablet t.i.d., Xanax ½ tablet q.4h. as needed, and Theo-Dur b.i.d.

94. Vanceril is the trade name for a corticosteroid.
The patient's current medications are Proventil metered-dose inhaler 2 puffs t.i.d. and Vanceril 2 puffs q.i.d.

95. Vasotec is the trade name for an antihypertensive.
The patient's current medications include Lopressor 50 mg q. a.m., Bumex 2 mg q. a.m., Zantac 150 mg b.i.d., Vasotec 10 mg p.o. b.i.d., isosorbide 10 mg p.o. q.i.d., and Mevacor 20 mg p.o. daily.

96. Ventolin is the trade name for a bronchodilator.
The patient was using several bronchodilators, including Ventolin 2 puffs q.i.d., Serevent 2 puffs b.i.d., and Azmacort 4 puffs b.i.d.

97. Xanax is the trade name for an antianxiety agent.
She was taking Xanax ½ tablet q.4h. as needed and Theo-Dur b.i.d.

98. Zantac is the trade name for an acid controller for heartburn and acid indigestion.
The patient's current medications include Lopressor 50 mg q. a.m., Bumex 2 mg q. a.m., Zantac 150 mg b.i.d., Vasotec 10 mg p.o. b.i.d., isosorbide 10 mg p.o. q.i.d., and Mevacor 20 mg p.o. daily.

1. b	26. c	51. c	76. a
2. b	27. a	52. d	77. c
3. d	28. d	53. b	78. c
4. a	29. b	54. b	79. b
5. d	30. d	55. a	80. b
6. c	31. c	56. d	81. c
7. b	32. a	57. b	82. a
8. b	33. a	58. c	83. b
9. c	34. b	59. a	84. d
10. b	35. a	60. c	85. a
11. b	36. c	61. d	86. c
12. c	37. b	62. c	87. a
13. b	38. b	63. a	88. b
14. d	39. a	64. d	89. c
15. c	40. d	65. c	90. a
16. a	41. a	66. d	91. c
17. b	42. c	67. a	92. d
18. b	43. a	68. b	93. a
19. a	44. a	69. b	94. b
20. a	45. a	70. c	95. a
21. c	46. a	71. a	96. d
22. a	47. a	72. b	97. c
23. d	48. d	73. a	98. c
24. b	49. a	74. c	
25. a	50. b	75. a	

CHAPTER 8 / ACTIVITY 8-4

Errors are indicated in **bold italic**. Margins are formatted at 1 inch.

CONSULTATION REPORT

Patient Name: Calabretta, Gregory
File Number: 09451
Date of Birth: January 15, 19xx
Examination Date: *current date*
Requesting Physician: Izzy Sertoli, MD

HISTORY OF PRESENT ILLNESS
The patient is a *42-year-old* white male who presented to the *hospital* with some vague chest pain as well as a history of shortness of *breath*. The patient states to me that he has had shortness of *breath* for approximately a year and *a half*. The *dyspnea* is worse on *exertion*, especially when climbing stairs and doing his job as a janitor. He has had a dry cough, which on occasion was productive of clear *sputum* but has not been productive of blood or *pus*. *He* complains of vague, substernal, *left-sided* chest pain. The pain is worse with movement or *palpation* of the area.

PAST HISTORY
His past history is significant for asthma. He had a bilateral hernia repair 3 *years* ago.

REVIEW OF SYSTEMS
Negative.

PHYSICAL EXAMINATION
GENERAL: His blood pressure is *120/70*, pulse *70*, respirations *12/min*.
HEENT: Negative. Neck veins are not *distended*. Trachea is *midline*. There are no *nodes* in the *supraclavicular* or cervical chain.
CHEST: Breath sounds reveal some *crackles* at the *bases* but are otherwise negative.
HEART: Heart sounds are normal, but distant.
EXTREMITIES: No *clubbing*, cyanosis, or edema noted.LABORATORY DATA
Room air *ABG* shows a *PO2* of *59* without *CO2* retention. Chest x-ray reveals a diffuse *interstitial* process with no hilar *nodes*.

continued

CONSULTATION REPORT
Patient Name: Calabretta, Gregory
File Number: 09451
Page 2

IMPRESSION
I suspect that we are dealing with an inflammatory *process* in his lungs. *An* illness such as *sarcoid* is a *distinct* possibility, as we discussed on the phone last night. Additionally, this could be *CHF*, although clinically it does not look like it. We will have an answer if the next chest *x-ray* results show improvement with *diuresis*. If it does not, *then* a more *extensive work-up* shall take place. Clinically, I doubt an infection. I suspect we *will* end up doing a *bronchoscopy* with a biopsy.

PLAN
If there is no improvement on *tomorrow's* x-ray, we will proceed with a more *aggressive work-up*. The patient states *he* has no previous chest x-rays for comparison.

Quadruple space

_____
Allan Bolus, MD

Double Space

ab:xx
D: current date
T: current date

CHAPTER 8 / ACTIVITY 8-5

Errors are indicated in **bold italic**. Margins are formatted at 1 inch.

current date

Quadruple space

Charles P. Davis, MD
FedDes Wellness Center
Family Practice Division, Suite 300
101 Wellness Way Drive
New York, NY 10036

Re: Lawrence *A*. Rabia
    Date of Birth: *January* 20, 19xx

Dear Dr. Davis

Mr. *Rabia* is a *62-year-old* white male with a past history of smoking. He is 6 weeks status post aortic aneurysm repair. Postoperatively *he* did well and was discharged. At home, *he* has been fairly *homebound*, but not bedridden. He was in his usual state of health, without an upper respiratory illness, cough, congestion, or aches, when he developed the *acute onset* of *left-sided* pleuritic chest pain. The *pleuritic* component of the pain has *intensified* and is actually positional at this time. He denied any *hemoptysis*. He has some mild shortness of *breath* and mild *dyspnea on* exertion. He has no history of ankle edema or deep vein *thrombosis, although* he has had coronary artery *bypass* grafting and a *saphenous* vein harvest on the left side.

On physical examination, the *patient's* temperature was *99*. His other vital signs were stable. *HEENT* was benign. Neck showed no mass or *adenopathy*. Lungs showed diminished *breath* sounds bilaterally, with *scratchy, rub-like* sounds on the left side. Cardiovascular exam shows *S1, S2* within normal limits and grade *1/6* systolic *ejection* murmur at the lower left sternal border. There was no cardiac rub. *Abdomen* was soft. Extremities showed no edema. *Calves* were benign and *nontender*.

Chest *x-ray* showed no evidence of **pneumothorax** with some **hyperinflation** and chronic obstructive pulmonary disease changes. **His** ventilation **perfusion** scan showed an abnormal perfusion study with 3 matched defects.

Lawrence **A.** Rabia
current date
Page **2**

IMPRESSION: Pleuritic **left-sided** chest pain 6 weeks **postoperative** and an abnormal perfusion scan. Given the indeterminate scan, I suspect there is a substantial chance this may yet be a pulmonary **embolus.** I would empirically **heparinize** at this time and **proceed** with pulmonary **angiography.** I have discussed this with the patient, and he understands and agrees.

Thank you for this referral.

Sincerely

Allan Bolus, MD

xx

CHAPTER 9 / TERMINOLOGY PRETEST

1. c	27. d	53. b	79. d
2. b	28. c	54. b	80. a
3. d	29. a	55. d	81. a
4. d	30. c	56. c	82. b
5. a	31. a	57. a	83. d
6. b	32. a	58. c	84. b
7. a	33. d	59. a	85. c
8. c	34. c	60. a	86. d
9. c	35. c	61. a	87. c
10. a	36. d	62. c	88. a
11. b	37. c	63. d	89. b
12. a	38. b	64. b	90. c
13. b	39. a	65. d	91. b
14. a	40. d	66. c	92. d
15. c	41. b	67. a	93. a
16. a	42. a	68. d	94. c
17. c	43. b	69. a	95. a
18. a	44. b	70. a	96. c
19. b	45. a	71. c	97. d
20. a	46. a	72. c	98. a
21. d	47. d	73. b	99. c
22. a	48. a	74. a	100. b
23. c	49. b	75. b	101. d
24. b	50. a	76. c	
25. b	51. a	77. b	
26. c	52. a	78. c	

CHAPTER 9 / ACTIVITY 9-3 (9T-1)

1. Adenomatous relates to some types of glandular hyperplasia.
   Given his history of large adenomatous polyps, a repeat colonoscopy is recommended in 3 years.
2. Anastomosis is an opening created by surgery, disease, or trauma between two or more organs or structures.
   A vascular anastomosis was performed to bypass an aneurysm.
3. Arteriogram is a radiographic record of an artery after injection of a contrast medium into it.
   The patient had a normal coronary arteriogram in 1994.
4. Biliary relates to bile or the biliary tract.
   The physician ruled out biliary disease such as gallstones or other cholestatic liver diseases.
5. Cecum is the cul-de-sac about 6 cm in depth, lying below the terminal ileum, forming the first part of the large intestine.
   The scope was easily advanced to the cecum, with good visualization of all areas.
6. Cholecystectomy is the surgical removal of the gallbladder.
   In addition, her history is remarkable for rectocele and cystocele repair and cholecystectomy.
7. Colitis is the inflammation of the colon.
   A biopsy was taken for microscopic colitis.
8. Colonoscope is an elongated endoscope, usually fiberoptic.
   The physician used the Olympus video colonoscope.
9. Colonoscopy is the visual examination of the inner surface of the colon by means of a colonoscope.
   The patient underwent a colonoscopy using the Olympus video colonoscope.
10. Colostomy is the establishment of an artificial opening into the colon.
    There is a colostomy in the left lower quadrant, which appears healthy.
11. Creatinine is a normal component of urine.
    Pertinent laboratory tests included electrolytes and creatinine, which were normal.
12. Cystocele is a hernia of the bladder, usually into the vagina and introitus.
    The patient's history is remarkable for cystocele repair and cholecystectomy.
13. Decubitus is a recumbent or horizontal position.
    The patient was placed in the left lateral decubitus position.
14. Dysphagia is the difficulty in swallowing.
    He denies any regular symptoms of dysphagia.
15. Electrolyte is any solution compound that conducts electricity.
    Pertinent laboratory tests included electrolytes and creatinine, which were normal.
16. Emesis is to vomit.
    She denies emesis.
17. Endoscopy is the examination of the interior of a canal or hollow viscus by means of endoscope.
    The gastroenterologist will perform an upper endoscopy later this morning.
18. Erythema is the redness of the skin due to capillary dilatation.
    An abdominal exam revealed that the PEG tube site is somewhat erythematous, with a fungal-appearing rash.
19. Exacerbation is an increase in the severity of a disease or symptoms.
    My impression is that this patient has classic symptoms of colitis with recent exacerbation.
20. Folate is folic acid.
    Her medications included folate 1 mg daily.
21. Formalin is a 37% aqueous solution of formaldehyde.
    The liver biopsy was sent in a formalin jar for pathological analysis.
22. Gastritis is an inflammation of the stomach, especially the mucosa.
    She was noted to have some chronic gastritis, but no evidence of ulcer disease.
23. Gastroesophageal relates to both the stomach and the esophagus.
    He denies any regular symptoms of dysphagia or gastroesophageal reflux.
24. Gastrointestinal relates to the stomach and the intestines.
    The patient's transient gastrointestinal distress has since resolved.

25. Gastroparesis is a slight degree of gastroparalysis.
The patient's past medical history is notable for diabetes mellitus, diabetic neuropathy, diabetic gastroparesis, diabetic retinopathy, and amputation of several toes.

26. Gastrostomy is the establishment of a new opening into the stomach.
The gastroenterologist replaced the PEG tube with a new replacement balloon gastrostomy kit.

27. Hematemesis is to vomit blood, indicating upper gastrointestinal bleeding.
The patient had no prior history of ulcer disease or hematemesis.

28. Hematochezia is the passage of bloody stools.
He presents today with 4 days of increasing, painless hematochezia.

29. Heme is the oxygen-carrying, color-furnishing group of hemoglobin.
She has heme-positive emesis.

30. Hemicolectomy is the removal of the right or left side of the colon.
This 79-year-old white lady presents for a 4-year follow-up colonoscopy evaluation of a right hemicolectomy performed on November 4, 1999.

31. Heparin is a generic name for an anticoagulant.
With the colonoscopy, she would have to stop her current medication, go on heparin, get the colonoscopy done, then go back on the medication.

32. Hepatosplenomegaly is the enlargement of the liver and spleen.
Soft and nontender abdomen, with no hepatosplenomegaly.

33. Hydrocortisone is a generic name for a corticosteroid.
Her current medications include hydrocortisone and aspirin.

34. Icterus is jaundice.
There is no scleral icterus.

35. Ketone is any compound containing carbon oxide.
Urinalysis shows trace ketones and a small amount of blood.

36. Labyrinthitis is the inflammation of the otitis interna.
The patient's past medical history was remarkable for an episode of labyrinthis.

37. Laminectomy is the surgical excision of the lamina.
This is a 45-year-old black female who 3 weeks ago underwent a cervical laminectomy of C5 and C6.

38. Lidocaine is a generic name for a local anesthetic; used as a cardiac antiarrhythmic.
Lidocaine 1% was used for topical anesthesia of the skin, - subcutaneous tissue, and down to the intercostal space.

39. Lumen is the cavity or channel within a tube.
There were no polyps or other lesions noted upon careful inspection of the lumen upon withdrawal of the endoscope.

40. Lymphadenopathy is the disease of the lymph nodes.
He had no lymphadenopathy.

41. Malaise is a feeling of uneasiness.
She also has anorexia with severely decreased oral intake, as well as malaise and severe fatigue.

42. Meclizine is a generic name for an antinauseant.
The patient was admitted for symptomatic therapy with meclizine as well as for intravenous therapy.

43. Melena is the darkening of the feces by blood pigments.
She denies any fever, chills, diarrhea, melena, hematemesis, hematochezia, or abdominal pain.

44. Motility is the ability to move spontaneously.
The patient is a very pleasant 48-year-old white female who I have previously seen for constipation that was due to a motility-related disturbance as a complication of her polio.

45. Myalgia is muscular pain.
She has had episodic fevers and chills, as well as myalgia over the last 3 weeks.

46. Nitroglycerin is a generic name for a vasodilator and is used to relieve certain types of pain.
Her current medications include hydrocortisone and nitroglycerin paste.

47. Nystagmus is the involuntary, rapid, rhythmic movement of the eyeball.
The patient's extraocular movements were intact, except for horizontal nystagmus of 3-4 beats.

48. Occult is specimen hidden from view.

A rectal exam reveals heme-negative brown stool, which tests negative for occult blood.

49. Odynophagia is the burning, squeezing pain while swallowing.
He denies any regular symptoms of dysphagia, odynophagia, or gastroesophageal reflux.

50. Pinna is the projecting part of the ear lying outside the head.
Pinna is normal.

51. Polyp is any growth or mass protruding from a mucous membrane.
The patient had a past history of multiple polyps.

52. Postprandial is after a meal.
He has a long history of postprandial heartburn and indigestion.

53. Prednisone is a generic name for an anti-inflammatory and antiallergic agent.
The patient was treated with prednisone and antibiotics.

54. Proctitis is the inflammation of the rectum.
He does have occasional red blood mixed in with his stool, which has been attributed to radiation proctitis.

55. Prophylactic is an agent that tends to ward off disease.
The patient was prescribed prophylactic treatments for her asthma.

56. Prostate is a gland in the male that surrounds the neck of the bladder and urethra.
The patient has an enlarged prostate.

57. Pyridoxine is one of the forms of vitamin B6.
Her medication included pyridoxine 250 mg daily.

58. Rectocele is the hernial protrusion of part of the rectum into the vagina.
The patient's history is remarkable for rectocele and cystocele repair and cholecystectomy.

59. Reflux is a backward or return flow.
He denies any regular symptoms of dysphagia, odynophagia, or gastroesophageal reflux.

60. Retroflexion is the bending of an organ so that its top is thrust backward.
There were no abnormalities noted, and retroflexion in the rectum was unremarkable.

61. Sclera is the tough white outer coat of the eyeball.
There is no scleral icterus.

62. Sigmoidoscope is an endoscope for use in sigmoidoscopy.
The patient had a normal sigmoidoscope examination.

63. Sigmoidoscopy is the direct examination of the interior of the sigmoid colon.
Sigmoidoscopy was completed to 60 cm into the descending colon.

64. Stenosis is the narrowing of a body passage or opening.
She has been in excellent health until approximately 1 month ago, when she underwent aortic valve replacement due to aortic stenosis.

65. Stent is a mold for keeping a skin graft in place.
He has a history of coronary artery disease and has had stenting in the past.

66. Thyromegaly is the enlargement of the thyroid gland.
He had no thyromegaly or lymphadenopathy.

67. Titrate is to analyze a given solution component by adding a liquid reagent.
We will then titrate his dose to the lowest possible dose required to control his reflux symptoms.

68. Turgor is the condition of fullness; the expected resiliency of the skin.
Skin color, turgor, and texture are normal for her age.

69. Ativan is the trade name for an antianxiety agent.
Her medications included Ativan.

70. Axid is the trade name for an antagonist for the treatment of gastric and duodenal ulcers.
He has been on Axid.

71. Bumex is the trade name for a loop diuretic.
Her current medications include hydrocortisone, Bumex, and nitroglycerin paste.

72. Chem-7 is the trade name for a profile of seven different chemical laboratory tests.
The gastroenterologist ordered a Chem-7, RBC, WBC, and partial thromboplastin time.

73. Coumadin is the trade name for an anticoagulant.
    With the colonoscopy, she would have to stop her Coumadin, go on heparin, get the colonoscopy done, then go back on the heparin and Coumadin.
74. Demerol is the trade name for a synthetic narcotic analgesic.
    The anesthesia administered was Demerol 25 mg IV.
75. Dilantin is the trade name for an anticonvulsant used in the treatment of epilepsy.
    Her current medications include hydrocortisone, Bumex, Dilantin, and nitroglycerin paste.
76. Elavil is the trade name for an antidepressant.
    Her medications included Elavil.
77. Hemoccult is the trade name for a guaiac test for occult blood.
    A rectal exam showed no stool available for Hemoccult evaluation.
78. Humulin is the trade name for an antidiabetic.
    The patient is diabetic and currently being treated with Humulin 45 units daily in the morning.
79. Hytrin is the trade name for an antihypertensive used in the treatment of benign prostatic hyperplasia.
    His only past medical history is that of benign prostatic hypertrophy, for which he takes Hytrin.
80. Indocin is the trade name for a nonsteroidal anti-inflammatory agent.
    Her medications included Indocin daily, nitroglycerin patch 0.4 mg/hr daily, and aspirin every other day.
81. K-Dur is the trade name for a potassium supplement.
    Her current medications include hydrocortisone, K-Dur, Bumex, Dilantin, and nitroglycerin paste.
82. Lopressor is the trade name for an antihypertensive.
    Her current medications include hydrocortisone, K-Dur, Bumex, Lopressor, Dilantin, and nitroglycerin paste.
83. Macrobid is the trade name for an urinary bacteriostatic.
    She has been taking Macrobid for the past 5 days for a urinary tract infection.
84. Maxzide is the trade name for a diuretic and antihypertensive.
    Her only medication has been Maxzide for hypertension.
85. Metamucil is the trade name for a bulk laxative.
    Her medications included Indocin daily, nitroglycerin patch 0.4 mg/hr daily, aspirin every other day, and Metamucil.
86. Naprosyn is the trade name for a nonsteroidal anti-inflammatory agent.
    She has been taking Naprosyn on a chronic basis, and over the last 4-5 days she has been having melenic stools.
87. Norvasc is the trade name for an antianginal and antihypertensive.
    Her medications included Norvasc 25 mg daily, aspirin daily, folate 1 mg daily, and pyridoxine 250 mg daily.
88. Paxil is the trade name for an antidepressant.
    Her medications included Paxil for her anxiety attacks.
89. Pepcid is the trade name for an acid controller for heartburn and acid indigestion.
    He had been placed originally on Pepcid 20 mg t.i.d. with initial relief.
90. Prilosec is the trade name for a gastric acid secretion inhibitor.
    Her medications included Norvasc 25 mg daily, aspirin daily, folate 1 mg daily, pyridoxine 50 mg daily, and most recently, Prilosec 20 mg daily.
91. Procardia is the trade name for a coronary vasodilator.
    The patient was taking Procardia 30 mg t.i.d.
92. Reglan is the trade name for a gastrointestinal stimulant, antiemetic.
    He reports that this problem was treated in the past with Reglan with some improvement.
93. Ritalin is the trade name for a mild central nervous system stimulant and antidepressant.
    Current medications are Ritalin, which he is taking for attention deficit disorder.
94. Synthroid is the trade name for a thyroid hormone.
    Her current medications include Synthroid, hydrocortisone, K-Dur, Bumex, Lopressor, Dilantin, Prilosec, and nitroglycerin paste.
95. Tenormin is the trade name for an antihypertensive.
    The patient's medications include Tenormin and Pepcid.
96. Terramycin is the trade name for an antibiotic.
    The patient is allergic to PENICILLIN and TERRAMYCIN.
97. Tigan is the trade name for an antiemetic.
    The patient was admitted for symptomatic therapy with meclizine and Tigan as well as for intravenous therapy.
98. Timoptic is the trade name for a beta blocker, antiglaucoma agent.
    The patient is currently on Coumadin and Timoptic.
99. Vasotec is the trade name for an antihypertensive.
    Her current medications include Synthroid, hydrocortisone, K-Dur, Bumex, Lopressor, Vasotec, Dilantin, Prilosec, and nitroglycerin paste.
100. Versed is the trade name for a short-acting benzodiazepine general anesthetic adjunct for preoperative sedation.
    The anesthesia administered was Demerol 25 mg IV and Versed 2 mg IV.
101. Zocor is the trade name for a reductase inhibitor for hypercholesterolemia and coronary heart disease.
    Her medications included Norvasc 25 mg daily, Zocor 20 mg at bedtime, aspirin daily, folate 1 mg daily, pyridoxine 250 mg daily, and most recently, Prilosec 20 mg daily.

CHAPTER 9 / TERMINOLOGY CHECK YOUR PROGRESS

1. b	27. c	53. d	79. d
2. d	28. b	54. c	80. b
3. c	29. d	55. a	81. c
4. a	30. d	56. c	82. d
5. d	31. a	57. a	83. c
6. a	32. b	58. a	84. a
7. a	33. a	59. d	85. b
8. c	34. d	60. c	86. c
9. a	35. c	61. c	87. b
10. c	36. a	62. d	88. d
11. a	37. b	63. c	89. a
12. a	38. a	64. a	90. c
13. b	39. b	65. b	91. a
14. b	40. a	66. a	92. a
15. d	41. c	67. a	93. c
16. c	42. a	68. a	94. c
17. b	43. c	69. c	95. b
18. a	44. a	70. d	96. a
19. d	45. b	71. a	97. b
20. b	46. a	72. c	98. c
21. a	47. d	73. b	99. b
22. b	48. a	74. d	100. c
23. b	49. c	75. d	
24. a	50. b	76. a	
25. a	51. b	77. a	
26. d	52. c	78. b	

CHAPTER 9 / ACTIVITY 9–4

Errors are indicated in **bold italic**. Margins are formatted at 1 inch.

HISTORY AND PHYSICAL EXAMINATION

Patient Name: Schupp, Lacey

File Number: 00841

Date of Birth: November 2, 19xx

Examination Date: *current date*

Physician: Anna Bolism, MD

HISTORY

Double space
CHIEF COMPLAINT
Melenic stools.

Double space
HISTORY OF ***PRESENT*** ILLNESS
The patient is a very pleasant ***48-year-old*** white ***female*** who I have previously ***seen*** for constipation that was due to a ***motility-related*** disturbance as a complication of her polio. ***She*** has been taking ***Naprosyn*** on a chronic ***basis***, and over the last ***4-5*** days she has been having melenic stools. During the same time frame, she has ***noted*** progressive fatigue and weakness. A ***hemoglobin*** study performed in Dr. Geiger's office showed that her ***hemoglobin*** was in the ***6.5*** range, and she was admitted to University Hospital. She denies any ***abdominal*** pain. There is ***no*** prior history of ulcer disease or ***hematemesis***. She has lost about ***3-5 pounds*** over this same time frame.

Double space
PAST MEDICAL HISTORY
She has had numerous postpolio complications, including a neurogenic bladder and constipation. She has had several back ***surgeries*** as well as a wrist operation. ***She*** does not smoke or drink.

Double space
MEDICATIONS
1. ***Naprosyn.***
2. ***Paxil.***
3. ***Elavil.***
4. Ativan.

Double space
FAMILY HISTORY
Noncontributory.

Double space
PHYSICAL ***EXAMINATION***

GENERAL: A pale white female who is in no acute distress.

HEART: Negative.

LUNGS: Negative.

ABDOMEN: Negative.

RECTAL: A rectal exam showed ***no*** stool available for ***Hemoccult*** evaluation.

continued

HISTORY AND PHYSICAL EXAMINATION
Patient Name: Schupp, Lacey
File Number: 00841

Page 2

LABORATORY DATA
Lab studies show a BUN elevated at ***33*** with a ***creatinine*** of ***0.4***. ***Her electrolytes*** were normal, as were her platelet count and ***coagulation*** time. ***Hemoglobin*** was ***6.9***.

IMPRESSION
GI bleed. ***It is*** almost certainly upper GI bleeding due to nonsteroid use.

PLAN
Transfuse 2 units of packed ***cells***.
Perform an upper ***endoscopy*** later this morning. We will make ***further recommendations*** after the ***endoscopy***.

Quadruple space

_____
Anna Bolism, ***MD***
ab:xx
D: current date
T: current date

CHAPTER 9 / ACTIVITY 9–5

Errors are indicated in **bold italic.** Margins are formatted at 1 inch.

OPERATIVE REPORT
Patient Name: Artemis, Jacob

File Number: 00864

Date of Birth: December 12, 1958

Operation Date: current date

PREOPERATIVE DIAGNOSIS
Hepatitis C and mildly elevated liver enzymes.

POSTOPERATIVE DIAGNOSIS
Hepatitis C and mildly elevated liver enzymes.

OPERATION
Percutaneous liver biopsy under ultrasound guidance.

PROCEDURE
The patient was ***counseled***. Potential complications were explained. ***Consent*** was obtained. The patient was ***placed*** supine on the exam table. ***Ultrasound*** was used to scan in the midaxillary line. The liver margins were identified, and the best location for the liver ***biopsy*** was selected along the ***midaxillary*** line at ***approximately*** the ***10th intercostal*** space. The skin was then ***prepped*** and draped in the usual sterile manner. ***Lidocaine 1%*** was used for topical anesthesia of the skin, ***subcutaneous*** tissue, and down to the ***intercostal*** space. A ***#22***-gauge spinal needle was used to sound the depth of the liver.

Because of the ***patient's*** obesity, the liver was found to be approximately ***5 cm*** from the skin surface. The Klatskin needle was then attached to a glass syringe filled with sterile saline. The ***Klatskin*** needle was inserted into the intercostal space and then subsequently into the liver for a quick suction biopsy. The first ***pass*** yielded only a ***5 mm*** fragment of tissue. A second pass was therefore performed, which yielded a much larger ***4 cm piece*** of ***tan-appearing*** liver. The liver biopsy was ***sent*** in a ***formalin*** jar for pathological ***analysis***. The skin was then dressed and ***taped***. The patient was then observed ***for 4*** hours. No immediate complications were observed. Postbiopsy vital signs were normal. The patient tolerated the procedure well, ***without*** any complications.

IMPRESSION
Hepatitis C and mildly elevated liver enzymes.

Quadruple space

_____
Kate Cobalamin, ***MD***
kc:xx
D: current date
T: current date

1. a	24. d	47. a	70. a
2. c	25. a	48. b	71. a
3. b	26. d	49. c	72. d
4. c	27. b	50. a	73. b
5. b	28. d	51. a	74. a
6. d	29. a	52. a	75. c
7. c	30. c	53. a	76. a
8. a	31. b	54. c	77. c
9. a	32. b	55. d	78. b
10. b	33. d	56. d	79. a
11. a	34. a	57. a	80. d
12. d	35. a	58. b	81. a
13. a	36. a	59. a	82. a
14. b	37. b	60. d	83. b
15. d	38. c	61. d	84. d
16. b	39. a	62. b	85. c
17. b	40. b	63. c	86. c
18. a	41. a	64. a	87. b
19. b	42. d	65. a	88. b
20. b	43. b	66. c	89. d
21. a	44. a	67. d	90. a
22. c	45. c	68. b	91. b
23. d	46. b	69. c	92. c

CHAPTER 10 / ACTIVITY 10-3 (10T-1)

1. Afebrile is without fever.
He is palpably afebrile.
2. Amaurosis is the loss of sight without the apparent lesion of the eye.
She has noted some intermittent visual symptoms in her left eye; however, I would not clearly call it amaurosis fugax.
3. Aneurysm is a localized abnormal dilatation of the wall of a blood vessel.
The physician felt no abdominal aortic aneurysm.
4. Angiography is the radiographic visualization of a blood vessel after injecting a contrast agent.
The patient requires a coronary angiography.
5. Arrhythmia is the variation from the normal rhythm of the heartbeat.
She has a history of hypertension, glaucoma, and arrhythmia.
6. Arteriography is the radiography of an artery after injection of a contrast medium in the bloodstream.
Combined coronary arteriography with cerebral angiography would be appropriate.
7. Atherosclerotic is the hardening of an artery due to deposits of plaque within the vessel.
She has a family history of atherosclerotic disease.
8. Atrial pertains to the atrium.
She has a history of chronic atrial fibrillation and sleep apnea.
9. Bradycardia is a slow heartbeat.
An electrocardiogram revealed bradycardia, and a junctional rhythm was documented.
10. Bruit is a sound or murmur heard in auscultation.
The abdomen contains no masses and no bruits.
11. Cardiomyopathy is the disease process of the heart muscle.
The patient is a 35-year-old with documented cardiomyopathy.
12. Cardioverter is a device used to administer electrical shocks to the heart.
The patient was given intravenous diuretics and readjusted her medicines to try to medically or electrically cardiovert her.
13. Carotid relates to the principal artery of the neck.
Carotid bruits are not heard.
14. Cholecystectomy is the surgical removal of the gallbladder.
She is scheduled next Wednesday morning for a laparoscopic cholecystectomy and possible open cholecystectomy.
15. Claudication is the cramp-like pains in the calf; limping.
She has a history of peripheral vascular disease and is status post left iliac angioplasty with good results and no residual claudication.
16. Collateral is a secondary or accessory blood pathway.
This is a 68-year-old male with single vessel coronary involving the left circumflex and bridging collaterals on the right coronary artery.
17. Cyanosis is a dark-bluish or purplish coloration of the skin due to deficient oxygenation of the blood.
No cyanosis or edema noted.
18. Diaphoresis is perspiration.
He developed chest pain suddenly 2 hours ago with diaphoresis and nausea.
19. Digoxin is a generic name for a cardiotonic.
Her medications included digoxin 0.125 mg daily and a laxative.
20. Diltiazem is a generic name for a coronary vasodilator.
She denies hypertension, although she is on diltiazem at the time of her arrival in my office.
21. Dobutamine is a generic name for a cardiotonic agent.
He was recently hospitalized several weeks ago for intravenous dobutamine therapy.
22. Duodenal relates to the duodenum, the first division of the small intestine.
She has a history of peptic ulcer disease and a bleeding duodenal ulcer.
23. Dysrhythmia is a defective rhythm.
She has a history of cardiac dysrhythmia in the past.
24. Echocardiogram is a diagnostic procedure using ultrasound to study heart structure and motion.
She had an echocardiogram and Holter monitor exam at that time.
25. Endarterectomy is a surgical procedure done to clear a blocked artery.
The patient underwent coronary artery bypass grafting on August 18, 1996, with right carotid endarterectomy at the same time.
26. Epiphysis is the center for the ossification at the proximal and distal ends of a long bone.
The patient's past medical history was significant for open reduction internal fixation of the right hip for what sounds like slipped capital femoral epiphysis disease.
27. Erythema is the redness of the skin due to capillary dilatation.
There is minimal erythema.
28. Expiratory relates to exhalation.
There is a moderately slight prolonged expiratory phase.
29. Fibrillation is the exceedingly rapid contractions of muscular fibrils.
She has a history of chronic atrial fibrillation and sleep apnea.
30. Gallop is a triple cadence to the heart sounds.
There are no significant murmurs or gallops.
31. Gout is a disorder associated with an inborn error of uric acid metabolism that increases production or interferes with the excretion of uric acid.
The patient also has a history of gout.
32. Hemiblock is the failure to conduct an impulse down one division of the left bundle branch.
The electrocardiogram shows a left anterior hemiblock, normal sinus rhythm, and premature arterial contractions.
33. Hemoptysis is the coughing or spitting of blood from the respiratory tract.
Negative for cough sputum or hemoptysis.
34. Heparin is a generic name for an anticoagulant.
The patient is refusing to consider intravenous heparin or any form of IV therapy or blood work.
35. Hypercholesterolemia is the presence of an abnormally large amount of cholesterol in the cells and plasma of the blood.
The patient is a 56-year-old gentleman with a history of chest pain, with negative evaluation in the past, and hypercholesterolemia.

36. Hyperkalemia is the greater than normal concentration of potassium ions in the blood.
He has hyperkalemia with an elevated potassium at 7.7.

37. Hyperlipidemia is a condition of elevated lipid levels in the blood.
The patient also has a history of mild hyperlipidemia and gout.

38. Hypotensive is characterized by low blood pressure or causing a reduction in blood pressure.
The patient would get so weak, dehydrated, and hypotensive that her diuretics would be cut back.

39. Idiopathic is a disease of unknown cause.
The patient is a 35-year-old with documented idiopathic cardiomyopathy.

40. Iliac relates to the ilium.
She has a history of peripheral vascular disease and is status post left iliac angioplasty with good results and no residual claudication.

41. Infarction is the sudden insufficiency of arterial or venous blood supply.
He presented to the University Hospital Emergency Room, and an acute inferior infarction was noted by the ECG.

42. Inferolateral pertains to a location situated below and to the side.
Testing shows anteroapical and inferolateral anemia.

43. Inotropic pertains to the force of muscular contractions.
Parenteral inotropic agents will again be employed.

44. Intimal relates to the inner coat of a vessel.
In August 1994, the patient did have a heart catheterization that demonstrated decreased left ventricular function and intimal coronary artery disease.

45. Ischemia is the decreased supply of oxygenated blood to a body part.
His 12-lead ECG shows no evidence of transmural ischemia.

46. Mediastinum is the mass of tissues and organs separating the sternum in front and the vertebral column behind.
Mediastinum looks normal size.

47. Myocardial pertains to the muscular tissue of the heart.
The patient's chest discomfort could certainly be attributed to myocardial ischemia and infarction, and this should be excluded.

48. Normocephalic is the normal size of the head.
The head is normocephalic, atraumatic.

49. Nortriptyline is a generic name for an antidepressant.
The patient's medications included nortriptyline 50 nightly.

50. Paroxysm is the sudden recurrence or increase in intensity of symptoms.
She has a history of paroxysmal atrial fibrillation and chronic atrial fibrillation.

51. Pectoralis pertains to the chest or breast.
There has been no definite angina pectoralis nor definite symptoms related to his right carotid lesion.

52. Pedal pertains to the foot or feet.
There is 1+ pedal edema.

53. Pitting is the formation of a small depression.
She has 4+ pitting edema of her lower extremities bilaterally.

54. Pleura is the serous membrane investing the lungs and lining the walls of the thoracic cavity.
She denies shortness of breath or pleuritic chest pain.

55. Polycythemia is an increase in the total red cell mass of the blood.
The patient has a history of polycythemia secondary to her COPD.

56. Quinidine is a generic name for an antiarrhythmic agent used in the treatment of atrial flutter, atrial fibrillation, premature ventricular contractions, and tachycardias.
The patient was medically converted with quinidine, and she improved.

57. Rhonchus is a continuous dry rattling in the throat or bronchial tube due to a partial obstruction, heard on auscultation.
Occasional rhonchi are present in the chest

58. Sinus is a cavity or channel.
ECG was done and appears to be normal sinus rhythm.

59. Stenosis is the narrowing or contraction of a body passage.
A carotid sonogram documents an 80%- 99% stenosis in the left internal carotid artery.

60. Syncope is a temporary suspension of consciousness; fainting.
The patient denies dizziness, lightheadedness, or syncope.

61. Tachycardia is an abnormal rapid heart rate.
The physician ruled out supraventricular tachycardia.

62. Thrombosis is the formation of a blood clot within the vascular system.
The question of deep venous thrombosis has been raised.

63. Venous pertains to the veins.
Venous pulses are unremarkable.

64. Verapamil is a generic name for a coronary vasodilator.
He has been on verapamil therapy.

65. Capoten is the trade name for an antihypertensive.
The patient's medications included Capoten 12.5 mg t.i.d.

66. Cardiolite is the trade name for myocardial perfusion agent for cardiac SPECT imaging.
Persantine IV Cardiolite shows anteroapical and inferolateral ischemia.

67. Cardizem is the trade name for a calcium channel blocker for atrial fibrillation.
His medications include Cardizem 60 t.i.d. and aspirin.

68. Coumadin is the trade name for an anticoagulant.
She has a history of paroxysmal atrial fibrillation, chronic atrial fibrillation, and is on Coumadin at home.

69. Cytotec is the trade name for an antisecretory, gastric protectant for the prevention of nonsteroidal anti-inflammatory drug–induced gastric ulcers.
The patient's current medication is Cytotec 100 mg daily.

70. Ecotrin is the trade name for an analgesic, anti-inflammatory.
Her medications include Ecotrin 1 daily.

71. Indocin is the trade name for nonsteroidal anti-inflammatory drug.
The patient's current medications are Indocin 25 mg daily and Cytotec 100 mg daily.

72. Isordil is the trade name for an antianginal.
His medications included Cardizem 60 mg t.i.d., Isordil 20 mg t.i.d., and aspirin.

73. K-Dur is the trade name for a potassium supplement.
The patient's current medications are Capoten 12.5 mg t.i.d., K-Dur 20 mEq b.i.d., and digoxin 0.125 mg daily.

74. Lanoxin is the trade name for a cardiac glycoside to increase cardiac output.
The patient's medications included Coumadin per prothrombin times at home and Lanoxin 0.25 mg daily.

75. Lasix is the trade name for a diuretic.
She will have her Lasix increased, and start on nitrates.

76. Lescol is the trade name for a reductase inhibitor for hypercholesterolemia.
The patient's medications included Ecotrin, 1 mg daily, Lescol, 20 mg daily, and nortriptyline, 50 mg nightly.

77. Lotensin is the trade name for an antihypertensive.
The patient was prescribed Lotensin 1 tablet daily.

78. Mevacor is the trade name for a reductase inhibitor for hypercholesterolemia.
The patient's current medications included Cardizem 60 mg t.i.d., Mevacor 20 mg, Isordil 20 mg t.i.d., and aspirin, which was stopped 6 days prior to surgery.

79. Persantine is the trade name for a coronary vasodilator.
Persantine IV Cardiolite shows anteroapical and inferolateral ischemia.

80. Premarin is the trade name for estrogen replacement therapy.
Her current medications include Premarin.

81. Provera is the trade name for progestin for secondary amenorrhea and abnormal uterine bleeding.
Her current medications include Premarin and Provera.

82. Quinidex is the trade name for an antiarrhythmic.
The patient's current medications include Capoten 12.5 mg t.i.d., K-Dur 20 mEq b.i.d., Quinidex 300 mg b.i.d., and digoxin 0.125 mg daily.

83. Reglan is the trade name for a gastrointestinal stimulant; antiemetic.
The patient had a history of intolerance to Reglan.

84. Senokot is the trade name for a laxative.
Her medications included digoxin 0.125 mg daily and Senokot.

85. Synthroid is the trade name for a thyroid hormone.
The patient's medications included Synthroid 0.1 mg daily, Ecotrin 1 mg daily, Lescol 20 mg daily, and nortriptyline 50 mg nightly.
86. Tenormin is the trade name for a beta blocker; antihypertensive agent.
The patient's current medications are Tenormin 12.5 mg b.i.d., Indocin 25 mg daily, and Cytotec 100 mg daily.
87. Terramycin is the trade name for an antibiotic.
The patient is allergic to TERRAMYCIN.
88. Theo-Dur is the trade name for a bronchodilator.
The patient's medications included Coumadin per prothrombin times at home, Lanoxin 0.25 mg daily, and Theo-Dur 300 mg b.i.d.
89. Trental is the trade name for an oral hemorheologic drug.
The patient's current medications are vitamin E, vitamin C, Trental, beta carotene, and Centrum Silver 1 tablet daily.
90. Vasotec is the trade name for an antihypertensive agent.
She will be continued on her Vasotec, have her Lasix increased, and start on nitrates.
91. Xanax is the trade name for an antianxiety agent.
Her current medications include Xanax, Premarin, and Provera.
92. Zyloprim is the trade name for an antigout agent.
The patient's current medications are vitamin E, vitamin C, Trental, beta carotene, Centrum Silver 1 tablet daily, and Zyloprim.

CHAPTER 10 / TERMINOLOGY CHECK YOUR PROGRESS

1. a	24. a	47. a	70. a
2. c	25. b	48. b	71. a
3. b	26. a	49. b	72. d
4. d	27. c	50. d	73. b
5. d	28. b	51. b	74. a
6. a	29. a	52. a	75. c
7. b	30. a	53. d	76. a
8. a	31. a	54. a	77. c
9. d	32. b	55. b	78. b
10. d	33. b	56. a	79. a
11. c	34. b	57. a	80. d
12. a	35. c	58. c	81. a
13. a	36. a	59. d	82. a
14. a	37. d	60. b	83. b
15. a	38. b	61. c	84. d
16. c	39. d	62. b	85. c
17. b	40. a	63. c	86. c
18. a	41. d	64. a	87. b
19. b	42. d	65. a	88. a
20. c	43. c	66. c	89. d
21. a	44. a	67. d	90. a
22. b	45. b	68. b	91. b
23. d	46. b	69. c	92. c

CHAPTER 10 / ACTIVITY 10–4

Errors are indicated in **bold italic**. Margins are formatted at 1 inch.

current date
Charles P. Davis, MD
FedDes Wellness Center
Family Practice Division, Suite 300
101 Wellness Way Drive
New York, NY 10036

Double space
Re: George Niehls
      Date of Birth: January 16, 19xx

Dear Dr. Davis

George Niehls is a ***62-year-old*** man who was admitted for a cystectomy because of carcinoma of the bladder. ***He*** has a history of ***intermittent*** visual ***blurring***. A routine physical examination revealed a right carotid bruit. A carotid ***sonogram*** was obtained***,*** which suggested ***high-grade*** stenosis of the ***right*** internal carotid. He is a ***long-time*** cigarette smoker and has moderate exertional ***dyspnea***. There has been no definite angina ***pectoralis*** nor definite symptoms related to his right ***carotid lesion***. There is a long history of hypotension***,*** but drug therapy was ***discontinued*** in 1990.

Physical examination ***shows*** a blood pressure of ***180/100*** and a pulse of 80 and regular. Venous pulses are unremarkable. There is a long ***right*** carotid ***bruit***. ***Occasional rhonchi*** are present in the chest***,*** and there is a moderately slightly***,*** prolonged ***expiratory phase***. The heart is not ***enlarged***. ***There*** are no significant ***murmurs*** or gallops. The ***abdomen*** contains no ***masses*** and no bruits. There is no ***peripheral*** edema.

Mr. Niehls would appear to have ***high-grade*** carotid artery ***stenosis***. With contemplated major surgery***,*** this should presumably be repaired ***preoperatively*** despite ***its*** essentially ***asymptomatic*** state. In addition***,*** combined coronary ***arteriography*** with cerebral angiography would be ***appropriate***. With his long history of hypertension***,*** it would seem reasonable to also perform a renal ***arteriogram*** during the same procedure.

George Niehls
Current date
Page 2

We will arrange these studies***,*** and subsequent ***recommendations*** will be based on the results of the diagnostic findings. We appreciate the opportunity to participate in ***his care***.

Sincerely

Quadruple space

_____

Lucas Site***,*** MD
xx

Errors are indicated in **bold italic**. Margins are formatted at 1 inch.

HISTORY AND PHYSICAL EXAMINATION REPORT

Patient Name: Rolf, Nathan

File Number: 59025

Date of Birth: February 21, 19xx

Examination Date: *current date*

Physician: Adam Valence, MD

HISTORY

CHIEF COMPLAINT
Shortness of **breath**.

HISTORY OF PRESENT ILLNESS
Nathan Rolf is a **35-year-old** male with documented **idiopathic cardiomyopathy**. **He** became symptomatic in 1995**,** and a subsequent cardiac catheterization was performed in 1997**,** at which time an ejection **fraction** of 25 was documented. His symptoms have progressed**,** and **he** was recently hospitalized several weeks ago for intravenous **dobutamine** therapy. He symptomatically improved**,** but in the past week he developed increasing **dyspnea** and **orthopnea**.

PHYSICAL EXAMINATION

VITAL SIGNS: Physical examination shows a blood pressure of **130/73** and a pulse of 112 and irregular.

NECK: Jugular **venous** pulse is slightly prominent.

CHEST: The chest is fairly clear.

HEART: The heart is moderately **enlarged** with an **S3** gallop. No significant murmurs.

IMPRESSION
Mr. Rolf has severe cardiomyopathy. **Parenteral inotropic** agents will again be **employed**. Presumably his gastrointestinal symptoms **are** also indicative of congestive heart failure**,** but a complicating **factor** needs to be **excluded** as well.

PLAN
Admit to **University** Hospital due to **his** increasing **dyspnea** and **orthopnea**. He will again be **assessed** for a possible cardiac transplantation.

_____

Adam Valence, MD
av:xx
D: *current date*
T: *current date*

CHAPTER 11 / TERMINOLOGY PRETEST

1. a	11. a	21. a	31. c
2. b	12. c	22. c	32. b
3. c	13. d	23. c	33. a
4. d	14. b	24. a	34. a
5. b	15. a	25. c	35. d
6. a	16. c	26. b	36. c
7. c	17. c	27. a	37. a
8. c	18. c	28. c	38. b
9. d	19. b	29. c	39. d
10. a	20. a	30. b	40. a

1. Acromioclavicular describes the articulation between the acromial process of the scapula and the clavicle.
   Mild degenerative changes are present at the acromioclavicular joint, characterized by mild inferior marginal spurring.
2. Amorphous is having no definite form, or shapeless.
   There is an amorphous calcific deposit in the right side of the pelvis measuring 2.3 x 0.8 cm, of which the exact etiology is not determined.
3. Anteverted is the abnormal forward tilting of an organ.
   Real-time ultrasound examination demonstrates a normal-size anteverted uterus, 10.3 cm in length, 4.1 cm in AP dimension.
4. Ascites is the effusion and accumulation of serous fluid in the abdominal cavity.
   There is no sonographic evidence of intra-abdominal mass, lymphadenopathy, or ascites.
5. Asymmetry is without symmetry, lacking similar form or relationship of parts.
   Asymmetry is therefore probably due to the superior position of unopacified bowel over the adnexa.
6. Bilateral is affecting both sides.
   Bilateral low-dose film screen mammography is compared to the study of October 12, 1999.
7. Calculus is a stone.
   I believe there is a 4 x 2-mm nonobstructing calculus in the proximal right ureter at the level of L3.
8. Carpometacarpal is the joint spaces between the carpal and metacarpal bones.
   Examination of the hands and wrists demonstrate degenerative changes at the 1st carpometacarpal joints bilaterally.
9. Centrum semiovale is the white matter of the cerebral hemispheres that has an almost oval shape.
   The lesions are contained to the deep white matter of the cerebrum and predominate in the centrum semiovale, bilaterally.
10. Contraindicate is a factor that makes it undesirable to treat a patient in the usual manner.
    A regular exercise program to include weightbearing exercise is also to be encouraged if not clinically contraindicated.
11. Contrast medium is the pharmaceutical given to the patient to allow radiographic visualization of a body structure.
    Computerized tomography was performed from the diaphragm to the symphysis pubis with the use of oral and intravenous contrast medium.
12. Cricopharyngeal is pertaining to the cricoid cartilage and the pharynx.
    Cricopharyngeal function is normal.
13. Demarcated is to set limits or boundaries.
    An 18 x 8 x 20-mm well-demarcated simple cyst is demonstrated within the central 12 o'clock position of the right breast corresponding to the well-demarcated density noted on mammography in this region.
14. Etiology is the science concerned with the causes or origin of a disease or disorder.
    There is an amorphous calcific deposit in the right side of the pelvis measuring 2.3 x 0.8 cm, of which the exact etiology is not determined.
15. Hiatus hernia is the herniation of an abdominal organ through the esophageal opening of the diaphragm.
    There is a tiny sliding hiatus hernia measuring 2 cm, which is not associated with reflux.
16. Hydronephrosis is the distention of the renal pelvis and calices with urine, often as a result of obstruction of the ureter.
    A survey of the kidneys reveals no left or right hydronephrosis.
17. Infarction is the death of a tissue due to lack of blood flow to the area.
    There is no evidence of hemorrhage or signs of infarction.
18. Intrahepatic is within the liver.
    The common bile duct and intrahepatic and extrahepatic biliary ducts are normal.
19. Ischemic is the lack of blood in a body part.
    Small vessel ischemic changes are seen in the convexity regions bilaterally, particularly on the right.

20. Jejunum is the second section of the small intestine.
    The stomach emptied in normal fashion with visualization of the jejunum.
21. Joint mouse is the loose bodies in synovial joints.
    A 2-mm oval osseous density is identified in the medial patellofemoral joint space consistent with a small joint mouse.
22. Lacuna is the small cavity within or between other body structures.
    An old lacunar infarct is present in the basal ganglia on the right side and the thalamus on the left side.
23. Lymphadenopathy is the disease of the lymph nodes.
    There is no retroperitoneal lymphadenopathy or pelvic lymphadenopathy.
24. Osteopenia is the decrease in bone mass below the normal.
    The degree of osteopenia is worse in the left hip with the reading at 2.19 standard deviations below the mean.
25. Parenchyma is the general anatomical term to describe the functional elements of an organ, as distinguished from its structure.
    The remainder of the testicular parenchyma has an inhomogeneous texture.
26. Paresthesia is the sensation of tingling and numbness.
    The patient reports a spastic bladder over the past 3 years with paresthesia involving the right leg over the past 6 years.
27. Passavant's cushion is a ridge appearing on the posterior wall of pharynx during swallowing due to contraction of palatopharyngeal sphincter.
    During swallowing, there is sufficient inferior motion of the soft palate and anterior movement of Passavant's cushion to prevent reflux into the nasopharynx.
28. Periarticular is situated around a joint.
    There are no periarticular calcifications.
29. Pericholecystic fluid is a coined term, meaning fluid around the gallbladder.
    I see no visible gallstones or pericholecystic fluid.
30. Reflux is a backward flow.
    There is no evidence of reflux or esophagitis.
31. Retroperitoneal is behind the peritoneum.
    There is no retroperitoneal adenopathy or ascites.
32. Stricture is an abnormal narrowing of a duct or passage.
    The ureter in the region appears mildly narrowed and somewhat variable, suggesting mild stricture or spasm.
33. Subluxation is a partial dislocation.
    There is no evidence of fracture or subluxation.
34. Thrombosis is a formation of a blood clot.
    There is no sonographic evidence of deep venous thrombosis.
35. Transducer is a device that translates one form of energy to another.
    The transducer was repositioned to allow determination of fetal age.
36. Vertex is the top or crown of the head.
    Transverse and longitudinal sonograms of the maternal abdomen were performed, revealing a single intrauterine gestation in vertex presentation.
37. Isovue is the trade name for a drug used as a contrast medium.
    Isovue was administered via intrathecal injection.
38. Lescol is the trade name for a drug that decreases LDL cholesterol.
    She lists her current medications and supplements as Synthroid and Lescol.
39. Provera is the trade name for a drug used in restoring hormonal imbalance.
    The patient lists her current medications as Estrace and Provera.
40. Synthroid is the trade name for a drug used as a replacement in decreased or absent thyroid function.
    She lists her current medications as Synthroid and pain medication, which she takes only as needed.

CHAPTER 11 / TERMINOLOGY CHECK YOUR PROGRESS

1. a	11. c	21. c	31. d
2. a	12. a	22. d	32. c
3. a	13. c	23. c	33. a
4. c	14. a	24. b	34. b
5. d	15. a	25. a	35. a
6. c	16. b	26. c	36. c
7. d	17. b	27. a	37. d
8. c	18. c	28. c	38. a
9. c	19. b	29. b	39. b
10. a	20. a	30. c	40. a

CHAPTER 11 / ACTIVITY 11–4

Errors are indicated in **bold italic**. Margins are formatted at 1 inch.

current date
P.H. Waters, MD
FedDes Wellness Center
Family Practice Division, Suite 300
101 Wellness Way Drive
New York, NY 10036

Re: Robin Hatherode
   Date of Birth: **December 19, 1953**
   Examination: LEFT WRIST **ARTHROGRAM**.

Dear Dr. Waters

Scout films are unremarkable.
Following appropriate preparation of the skin, a #22-**gauge** needle was inserted into the **radionavicular** joint and 2 mL of iodinated **contrast** media was injected. Films were then obtained after minimal manipulation of the wrist. **An** additional group of films **were** obtained following further manipulation of the wrist. Contrast is present in the distal radioulnar joint**,** indicating a tear of triangular fibrocartilage.
There is no evidence of contrast in the midcarpal joints to suggest the presence of a **ligamentous** tear. No additional findings of **significance** are seen.

IMPRESSION: Findings consistent with a tear of the triangular fibrocartilage.

Thank you for referring this patient to us.

Yours **truly**

_____
Hounsfield T. Scanner, MD
xx

Errors are indicated in **bold italic**. Margins are formatted at 1 inch.

current date
Ida Gundrum, MD
Railroad Station Health Center
321 Trainmaster Boulevard
Reading, PA 19604

Re: Tonya Guerrero
    Date of Birth: **May 24, 1981**
    Examination: CT **ABDOMEN** AND PELVIS.

Double space

Dear Dr. Gundrum
Computerized tomography was performed from the **diaphragm** to
the symphysis **pubis** with the use of oral and intravenous **contrast**
medium.

The liver and spleen are normal. I see no visible gallstones or
pericholecystic fluid. There is no pancreatic **mass** or calcifications.
The kidneys are both functional and **unobstructed**. There is no
retroperitoneal lymphadenopathy or pelvic **lymphadenopathy**.
The uterus is **midline**. There is some slight fullness in the right
adnexa. An ultrasound was performed on June **9, 20xx,** that showed
no **adnexal** pathology. **Asymmetry** is**,** therefore**,** probably due to
the **superior** position of unopacified **bowel** over the adnexa. No
other pelvic abnormality is seen.

IMPRESSION: Negative exam.
Thank you for referring this patient to us.

Yours **truly**

_____
Hounsfield T. Scanner, MD
xx

Glossary

Medical Terminology

Abduction (ab-<u>duk</u>-shun) is the movement of an extremity away from the midline.

Acromioclavicular (<u>ah</u>-kro-me-o-klah-<u>vik</u>-u-lar) describes the articulation between the acromial process of the scapula and the clavicle.

Acromion (ah-<u>kro</u>-me-on) is a spinous projection off the scapula.

Adduction (ad-<u>duk</u>-shun) is the movement of an extremity toward the midline.

Adenocarcinoma (ade-no-kar-si-<u>no</u>-mah) is a malignant tumor of the glands.

Adenoma (ad-ah-<u>no</u>-mah) is a benign tumor in which cells are derived from glandular epithelium.

Adenomatous (ad-e-<u>no</u>-ma-tus) relates to some types of glandular hyperplasia.

Adenopathy (ad-ah-<u>nop</u>-ah-the) is enlargement of the glands, especially the lymph nodes.

Adnexa (ad-<u>nek</u>-sa) are the tissues or body parts that are near, next to or connected to one another.

Aeration (aer-<u>a</u>-shun) is the exchange of carbon dioxide for oxygen by the blood in the lungs.

Afebrile (a-<u>feb</u>-ril) is without fever.

Amaurosis (am-aw-<u>ro</u>-sis) is the loss of sight without an apparent lesion of the eye.

Amenorrhea (ah-men-o-<u>re</u>-ah) is the absence of the menses.

Amorphous (ah-<u>mor</u>-fus) is having no definite form, or shapeless.

Anastomosis (a-nas-to-<u>mo</u>-sis) is an opening created by surgery, disease, or trauma between two or more organs or structures.

Aneurysm (<u>an</u>-u-rizm) is a localized dilatation of the wall of a blood vessel.

Angiography (an-je-<u>og</u>-rah-fe) is radiography of a blood vessel after injecting a contrast agent.

Anteverted (<u>an</u>-te-<u>vert</u>-ed) is the abnormal forward tilting of an organ.

Apophysis (ah-<u>pofi</u>-sis) is any outgrowth or swelling; a process or projection of a bone.

Arrhythmia (ah-<u>rith</u>-me-ah) is the variation from the normal rhythm of the heartbeat.

Arteriogram (ar-<u>te</u>-re-o-gram) is the radiographic visualization of an artery after injection of a contrast medium.

Arteriography (ar-te-re-<u>og</u>-rah-fe) is radiography of an artery after injection of a contrast medium into the bloodstream.

Arthroplasty (ar-<u>thro</u>-plas-te) is reconstructive surgery to repair or reshape a diseased joint.

Arthroscopy (ar-<u>thros</u>-ko-pe) is examination of the interior of a joint with an arthroscope.

Ascites (ah-<u>si</u>-teez) is the effusion and accumulation of serous fluid in the abdominal cavity.

Aspirate (as-<u>pi</u>-rat) is to draw in or out by suction.

Asymmetry (a-<u>sim</u>-e-tre) is without symmetry, lacking similar form or relationship of parts.

Asymptomatic (a-<u>simp</u>-to-mat-ik) is without symptoms.

Atelectasis (ate-<u>lek</u>-tah-sis) is the collapse of a portion of the lung.

Atherosclerosis (ath-er-o-skle-<u>ro</u>-sis) is hardening of an artery caused by deposits of plaque within the vessel.

Atrial (<u>a</u>-tre-al) pertains to the atrium.

Atrioventricular (a-tre-o-ven-<u>trik</u>-u-lar) pertains to an atrium and ventricle of the heart.

Auscultation (aw-skul-<u>ta</u>-shun) is the act of listening for sounds produced within the body with an unaided ear or with a stethoscope.

Avulsion (ah-<u>vul</u>-shun) is a tearing away or ripping of a part or structure.

Bilateral (bi-<u>lat</u>-er-al) is affecting or relating to two sides.

Biliary (<u>bil</u>-e-ar-e) relates to bile or the biliary tract.

Bimanual (bi-<u>man</u>-u-al) is using both hands.

Bleb (bleb) is a bulla or blister.

Blepharospasm (<u>blef</u>-ah-ro-spazm) is a spasm of the orbicular muscle of the eyelid.

Bradycardia (brad-e-<u>kar</u>-de-ah) is the slowness of the heartbeat.

Bronchodilator (brong-ko-di-<u>la</u>-tor) is any drug that has the capability to increase the capacity of the pulmonary air passages and improve ventilation to the lungs.

Bruit (<u>broo</u>-e) is a sound or murmur heard on auscultation.

Buccal (<u>buk</u>-al) pertains to the cheek.

Calcaneus (kal-<u>kay</u>-nee-us) is the heel bone or os calcis.

Calculus (kal-ku-lus) is an abnormal concretion; stone.

Callus (kal-us) is the new growth of bony tissue surrounding the bone ends in a fracture; part of the repair process of a fractured bone.

Cardiomyopathy (kar-de-o-mi-op-ah-the) is disease of the myocardium caused by a primary disease of the heart muscle.

Cardioverter (kar-de-o-ver-ter) is a device used to administer electrical shocks to the heart.

Caries (kar-ez) is the condition of decay and destruction of a tooth.

Carotid (kah-rot-id) relates to the principal artery of the neck.

Carpometacarpal (kar-po-met-ah-kar-pal) is the joint space between the carpal and metacarpal bones.

Cecum (se-kum) is the cul-de-sac about 6 cm in depth lying below the terminal ileum, forming the first part of the large intestine.

Centrum semiovale (sen-trum sem-i-o-val) is the white matter of the cerebral hemispheres that has an almost oval shape.

Chlamydia (klah-mid-e-ah) is a member of a widespread sexually transmitted genus (*Chlamydia*) of gram-negative, nonmotile bacteria.

Cholecystectomy (ko-le-sis-tek-to-me) is surgical removal of the gallbladder.

Cholecystitis (ko-le-sis-ti-tis) is inflammation of the gallbladder.

Claudication (klaw-di-ka-shun) is cramping pains of the calves caused by poor circulation to the leg muscles.

Coapt (ko-apt) is to bring together, as in suturing a laceration.

Colitis (ko-li-tis) is inflammation of the colon.

Collateral (ko-lat-er-al) is a secondary or accessory blood pathway.

Colonoscope (ko-lon-o-skop) is an elongated endoscope, usually fiberoptic.

Colonoscopy (ko-lon-os-ko-pe) is the visual examination of the inner surface of the colon by means of a colonoscope.

Colostomy (ko-los-to-me) is the establishment of an artificial opening into the colon.

Colporrhaphy (kol-por-ah-fe) is suturing of the vagina.

Concomitant (kon-kom-i-tant) refers to taking place at the same time.

Continent (kon-ti-ent) is the ability to control urination and defecation urges.

Contraindication (kon-trah-in-di-ka-shun) is a factor that makes it undesirable to treat a patient in the usual manner.

Contrast medium (kon-trast med-e-um) is the pharmaceutical given to the patient to allow radiographic visualization of a body structure.

Contusion (kon-to-shun) is commonly called a *bruise*, with trauma to a body part but no break in the skin surface.

Cor pulmonale (kor pul-mo-na-le) is an abnormal heart condition characterized by increased size of the right ventricle.

Coudé (koo-dae) is bent or elbowed.

Creatine kinase (kre-a-tin ki-nas) is an enzyme that strongly indicates a recent myocardial infarction when present in the blood.

Creatinine (kre-at-i-nin) is a normal alkaline constituent of urine and blood.

Crepitus (krep-i-tus) is the grating sound of bone fragments rubbing together.

Cricopharyngeal (kri-ko-fah-rin-je-al) pertains to the cricoid cartilage and the pharynx.

Crohn's disease (kronz) is inflammation of the terminal portion of the ileum.

Cyanosis (si-ah-no-sis) is the bluish purple discoloration of the skin resulting from lack of oxygenated blood.

Cystitis (sis-ti-tis) is inflammation of the urinary bladder.

Cystocele (sis-to-sel) is a hernia of the bladder, usually into the vagina and introitus.

Cystometrography (sis-to-me-trog-ra-fe) is the graphic record of the pressure in the bladder at varying stages of filling.

Cystoscope (sis-to-skop) is an endoscope specially designed for passing through the urethra into the bladder to permit visual inspection of its interior.

Cystourethroscope (sis-to-u-re-thro-skop) is an instrument for examining the posterior urethra and bladder.

Debridement (da-breed-ment) is the removal of dead or damaged tissue.

Decubitus (de-ku-bi-tus) is the state of lying down.

Demarcated (de-mar-ka-ted) refers to set limits or boundaries.

Dentition (den-tish-un) refers to the position and condition of the teeth.

Diaphoresis (di-a-fo-re-sis) is perspiration, especially when profuse.

Digit (dij-it) is a finger or toe.

Distal (dis-tal) is farther from any point of reference; remote.

Diuresis (di-u-re-sis) is increased excretion of urine.

Diuretic (di-u-ret-ik) is a substance that promotes the excretion of urine.

Diverticulitis (di-ver-tik-u-li-tis) is inflammation of the diverticula of the colon.

Diverticulum (di-ver-tik-u-lum) is a sac or pouch in the walls of a canal or organ.

Doppler (dop-ler) is an ultrasound scanning technique used to analyze blood flow and the heart and to study intermittent claudication, thrombus obstruction of deep veins, and other abnormalities.

Dorsiflexion (dor-si-<u>flek</u>-shun) is bending or flexion backward.

Duodenal (du-o-<u>de</u>-nal) relates to the duodenum, the first division of the small intestine.

Dysmenorrhea (dis-men-o-<u>re</u>-ah) is painful menstruation.

Dysphagia (dis-<u>fa</u>-je-a) is difficulty in swallowing.

Dyspnea (<u>disp</u>-ne-ah) is labored or difficult breathing.

Dysrhythmia (dis-<u>rith</u>-me-ah) is a disordered rhythm.

Dysuria (dis-<u>u</u>-re-ah) is painful or difficult urination.

Ecchymosis (ek-i-<u>mo</u>-sis) is a skin discoloration caused by a hemorrhage.

Echocardiogram (eko-<u>kar</u>-de-o-gram) is a diagnostic procedure using ultrasound to study heart structure and motion.

Edema (e-de-mah) is the accumulation of excess fluid in the tissues of the body.

Effusion (e-<u>fu</u>-zhun) is the escape of fluid from blood vessels because of rupture or seepage, usually into a body cavity.

Electrolytes (e-<u>lek</u>-tro-lit) is any solution compound that conducts electricity.

Embolus (<u>em</u>-bo-lus) is a mass brought by the blood from another vessel, which that obstructs blood circulation.

Emesis (<u>em</u>-e-sis) is an act of vomiting.

Empiric (em-<u>pir</u>-ik) is treating a disease based on observation and experience rather than reasoning alone.

Endarterectomy (end-ar-ter-<u>ek</u>-to-me) is to excise the diseased endothelium and part or all of the media of an artery.

Endoscopy (en-<u>dos</u>-ko-pe) is the examination of the interior of a canal or hollow viscus by means of endoscope.

Epiphysis (e-<u>pif</u>-i-sis) is the center for ossification at the proximal and distal ends of a long bone.

Erythema (er-i-<u>the</u>-ma) is redness of the skin due to capillary dilatation.

Etiology (e-te-<u>ol</u>-oj-e) is the science concerned with the causes or origin of a disease or disorder.

Evert (e-<u>vert</u>) is to turn inside out.

Exacerbation (eg-zas-er-<u>ba</u>-shun) is an increase in the severity of a disease or symptoms.

Exostosis (ek-sos-<u>to</u>-sis) is an abnormal, benign growth on the surface of a bone; also called *hyperostosis*.

Expiratory (ek-<u>spi</u>-ra-to-re) relates to exhalation.

Extravasation (eks-trav-ah-<u>za</u>-shun) is a discharge or escape of fluid from a vessel into the tissues.

Exudate (<u>eks</u>-u-date) is an accumulation of fluid and cellular debris in the tissues.

Fasciculations (fa-sik-u-<u>la</u>-shuns) are the uncontrolled twitchings of a group of muscle fibers.

Fibrillation (fi-bri-<u>la</u>-shun) is the exceedingly rapid contraction of muscular fibrils.

Flank (flangk) is the side of the body between the ribs and ilium.

Flexion (<u>flek</u>-shun) is the movement by a joint that decreases the angle between the two adjoining bones; the bending of a joint.

Flora (<u>flo</u>-rah) are normally occurring microorganisms that live within the body and provide natural immunity against certain organisms.

Folate (<u>fo</u>-lat) is folic acid.

Formalin (<u>for</u>-ma-lin) is a 37% aqueous solution of formaldehyde.

Fossa (<u>fos</u>-ah) is a hollow or depressed area.

Fulguration (ful-gu-<u>ra</u>-shun) is the destruction of living tissue by electric sparks generated by a high-frequency current.

Fundus (<u>fun</u>-dus) is the bottom or base of an organ.

Fusiform (<u>fu</u>-zi-form) describes a spindle-shaped structure tapered at both ends.

Gallop (<u>gal</u>-op) is a disorder in the rhythm of the heart.

Ganglion (<u>gang</u>-gle-on) is a knot or knotlike mass.

Gastritis (gas-<u>tri</u>-tis) is inflammation of the stomach, especially the mucosa.

Gastroesophageal (<u>gas</u>-tro-e-sof-a-je-al) relates to both the stomach and the esophagus.

Gastrointestinal (<u>gas</u>-tro-in-tes-tin-al) relates to the stomach and the intestines.

Gastroparesis (gas-tro-pa-<u>re</u>-sis) is a slight degree of gastroparalysis.

Gastrostomy (gas-<u>tros</u>-to-me) is the establishment of a new opening into the stomach.

Gellhorn pessary (<u>pes</u>-ah-re) is an inflexible device of acrylic resin or plastic in the form of a large collar button with a canal through the stem that allows drainage of vaginal secretions.

Genitourinary (<u>jen</u>-i-to-<u>u</u>-ri-ner-e) pertains to the genitalia and urinary organs.

Genu varum (<u>je</u>-nu <u>va</u>-rum) is bowleg.

Gluteus medius (<u>gloo</u>-te-us <u>me</u>-de-us) is one of three muscles that form the buttocks, acting to abduct and rotate the thigh.

Gout (gowt) is a disorder associated with an inborn error of uric acid metabolism that increases production or interferes with the excretion of uric acid.

Granuloma (gran-u-<u>lo</u>-mah) is a small nodular tumor or growth.

Greater trochanter (tro-<u>kan</u>-ter) is the large projection at the proximal end of the femur.

Guaiac (<u>gwi</u>-ak) is a reagent used in tests for occult blood.

Guarding (<u>gahr</u>-ding) is a body defense method to prevent movement of an injured part.

Hematemesis (he-ma-<u>tem</u>-e-sis) is vomiting of blood, indicating upper gastrointestinal bleeding.

Hematochezia (<u>he</u>-ma-to-<u>ke</u>-ze-a) is the passage of bloody stools.

Hematuria (hem-ah-<u>tu</u>-re-ah) is the discharge of blood in the urine.

Heme (hem) is the nonprotein, insoluble, iron constituent of hemoglobin.

Hemiblock (<u>hem</u>-e-blok) is the failure to conduct an impulse down one division of the left bundle branch.

Hemicolectomy (<u>hem</u>-e-ko-<u>lek</u>-to-me) is the removal of the left or right side of the colon.

Hemoptysis (he-<u>mop</u>-ti-sis) is the coughing or spitting up of blood.

Heparin (<u>hep</u>-a-rin) is a generic name for an anticoagulant.

Hepatosplenomegaly (hep-ah-to-sple-no-<u>meg</u>-ah-le) is the enlargement of the liver and spleen.

Hiatus hernia (hi-<u>a</u>-tus <u>her</u>-ne-ah) is the herniation of an abdominal organ through the esophageal opening of the diaphragm.

Homans' sign (<u>ho</u>-manz sin) is a calf pain with dorsiflexion of foot.

Hydrate (<u>hi</u>-drate) is a compound containing water molecules.

Hydrocele (<u>hi</u>-dro-sel) is the accumulation of fluid in a saclike cavity.

Hydronephrosis (hi-dro-ne-<u>fro</u>-sis) is the distention of the renal pelvis and calyces with urine, often as a result of obstruction of the ureter.

Hypercholesterolemia (<u>hi</u>-per-ko-<u>les</u>-ter-ol-e-me-a) is the presence of an abnormally large amount of cholesterol in the cells and plasma of the blood.

Hyperkalemia (<u>hi</u>-per-kal-<u>e</u>-ma-a) is the greater than normal concentration of potassium ions in the blood.

Hyperlipidemia (<u>hi</u>-per-lip-i-<u>de</u>-me-ah) is the elevated concentrations of any or all lipids in the plasma.

Hypertrophy (hi-<u>per</u>-tro-fe) is an increase in the size of an organ or structure.

Hypotensive (<u>hi</u>-po-<u>ten</u>-siv) means characterized by low blood pressure or causing a reduction in blood pressure.

Icterus (<u>ik</u>-ter-us) is jaundice.

Idiopathic (<u>id</u>-e-o-<u>path</u>-ik) refers to a disease of unknown cause.

Iliac (<u>il</u>-e-ak) relates to the ilium.

Impingement (im-<u>pinj</u>-ment) is an abnormal contact or pressure between two structures.

Incontinence (in-<u>kon</u>-ti-nens) is the inability to control excretory functions.

Infarction (in-<u>farkt</u>-shun) is the death of a tissue caused by lack of blood flow to the area.

Inferolateral (in-fer-o-<u>lat</u>-e-ral) pertains to a location situated below and to the side.

Infiltrate (in-<u>fil</u>-trate) is to pass into tissue spaces, as by fluid, cells, or other substances.

Inotropic (in-o-<u>trop</u>-ik) means influencing the contractions of the muscular tissue.

Interarticular (in-ter-ar-<u>tik</u>-u-lar) means between two joints.

Interosseous (in-ter-<u>os</u>-e-us) is situated or occurring between bone.

Intimal (<u>in</u>-ti-mal) relates to the inner coat of a vessel.

Intrahepatic (in-trah-he-<u>pat</u>-ik) means within the liver.

Intrauterine (in-trah-<u>u</u>-ter-in) means within the uterus.

Ischemia (is-<u>ke</u>-me-ah) is decreased supply of oxygenated blood to a body part.

Jejunum (je-<u>joo</u>-num) is the second section of the small intestine.

Joint mouse (joint mows) is a loose body in synovial joints.

Ketone (<u>ke</u>-tone) is any compound containing carbon oxide.

Labyrinthitis (lab-i-rin-<u>thi</u>-tis) is inflammation of the internal ear, or otitis interna.

Lactic dehydrogenase (<u>lak</u>-tik de-<u>hi</u>-dro-jen-as) (LDH) is an enzyme present in elevated concentrations in blood serum when tissues are injured. Determining the pattern of LDH isoenzymes in serum helps to identify which tissue has been damaged.

Lacuna (lah-<u>ku</u>-nah) is the small cavity within or between other body structures.

Lamina (<u>lam</u>-i-nah) is a thin, flat layer.

Laminectomy (lam-i-<u>nek</u>-to-me) is surgical excision of the lamina.

Laparoscope (lap-ah-ro-skop) is an endoscope for examining the peritoneal cavity.

Leukocytes (<u>loo</u>-ko-sits) are colorless blood corpuscles.

Lingula (<u>ling</u>-gu-lah) is a small, tongue-shaped anatomic structure.

Lipoma (li-<u>po</u>-mah) is a benign tumor composed mostly of fat cells.

Lipomatous (li-<u>po</u>-mah-tus) is affected with or of the nature of lipoma.

Lithotomy (li-<u>thot</u>-o-me) is the incision of a duct or organ for the removal of calculi.

Lumen (<u>lu</u>-men) is the cavity or channel within a tube.

Lymphadenopathy (lim-fad-e-<u>nop</u>-ah-the) is disease of the lymph nodes.

Lymphedema (<u>lim</u>-fi-de-ma) is edema caused by obstruction of lymph vessels.

Malaise (mal-<u>az</u>) is a feeling of uneasiness.

Malleolus (mah-<u>lee</u>-o-lus) is either of the two rounded projections on each side of the ankle joint.

Marshall test (<u>mar</u>-shul test) is performed to determine stress-related urinary incontinence.

Meatus (me-<u>a</u>-tus) is an opening.

Mediastinum (me-de-ah-<u>sti</u>-num) is the mass of

tissues and organs separating the sternum in front and the vertebral column behind.

Melena (me-<u>le</u>-nah) is the darkening of the feces by blood pigments.

Meniscectomy (me-ni-<u>sek</u>-to-me) is surgical removal of a meniscus.

Meniscus (me-<u>nis</u>-kus) is the crescent-shaped fibrocartilage in the knee joint.

Metastasis (me-<u>tas</u>-tah-sis) is the transfer of disease from one organ or part to another not directly connected with it.

Metatarsus (met-a-<u>tar</u>-sus) is any of the five long bones of the foot between the ankle and the toes.

Motility (mo-<u>til</u>-i-te) is the ability to move spontaneously.

Mucosa (mu-<u>ko</u>-sah) is the mucous membrane.

Myalgia (mi-<u>al</u>-je-ah) is muscular pain.

Myocardial (mi-o-<u>kar</u>-de-al) pertains to the muscular tissue of the heart.

Myringotomy (mir-in-<u>got</u>-o-me) is an incision of the tympanic membrane.

Nebulization (neb-u-li-<u>za</u>-shun) is a treatment by a spray.

Nephrectomy (ne-<u>frek</u>-to-me) is surgical removal of the kidney.

Nocturnal (nok-<u>tur</u>-nal) means occurring at night.

Normocephalic (nor-mo-se-<u>fal</u>-ik) is having a normal-sized head; mesocephalic.

Nystagmus (nis-<u>tag</u>-mus) is the involuntary, rapid, rhythmic movement of the eyeball.

Occlude (o-<u>klood</u>) is to close tight.

Occlusion (o-<u>kloo</u>-zhun) is the act of closure or state of being closed.

Occult (o-<u>kult</u>) refers to a specimen hidden from view.

Odynophagia (o-din-o-<u>fa</u>-je-ah) is pain with the swallowing of food.

Oophorectomy (o-of-o-<u>rek</u>-to-me) is excision of one or both ovaries.

Orthopnea (or-thop-<u>ne</u>-ah) is the ability to breathe easily only in an upright position.

Os (os) is an opening, mouth, or bone.

Osteopenia (os-te-o-<u>pe</u>-ne-ah) is a decrease in bone mass below normal.

Osteophyte (<u>os</u>-te-o-fit) is an outgrowth of bone usually found around a joint.

Palpitation (pal-pi-<u>ta</u>-shun) is an unusually rapid, strong, or irregular heartbeat.

Panendoscope (pan-<u>en</u>-do-skop) is a cystoscope that gives a wide-angle view of the bladder.

Parenchyma (pah-<u>reng</u>-ki-mah) is the general anatomic term to describe the functional elements of an organ, as distinguished from its structure.

Paresthesia (par-es-<u>the</u>-ze-ah) is the sensation of tingling and numbness.

Parkinson's disease is a slowly progressive disease characterized by degeneration within the nuclear masses of the extrapyramidal system.

Paronychia (par-o-<u>nik</u>-e-ah) is the inflammation involving the folds of tissue surrounding the nail.

Paroxysm (<u>par</u>-ok-sism) is the sudden recurrence of symptoms.

Partial thromboplastin time is the period required for clot formation in recalcified blood plasma after contact and the activation and the addition of platelet substitutes; used to assess the pathways of coagulation.

Passavant's cushion (<u>pahs</u>-a-vahnts) is a ridge appearing on the posterior wall of pharynx during swallowing resulting from contraction of the palatopharyngeal sphincter.

Pectoralis (pek-to-<u>ra</u>-lis) pertains to the chest or breast.

Pedal (<u>ped</u>-al) pertains to the foot.

Periarticular (per-e-ar-<u>tic</u>-u-lar) is situated around a joint.

Pericholecystic fluid (per-i-ko-le-sis-<u>tic</u>) is a coined term for fluid around the gallbladder.

Peripheral (pe-<u>rif</u>-er-al) means occurring away from the center.

Perirectal (per-i-<u>rek</u>-tal) means around the rectum.

Periumbilical (per-e-um-<u>bil</u>-i-kal) means around the umbilicus.

Pessary (<u>pes</u>-ah-re) is an instrument placed in the vagina to support the uterus or rectum.

Phalanx (<u>fa</u>-langks) is the general term for any bone of a finger or toe.

Phallus (<u>fal</u>-us) is the penis.

Pinna (<u>pin</u>-ah) is the projecting part of the ear lying outside the head.

Pisiform (<u>pi</u>-si-form) is the smallest carpal bone; pea shaped.

Pitting (<u>pit</u>-ing) is the formation of a small depression.

Plantar (<u>plan</u>-tar) pertains to the sole of the foot.

Pleura (<u>ploo</u>-rah) is the serous membrane investing the lungs and lining the walls of the thoracic cavity.

Pneumonectomy (nu-mo-<u>nek</u>-to-me) is surgical removal of all or a segment of the lung.

Pneumothorax (nu-mo-<u>tho</u>-raks) is the presence of air or gas in the pleural cavity.

Polycythemia (pol-e-si-<u>the</u>-me-ah) is an increase in the total red cell mass of the blood.

Polyp (<u>pol</u>-ip) is any growth or mass protruding from a mucous membrane.

Polypoid (<u>pol</u>-y-poid) means resembling a polyp.

Postprandial (post-<u>pran</u>-de-al) means after a meal.

Postvoid film is a film of the bladder area taken after the patient has emptied the bladder.

Prevoid film is a film of the bladder area taken before the patient has emptied the bladder.

Proctitis (prok-<u>ti</u>-tis) is inflammation of the rectum.

Prophylactic (pro-fi-<u>lak</u>-tik) is an agent that tends to ward off disease.

Prostate (<u>pros</u>-tat) is the male gland that surrounds the neck of the bladder and urethra.

Prothrombin time is a test to measure the activity of factors I, II, V, VII, and X, which participate in the extrinsic pathway of coagulation.

Pruritus ani (proo-<u>ri</u>-tus <u>a</u>-ni) is intense chronic itching in the anal region.

Pulmonary toilet (<u>pul</u>-mo-ner-e) is the cleansing of the trachea and bronchial tree.

Purulent (<u>pu</u>-roo-lent) means containing pus.

Pyelogram (<u>pi</u>-e-lo-gram) is an x-ray study of the renal pelvis and ureters.

Pyelonephritis (pi-e-lo-ne-<u>fri</u>-tis) is inflammation of the kidney and renal pelvis.

Pyuria (pi-<u>u</u>-re-ah) is pus in the urine.

Radiation (ra-de-<u>a</u>-shun) is the divergence of pain from the site of injury to other areas of the body.

Radiculitis (rah-dik-u-<u>li</u>-tis) is inflammation of a spinal nerve root.

Rale (rahl) is an abnormal crackle sound heard on chest auscultation.

Raphe (<u>ra</u>-fe) is a seam or ridge noting the junction of two halves of a part.

Real-time ultrasound is a rapid imaging system that produces a video display of organ motion.

Rebound (<u>re</u>-bownd) is a reversed response occurring on withdrawal of a stimulus.

Rectocele (<u>rek</u>-to-sel) is a hernial protrusion of part of the rectum into the vagina.

Reflux (<u>re</u>-fluks) is a backward or return flow.

Resect (re-<u>sekt</u>) is to cut off or cut out a portion of a tissue or organ.

Retroflexion (ret-ro-<u>flek</u>-shun) is the bending of an organ so its top side is thrust backward.

Retroperitoneal (ret-ro-<u>per</u>-i-to-<u>ne</u>-al) means behind the peritoneum.

Rhinitis (ri-<u>ni</u>-tis) is inflammation of the mucous membrane of the nose.

Rhonchus (<u>rong</u>-kus) is an abnormal sound heard on chest auscultation that is caused by an obstructed airway.

Rub (rub) is an auscultatory sound caused by two surfaces rubbing together.

Saphenous (sah-<u>fe</u>-nus) pertains to the two main superficial veins of the lower leg.

Sclera (<u>skle</u>-rah) is the tough white outer coat of the eyeball.

Sequela (se-<u>kwel</u>-lah) is any abnormal condition that follows and is the result of a disease, treatment, or injury.

Sigmoidoscope (sig-<u>moi</u>-do-skop) is an endoscope for use in sigmoidoscopy.

Sigmoidoscopy (sig-moi-<u>dos</u>-ko-pe) is the direct examination of the interior of the sigmoid colon.

Sinus (<u>si</u>-nus) is a cavity or channel.

Somnolence (<u>som</u>-no-lens) is drowsiness.

Spironolactone (sper-o-no-<u>lak</u>-ton) is the generic name for a diuretic.

Sputum (<u>spu</u>-tum) is the mucous secretion from the lungs, bronchi, and trachea that is ejected through the mouth.

Staghorn (<u>stag</u>-horn) is the calculus of the renal pelvis usually extending into multiple calyces.

Stasis (<u>sta</u>-sis) is an abnormal slowing or stopping of fluid flowing through a vessel.

Stenosis (ste-<u>no</u>-sis) is the narrowing or contraction of a body passage.

Stent (stent) is a device placed within the lumen of a vessel to provide support and patency of the vessel.

Stricture (<u>strik</u>-chor) is an abnormal narrowing of a duct or passage.

Subluxation (sub-luk-<u>sa</u>-shun) is a partial dislocation.

Suprapubic (soo-prah-<u>pu</u>-bik) means above the pubis.

Supraventricular (soo-prah-ven-<u>trik</u>-u-lar) means situated or occurring above the ventricles.

Symptomatology (simp-to-mah-<u>tol</u>-o-je) is the combined symptoms of a specific disease.

Syncope (<u>sing</u>-ko-pe) is a temporary suspension of consciousness; fainting.

Synovia (si-<u>no</u>-ve-ah) is the lubricating fluid of joints.

Tachycardia (tak-e-<u>kar</u>-de-ah) is an abnormally fast heartbeat.

Tendinitis (ten-di-<u>ni</u>-tis) is inflammation of a tendon; also *tendonitis*.

Thoracentesis (tho-rah-sen-<u>te</u>-sis) is the aspiration of fluid from the chest cavity.

Thrombosis (throm-<u>bo</u>-sis) is the formation of a blood clot in the vascular system.

Thyromegaly (thi-ro-<u>meg</u>-ah-le) is enlargement of the thyroid gland.

Titrate (<u>ti</u>-trat) is to analyze a given solution component by adding a liquid reagent.

Trabeculation (trah-bek-u-<u>la</u>-shun) is a small beam or supporting structure.

Transducer (trans-<u>doo</u>-ser) is an ultrasound device that transforms sound waves into an electronically displayed image.

Trapezius (trah-<u>pee</u>-zee-us) is the muscle of the back of the neck and shoulder.

Trigone (<u>tri</u>-gon) is a triangular area.

Turgor (<u>tur</u>-gor) is the normal resiliency of the skin.

Ulna (<u>ul</u>-nah) is the long medial bone of the forearm.

Urethrocele (u-re-thro-sel) is the prolapse of the female urethra through the urinary meatus.

Urethrotrigonitis (u-re-thro-tri-go-ni-tis) is inflammation of the urethra and trigone of the bladder.

Urogram (u-ro-gram) is a radiograph of part of the urinary tract.

Urosepsis (u-ro-sep-sis) is the poisoning from retained and absorbed urinary substances.

Uvula (u-vu-lah) is a small, soft structure hanging from the free edge of the soft palate.

Valsalva's maneuver (val-sal-vahz) is an attempt to exhale forcibly with the glottis, nose, and mouth closed.

Vas deferens (vas def-er-ens) are the excretory ducts of the testis.

Vasculature (vas-ku-lah-tur) is the supply of vessels to a specific region.

Venous (ve-nus) pertains to the veins.

Vertex (ver-teks) is the top or crown of the head.

Verumontanum (ver-oo-mon-ta-num) is the elevation on the floor of the prostatic portion of the urethra where the seminal ducts enter.

Volar (vo-lar) pertains to the palm of the hand or sole of the foot.

Vulva (vul-vah) is the external genital organs in women.

Drugs

Aldactone (al-dak-ton) is a trade name for a diuretic.

Amoxicillin (ah-moks-i-sil-in) is a generic name for an aminopenicillin antibiotic.

Amoxil (ah-moks-il) is a trade name for a preparation of amoxicillin, an antimicrobial.

Ancef (an-sef) is a trade name for a cephalosporin antibiotic.

Ascriptin (ah-skrip-tin) is a trade name for a preparation of aspirin with aluminum, magnesium, and calcium; an analgesic and anti-inflammatory.

Aspirin is a generic name for an analgesic, antipyretic, and anti-inflammatory; an antirheumatic.

Ativan (at-i-van) is a trade name for an anxiolytic.

Atrovent (at-ro-vent) is a trade name for a bronchodilator and nasal spray.

Augmentin (awg-men-tin) is a trade name for a preparation of amoxicillin, an antimicrobial.

Axid (ak-sid) is a trade name for an antagonist used to treat gastric and duodenal ulcers.

Azmacort (az-ma-kort) is a trade name for a corticosteroid used to prevent and treat bronchial asthma.

Bacitracin (bas-i-tra-sin) is a generic name for an antibacterial.

Bactrim (bak-trim) is a trade name for an antibiotic.

Beta blocker is a generic name for a drug that blocks the action of epinephrine at beta-adrenergic receptors on cells of effector organs; used to treat angina pectoralis, hypertension, and cardiac arrhythmias.

Beta carotene (kar-ah-teen) is a vitamin A precursor and ultraviolet screen.

Betadine (bat-ah-din) is a trade name for a topical antibacterial and antiseptic.

Biaxin (bi-ak-sin) is a trade name for an antibiotic.

Botox (bo-toks) is a trade name for a powder for extraocular muscle injection.

Bumex (bu-meks) is a trade name for a loop diuretic.

Calan (kal-an) is a trade name for an antianginal, antiarrhythmic, and antihypertensive.

Capoten (kap-o-ten) is a trade name for an antihypertensive.

Captopril (kap-to-pril) is a generic name for an angiotensin-converting enzyme inhibitor.

Cardiolite (kar-de-o-lit) is a trade name for a myocardial perfusion agent for cardiac imaging.

Cardizem (kar-di-zem) is a trade name for a calcium channel blocker used for atrial fibrillation.

Cardura (kar-du-rah) is a trade name for an antihypertensive and antiadrenergic.

Cephalosporin (sef-ah-lo-spor-in) is a generic name for any of a large group of broad-spectrum antibiotics.

Chem-7 is a trade name for a profile of seven different chemical laboratory tests.

Cipro (si-pro) is a trade name for a fluoroquinolone antibiotic and antibacterial.

Claritin (klar-i-tin) is a trade name for a nonsedating antihistamine.

Codeine (ko-deen or ko-dean) is a generic name for an opioid analgesic.

Colace (ko-las) is a trade name for a stool softener.

Compazine (kom-pah-zen) is a trade name for a tranquilizer and antiemetic.

Copolymer (ko-pol-i-mer) is a trade name for one of the immune-modulating drugs.

Cortisone (cor-ti-son) is a generic name for a corticosteroid used to treat inflammation.

Coumadin (koo-mah-din) is a trade name for an anticoagulant.

Cytotec (si-to-tek) is a trade name for a drug used for the prevention of NSAID-induced gastric ulcers.

Darvocet (dar-vo-set) is a trade name for a preparation of acetaminophen and propoxyphene, a narcotic analgesic.

Darvon (dar-von) is a trade name for a narcotic analgesic.

Demerol (dem-er-ol) is a trade name for meperidine, a narcotic analgesic.

Digoxin (di-jok-sin) is a generic name for a cardiotonic.

Dilantin (di-lan-tin) is a trade name for an anticonvulsant used to treat epilepsy.

Diltiazem (dil-ti-a-zem) is a generic name for a coronary vasodilator.

Ditropan (di-tro-pan) is a trade name for a urinary antispasmodic.

Dobutamine (do-byu-ta-men) is a generic name for a cardiotonic agent; a synthetic catecholamine administered parenterally for inotropic support in short-term treatment of adults with cardiac decompensation.

Dolobid (do-lo-bid) is a trade name for a drug classified as an NSAID, a nonsteroidal anti-inflammatory drug.

Doxepin (dok-se-pin) is a generic name for an antidepressant.

Doxycycline (dok-se-si-klen) is a generic name for a broad-spectrum antibiotic active against a wide range of gram-positive and gram-negative organisms.

E.E.S. is a trade name for an antibiotic.

Ecotrin (ek-o-trin) is a trade name for an analgesic and anti-inflammatory.

Elavil (el-ah-vil) is a trade name for an antidepressant.

Erythromycin (e-rith-ro-mi-sin) is a generic name for a broad-spectrum antibiotic.

Estrace (es-tras) is a trade name of an estrogen classified as an antineoplastic.

Evista (e-vis-ta) is a trade name for a selective estrogen receptor modulator used to prevent postmenopausal osteoporosis.

FiberCon (fi-ber-kon) is a trade name for a bulk-forming laxative.

Heparin (hep-ah-rin) is a generic name for an anticoagulant.

Humulin (hu-mu-lin) is a trade name for an antidiabetic.

Hydrochlorothiazide (hi-dro-klor-o-thi-a-zide) is a generic name for a diuretic, antihypertensive agent.

Hydrocortisone (hi-dro-kor-ti-son) is a generic name for a corticosteroid.

Hytrin (hi-trin) is a trade name for an antihypertensive used to treat benign prostatic hyperplasia.

Imodium (i-mo-de-um) is a trade name for an antidiarrheal.

Indocin (in-do-sin) is a trade name for a nonsteroidal anti-inflammatory drug, NSAID.

Isordil (i-sor-dil) is a trade name for an antianginal.

Isosorbide (i-so-sor-bid) is a generic name for a nitrate-based antianginal agent.

Isovue (i-so-vu) is a trade name for a drug used as a contrast medium.

K-Dur is a trade name for a potassium supplement.

Keflex (kef-leks) is a trade name for an antibiotic.

Klonopin (klon-o-pin) is a trade name for an anticonvulsant, antianxiety drug.

Lanoxin (lah-nok-sin) is a trade name for a cardiac glycoside used to increase cardiac output.

Lasix (la-ziks) is a trade name for a diuretic.

Lescol (le-zkol) is a trade name for a lipid-lowering agent.

Lidocaine (li-do-kan) is a generic name for a local anesthetic and antiarrhythmatic.

Lipitor (lip-i-tor) is a trade name for an antihyperlipidemic used for hypercholesterolemia.

Lo-Ovral (lo-ov-ral) is a trade name for an oral contraceptive.

Lopressor (lo-pres-or) is a trade name for a beta-adrenergic blocker, an antihypertensive.

Lorazepam (lor-az-e-pam) is a generic antianxiety drug.

Lotensin (lo-ten-sin) is a trade name for an antihypertensive.

Macrobid (mak-ro-bid) is a trade name for a urinary bacteriostatic.

Maxaquin (mak-sa-kwin) is a trade name for a fluoroquinolone antibiotic and antibacterial.

Maxzide (mak-sid) is a trade name for a diuretic and antihypertensive.

Meclizine (mek-li-zen) is a generic name for an antiemetic and antihistamine, used for motion sickness relief.

Melatonex (mel-a-to-neks) is a trade name for a sleep aid.

Metamucil (met-ah-mu-sil) is a trade name for a bulk laxative.

Mevacor (mev-a kor) is a trade name for a reductase inhibitor for hypercholesterolemia.

Naprosyn (na-pro-sin) is a trade name for a nonsteroidal anti-inflammatory drug, NSAID.

Neosporin (ne-o-spor-in) is a trade name for a topical antibiotic.

Neptazane (nep-ta-zan) is a trade name for a diuretic and antiglaucoma agent.

Nifedipine (ni-fed-i-pen) is a generic name for a calcium channel blocker.

Nitroglycerin (ni-tro-glis-er-in) is a generic name for a coronary vasodilator and antianginal.

Noroxin (nor-o-sin) is a trade name for an antibacterial and urinary tract anti-infective.

Nortriptyline (nor-trip-ti-lin) is a generic name for an antidepressant.

Norvasc (nor-vask) is a trade name for an antianginal and antihypertensive.

NPH (neutral protamine Hagedorn) is a trade name for an insulin that decreases blood sugar.

Ophthetic (of-the-tik) is a trade name for proparacaine hydrochloride eye drops.

Ortho Tri-Cyclen (<u>or</u>-tho tri-<u>si</u>-klen) is a trade name for a triphasic oral contraceptive also used to treat acne vulgaris in women.

Paxil (<u>paks</u>-il) is a trade name for a selective serotonin reuptake inhibitor for depression, obsessive-compulsive disorder, and panic disorder.

Pencillin is a generic name for any of a large group of natural or semisynthetic antibacterial antibiotics.

Pepcid (<u>pep</u>-sid) is a trade name for an acid controller for heartburn and acid indigestion.

Percocet (per-<u>ko</u>-set) is a trade name for an opioid analgesic (Schedule II).

Persantine (per-<u>san</u>-ten) is a trade name for a coronary vasodilator and antiplatelet agent.

Phenergan (<u>fen</u>-er-gan) is a trade name for an antihistamine.

Prednisone (<u>pred</u>-ni-son) is a generic name for an anti-inflammatory and antiallergic agent.

Premarin (<u>prem</u>-ah-rin) is a trade name for an estrogen replacement.

Prilosec (<u>pril</u>-o-sek) is a trade name for a proton pump inhibitor for gastric and duodenal ulcers and other gastroesophageal disorders.

Procardia (pro-<u>kar</u>-de-ah) is a trade name for a coronary vasodilator.

Proctocream HC (<u>prok</u>-to-kreem) is a trade name for a topical corticosteroid anti-inflammatory used as anorectal cream.

Propine (<u>pro</u>-pine) is a trade name for an antiglaucoma agent; eye drops.

Proventil (pro-<u>ven</u>-til) is a trade name for a bronchodilator and metered-dose inhaler.

Provera (pro-<u>ver</u>-ah) is a trade name for progestin used for secondary amenorrhea and abnormal uterine bleeding.

Pyridoxine (pir-o-<u>dok</u>-sen) is one of the forms of vitamin B6.

Quinidex (<u>kwin</u>-i-deks) is a trade name for an antiarrhythmic.

Quinidine (<u>kwin</u>-i-den) is a generic name for an antiarrhythmic used to treat atrial flutter, atrial fibrillation, premature ventricular contractions, and tachycardia.

Reglan (<u>reg</u>-lan) is a trade name for a gastrointestinal stimulant and antiemetic.

Restoril (<u>res</u>-to-ril) is a trade name for a sedative-hypnotic.

Ritalin (<u>rit</u>-ah-lin) is a trade name for a mild central nervous system stimulant and antidepressant.

Senokot (se-<u>no</u>-kot) is a trade name for a laxative.

Serevent (<u>ser</u>-e-vent) is a trade name for an aerosol bronchodilator.

Skelaxin (skel-aks-in) is a trade name for a skeletal muscle relaxant.

Slo-bid is a trade name for an extended-release bronchodilator.

Sulfacetamide (sul-fah-<u>set</u>-ah-mid) is a generic name for an antibacterial sulfonamide and antibiotic.

Synthroid (<u>sin</u>-throid) is a trade name for a replacement hormone in decreased or absent thyroid function.

Tenormin (<u>ten</u>-or-min) is a trade name for a beta blocker.

Terpin (<u>ter</u>-pin) is a product used as an expectorant.

Terramycin (<u>ter</u>-ah-mi-sin) is a trade name for an antibiotic.

Tetracycline (te-trah-<u>si</u>-klen) is a generic name for an antibiotic.

Theo-Dur (<u>the</u>-o-dur) is a trade name for a bronchodilator.

Theophylline (the-o-<u>fil</u>-in) is a generic name for a bronchodilator.

Tigan (<u>ti</u>-gan) is a trade name for an antiemetic.

Timoptic (tim-<u>op</u>-tik) is a trade name for a topical antiglaucoma agent, antihypertensive, and beta blocker.

Tolinase (<u>tol</u>-i-nas) is a trade name for an antidiabetic agent.

Toradol (<u>tor</u>-a-dol) is a trade name for a nonsteroidal anti-inflammatory drug and analgesic for acute, moderately severe pain.

Trental (<u>tren</u>-tal) is a trade name for an oral hemorheologic drug.

Triamcinolone (tri-am-<u>sin</u>-o-lon) is a generic name for a corticosteroid.

Trimpex (<u>trimp</u>-eks) is a trade name for an antibacterial and antibiotic.

Vancenase (<u>van</u>-sen-az) is a trade name for a corticosteroid for bronchial asthma and pocket inhaler.

Vanceril (<u>van</u>-ser-il) is a trade name for a corticosteroid.

Vasotec (<u>vah</u>-o-tek) is a trade name for an angiotensin-converting enzyme inhibitor.

Ventolin (<u>ven</u>-to-lin) is a trade name for a bronchodilator.

Verapamil (ver-<u>ap</u>-a-mil) is a generic name for a coronary vasodilator.

Versed (<u>ver</u>-sed) is a trade name for a short-acting benzodiazepine and general anesthetic adjunct for preoperative sedation.

Vicodin (<u>vi</u>-ko-din) is a trade name for a preparation of acetaminophen and hydrocodone, an opioid analgesic.

Vicoprofen (vi-ko-<u>pro</u>-fen) is a trade name for a narcotic analgesic.

Vitamin C is ascorbic acid, used as an antiscorbutic and urinary acidifier.

Vitamin E is used as a nutritional supplement and topical emollient.

Xanax (<u>zan</u>-aks) is a trade name for an antianxiety agent.

Xylocaine (<u>zi</u>-lo-cane) is a trade name for an antiarrhythmic and local anesthetic.

Zantac (<u>zan</u>-tak) is a trade name for an acid controller for heartburn and acid indigestion.

Zocor (zo-<u>kor</u>) is a trade name for a reductase inhibitor for hypercholesterolemia and coronary heart disease.

Zyloprim (<u>zi</u>-lo-prim) is a trade name for an antigout agent.

Index

Initials, reference, in consultation/business letters, 23
Institute for Safe Medication Practices, 44
Intercostal arteries, 310f
Intestine, large, double-contrast posteroanterior radiographic view of, 275f

J

Jejunum, 276f
Joint Commission on Accreditation of Healthcare Organizations (JCAHO), 16, 74
    Do Not Use list, 43-44, 43t, 44t
Journal of the American Association for Medical Transcription (JAAMT), 69

K

Knee
    sagittal magnetic resonance scan of, 163f
    sagittal view of, 163f

L

Laboratory data, in history and physical examination report, 18b, 20
Lateral meniscus, 163f
Left lateral projection, 21
Lens, 343f
Letter(s)
    business, 22-23
    consultation, sample of, 6f
    diagnostic imaging, sample of, 5f
Ligaments, of wrist, 163f
Liver, 276f
Lumbar spine, 162f
Lunate, 163f
Lung exam, in history and physical examination report, 18b, 20
Lymphatic system, 342

M

Magazines, reference materials, 69
Magnetic resonance imaging (MRI) report, format of, 20
Mamillary body, 340f
Masseter muscle, 339f
Medical dictionaries, 68
    electronic, 69
Medical reports. *See* Reports, medical
Medical spellers, electronic, 69
Medical terms
    keyboarding
        in cardiology practice, 286-287
        in diagnostic imaging practice, 319
        in family practice transcription, 104-105
        in gastroenterology practice, 249-250
        in orthopedic practice, 139-140
        in pulmonary medicine practice, 209-211
        in urology practice, 174-175
    spelling
        in cardiology practice, 288
        in diagnostic imaging practice, 320
        in family practice transcription, 106
        in gastroenterology practice, 251
        in orthopedic practice, 141
        in pulmonary medicine practice, 212
        in urology practice, 176
Medical Transcription Guide Do's and Don'ts, 69
Medical transcriptionist
    career outlook of, 4
    demand for, 4
    Essentials of Medical Transcription and, 9
    knowledge needed by, 6
    personal attributes of, 6
    profile of, 4, 6
    skills needed by, 6

Medications, in history and physical examination report, 18b, 19
Medulla, 341f
Merck Manual, 68
Metacarpal bone, 163f
Mosby's Medical Drug Reference, 68
MRI. *See* Magnetic resonance imaging
Muscular system, 339f

N

Neck
    axial magnetic resonance imaging of, 339f
    axial computed tomography of, 339f
    muscles, 339f
Neck exam, in history and physical examination report, 18b, 19
Nervous system, 341f
Neurological exam, in history and physical examination report, 18b, 20
Nuclear medicine report, format of, 20
Number expression guidelines, 45-47

O

Occupational Outlook Handbook, 4
Online, reference materials, 69, 70b
Operative reports, statistical data in, 22
Optic chiasm, 340f
Optic nerve, 343f
Orbit
    axial computed tomography scan of, 343f
    axial magnetic resonance scan of, 343f
    axial view of, 343f
Orthopedic practice, office medical transcription from
    keyboarding medical terms and definitions and, 139-140
    proofreading and error analysis in, 149-155
    spelling medical terms in, 141
    transcribing medical sentences in, 142
    transcription tips for, 157-160
Orthopedic practice, overview of, 132
Outpatient facilities, medical reports used in, 4f-6f

P

Pancreas, 276f
Parotid gland, 276f
Past medical history (PMH), in history and physical examination report, 18b, 19
Patella, 163f
Patellar ligament, 163f
PDR. See Physicians' Desk Reference
Pelvic exam, in history and physical examination report, 18b, 20
Period, guidelines for use of, 42f, 47
Peroneal artery, 311f
Perspectives on the Medical Transcription Profession, 69
Pharmaceutical, reference materials, 68
Physical examination report, sample of, 5f
Physicians' Desk Reference (PDR), 68
Physiology textbooks, 69
Pineal gland, 341f
Pituitary gland, 340f, 341f
Plan of treatment, in history and physical examination report, 18b, 20
PMH. *See* Past medical history
Pons, 341f
Popliteal artery, 311f
Posterior horn, meniscus, 163f
Prepatellar bursa, 163f
Procedure codes (CPT), 16
Procedure reports, statistical data in, 21
Production for pay summary, 74, 74t
Profunda femoris artery, 311f
Projections, in diagnostic imaging letters, 20-21